PSYCHOPHYSIOLOGICAL MEASUREMENT AND MEANING

Psychophysiological Measurement and Meaning is a comprehensive resource for psychophysiological research on media responses, a new paradigm sweeping media research. It addresses the theoretical underpinnings, methodological techniques, and most recent research in this area. It goes beyond current volumes by placing the research techniques within a context of communication processes and effects as a field, and demonstrating how the real-time measurement of physiological responses enhances and complements more traditional measures of psychological effects from media.

This volume will introduce readers to the theoretical assumptions of psychophysiology as well as operational details of collecting psychophysiological data. In addition to discussing specific measures, it includes brief reviews of recent experiments that have used psychophysiological measures to study how the brain processes media. It will serve as a valuable reference for media researchers utilizing psychophysiological methodologies, or for other researchers needing to understand the theories, history, and methods in this area of research.

Robert F. Potter (Ph.D. Indiana University) is Associate Professor of Telecommunications at Indiana University, Bloomington. He is a member of Core Faculty-Cognitive Science Program and Director of the Institute for Communication Research. His research focuses on the impact of auditory elements on information processing of media, psychophysiological measures as indicators of cognitive and emotional responses to media, and the concept of advertising clutter and its influence on information processing. Additional information about Potter's work can be found at www.theaudioprof.com.

Paul D. Bolls (Ph.D. Indiana University) is Co-Director of the PRIME Lab and an Associate Professor of Strategic Communication at the Missouri School of Journalism. He conducts media psychophysiology research with a specific focus on examining mental processing of public health messages. He has been involved in building and running media psychophysiology labs for the past 15 years, having worked in labs at Indiana University, University of Missouri, and Washington State University.

PSYCHOPHYSIOLOGICAL MEASUREMENT AND MEANING

Cognitive and Emotional Processing of Media

Robert F. Potter

Paul D. Bolls

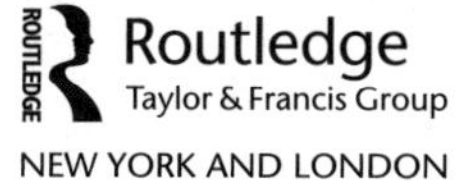

NEW YORK AND LONDON

First published 2012
by Routledge
711 Third Ave., New York, NY 10016

Simultaneously published in the UK
by Routledge
2 Park Square, Milton Park, Abingdon, Oxon OX14 4RN

Routledge is an imprint of the Taylor & Francis Group, an informa business

Library of Congress Cataloging in Publication Data
Potter, Robert F.
  Pyschophysiological measurement and meaning/Robert Potter,
  Paul Bolls.
    p. cm.
  Includes index.
  1. Mass media—Psychological aspects.   2. Communication—
  Psychological aspects.   3. Psychophysiology—Research.
  4. Psychometrics.   I. Bolls, Paul David, 1966–.   II. Title.
  P96.P75P68 2011
  302.2301′9—dc22   2010054570

ISBN13: 978–0–8058–6286–7 (hbk)
ISBN13: 978–0–415–99414–9 (pbk)
ISBN13: 978–0–203–18102–7 (ebk)

Typeset in Bembo and Stone Sans by
Florence Production Ltd, Stoodleigh, Devon

Printed and bound in the United States of America on acid-free paper by
Edwards Brothers, Inc.

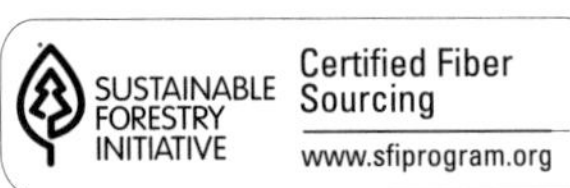

Dedication

Writing this book has been a long intellectual adventure. During it we were especially blessed with encouragement from two amazing women—our wives, Pam Potter and Val Bolls. They provided the love and support we needed to finish this project; one which has helped us to grow as scholars and individuals. We dedicate this book to them with many thanks and much love.

RFP & PDB

CONTENTS

FOREWORD

Reading this book makes me feel old.

I must be old because I remember when the first version of this book was published in 1994 more clearly than I remember yesterday, or last week, or last year. I must be old because it doesn't feel like more than two or three years ago. The memories are so clear I don't see how that book could be out of print or out of date.

I must be old because I do remember punching cards and feeding them into a card reader to do my master's thesis (1983). I must be old because I also remember slogging through the snow in Wisconsin to go to the computer center where one could actually type commands on a keyboard and see responses on a monitor and stand in line at the output window to get a great big printout that said "ERROR" (1985)!

And I must be old because I remember the monolithic pen recording moving chart polygraph on which I collected the data for my first psychophysiological study (1987). Hmmm. So, maybe it is time to update this book!

But how could it be Paul D. Bolls and Robert F. Potter writing this book? I remember when Paul Bolls ran his first study—ever—and recruited subjects before the study was ready to run—with predictable consequences (1993). I remember when Rob Potter was planning a career in cultural studies (1995). I also remember building a wall with Paul and Rob in the kitchen of a tumble-down house in Bloomington, IN, to separate the subjects from the equipment (1996). I remember them learning how to build a lab, and collect and analyze physiological data, and do studies, and write dissertations, and get jobs, and get tenure . . . so I guess they *can* write this book.

But it does make me feel old.

On the other hand, it also makes me feel proud, and hopeful, and excited about the future of the field. I remember when nobody in mass communication was doing psychophysiological research. I remember when only a few people were doing it and I pretty much knew all of them. Now there are plenty of people I don't know doing psychophysiological research in mass communication and a whole lot of people I do know because they are my colleagues, my academic children, and even my academic grandchildren.

Okay, so I'm old, and my academic children are now old and respected authorities who have written the book which you are about to read. What will you get out of it? A lot! Professors Bolls and Potter offer not just a compendium of measures but rather an integrated theoretical and methodological paradigm for studying communication as a complex embodied dynamic activity. The book begins with a careful consideration of how media researchers have historically used physiological measures (Chapter 1) followed by a comprehensive explication of the underpinnings of the field of psychophysiology (Chapter 2). In particular, they discuss the difference between measuring physiology in order to determine physiological responses and doing psychophysiology. Doing psychophysiology means that you are measuring real-time changes in the physiological system time-locked to some kind of stimulus in order to make inferences about psychological processes. Thus, it is not that we are looking for an increase or decrease in the activation of some physiological system or state, but rather, that we are looking for some specific, usually brief, and usually small change in a specific physiological measure, that has been shown, in a specific context, to be an indicator of a specific psychological event or process.

For example, careful work by psychophysiologists over two or three decades determined that three different kinds of attentional responses, the orienting response, the startle response, and the defensive response, could be differentiated by measuring very short-term change in heart rate (Graham, 1979). Specifically, it was shown that heart rate decelerated for about six beats following an orienting eliciting stimulus, but accelerated for six beats following a stimulus that elicited either a startle or a defensive response. This differentiation was shown to exist and to be valid when the stimuli which elicited the response were simple tones, white noise, and flashes in an equally simple context. In order to translate this finding into the media laboratory, studies were undertaken measuring heart rate time-locked to specific structural features of media that were thought to elicit orienting responses and checking to see if heart rate decelerated for six to seven beats following these features. Using this technique, it was determined that things like scene changes in TV, voice changes in radio, and animation in web content did indeed elicit orienting responses (Lang, 1990; Lang, Wise, Borse, & David 2002; Potter, 2000).

As can be seen, one of the things that needs to be done, in order to take these techniques for using physiological responses as indicators of psychological processes out of the psychophysiology lab and put them in the media researchers' arsenal, is the careful work of validating each measure as an indicator of the psychological process of interest within the context of a complex media message. One of the many strengths of this book is that it has gathered together all of this information, organized it, and laid it out in a way that will allow the reader who is new to psychophysiology to employ complex, theoretically based measures in a valid and appropriate way.

Another strength of this book is the way it straightforwardly addresses the fact that any given physiological measure can simultaneously be an indicator of multiple psychological processes and that which process is being indicated is determined by the way the measure was collected and analyzed. Thus, a single measure can be used as an indicator of multiple psychological processes during the same message. This is because, over time, the embodied brain is engaging in multiple emotional and cognitive processes in response to a single mediated message. These affective and cognitive responses are reflected (albeit dimly) in the physiological systems that support thinking and feeling. Thus, a given measure, analyzed second by second at time point A may tell you something about attention while examining the average, at time point B, may tell you something about motivational activation or direction of emotional response. Understanding which measures, and which analyses, indicate which processes in what contexts is a complex body of knowledge which this book lays out forthrightly for the reader (Chapters 4 and 5).

In addition, the book considers and discusses the whole range of possible psychophysiological measures from easy and common measures like heart rate and skin conductance, to probe measures like startle and the post-auricular response, and finally to complex brain-centered measures like electroencephalography (EEG) and functional magnetic resonance imaging (fMRI). As a result, the book will serve as an extremely up-to-date and comprehensive reference volume for all the measures that have so far been used to track mediated messages through the black box that is the human motivated processing system.

Finally, this book is different from most books which focus on psychophysiology, in that it connects psychophysiological measures to other measures of mediated message processing (Chapter 7). The use of these measures is integrated with core mass communication theory and measures, and examples illustrate how psychophysiology can add to the understanding provided by our more traditional measures. Readers are provided with multiple avenues to approach and become adept at using these measures (Chapter 9), concluding with suggestions from experienced users of these measures about the many areas of media research that seem ripe for further investigation by a new generation of *media-psychophysiologists*.

Enjoy the journey!

Annie Lang
Bloomington, IN, 2011

PREFACE

This is your brain on media! More than just a play on words—"borrowed" from a legendary anti-drug message—beginning this book with that statement reflects how the field of media research is in the process of an exciting paradigm shift. This paradigm shift is fueled by the efforts of researchers who work from an expanded methodological toolbox that includes a variety of psychophysiological measures enabling the observation of mental processes embodied in the brain that are engaged during media consumption. Data obtained from these measures, in essence, provide a view of the human brain "on" media. The growth in research examining how the brain processes media has reached a point where we believe it should be recognized as a new, specialized area of media research that, in this book, we have termed media psychology research. Media psychology researchers go far beyond insights provided by traditional media effects scholars to developing rich explanations of the dynamic mental processes that unfold across time as individuals consume and are impacted by media. Psychophysiology is part of the methodological core for media psychology research and this is the first book to exclusively focus on the application of psychophysiological measures to studying how the brain processes media content.

Our primary purpose in writing this book was to cover psychophysiological measures in a way that would be accessible and interesting to readers whose formal education is more likely to be in a media related field of study rather than psychophysiology. This objective makes it necessary to note up front that it is more accurate to consider this a book on media psychophysiology—the application of psychophysiological measures in media research—rather than a book that joins the ranks of excellent technical volumes on psychophysiology, such as the *Handbook of psychophysiology*. Those volumes are exclusively focused on psychophysiology, providing a more in-depth conceptual and operational discussion of a wider range of specific measures than we have included here. Readers who will be engaging in media psychophysiology research should not consider our book a substitute for reading more specialized volumes on psychophysiology. Within the field of media psychology research, this book is intended to complement the valuable edited volume by Annie Lang, *Measuring psychological responses to media*. That volume should be considered the first methods book in media psychology research and included a couple chapters on psychophysiological measures. Our work builds on Annie Lang's volume by providing an entire book focused on media psychophysiology. Ultimately our hope is that this book serves to promote media psychophysiology as a scientific endeavor among the community of scholars that are more generally interested in media psychology research.

We hope that a variety of scholars are intrigued by this book. We believe such scholars could include anyone who is curious about the nature of the exciting and dynamic interaction between media and the human brain, ranging from the scientist working in a media psychophysiology lab to interested students, professors, and media industry professionals. The effects of media content on individuals emerge from this interaction, making the topic of media and the human brain potentially relevant to anyone that has more than a passing interest in "media effects." However, this book is specifically for scholars whose intellectual interests create a need to learn more about the promises and pitfalls of applying psychophysiological measures to studying the fascinating and critically important ways individuals mentally process and are influenced by media content. This need could be driven by a desire to directly participate in the growing community of scholars conducting media psychophysiology research or simply an interest in being able to critically read the growing body of published research that includes psychophysiological data. We had both types of readers in mind when writing this book. That is why we have made a concentrated effort to include technical content that is critical to serving the practical needs of scientists who will incorporate these measures in their research labs as well as a more general discussion of the theoretical framework that has enabled psychophysiological measures to be more than a fleeting methodological fad in media psychology research.

The chapters in this book follow a logical progression starting with a focus on theoretical/conceptual background material before moving to a discussion of specific measures and the operational details of conducting media psychophysiology research. The first three chapters provide necessary background for understanding the current application of psychophysiological measures in media psychology research. Chapter 1 provides a historical review of media effects research, specifically highlighting early efforts to establish a link between human physiological responses and exposure to certain types of media content. In looking back at the history of media research one cannot help but appreciate the work of researchers who recognized the importance of a scientific approach to understanding media effects and pioneered that effort. Chapter 1 not only reviews this history but also showcases how media research moved from a field focused on behavioral effects of media exposure to adopting an information processing paradigm, focused on bursting open the black box of the human mind in order to investigate mental processes believed to underlie the effects of media on individuals. This sets the stage for Chapter 2 where we formally introduce psychophysiology as the theoretical framework that has led to what we believe is the permanent establishment of psychophysiological measures as part of the methodological toolbox used in media research. Chapter 2 outlines the theoretical assumptions of psychophysiology that are the very foundation of any effort to validly apply psychophysiological measures in studying how the brain processes media. Chapter 3 introduces a more technical discussion of psychophysiological measures, covering the basics of recording physiological signals and introducing key terms and concepts involved in understanding patterns of variation that can be found in psychophysiological data.

We move from discussion of important background material to covering specific psychophysiological measures in Chapters 4–6. Despite the fact that the theoretical approach presented in this book does not draw a sharp distinction between human cognition and emotion, psychophysiological measures can be broadly organized around a distinction between measures that primarily index mental processes involved in the operation of human attention and memory and measures that index mental processes involved in human emotion. The organization of Chapters 4 and 5 reflects this distinction. In Chapter 4 we discuss psychophysiological measures of cognitive processes. Chapter 5 covers psychophysiological measures of emotional processes. Both chapters cover two psychophysiological measures that are well-established in the media psychophysiology lab. Chapter 4 highlights cardiac activity and EEG while Chapter 5 showcases skin conductance and facial EMG. The first part of each chapter provides a theoretical background for using psychophysiological measures to study cognitive and emotional processing of media content while the second part focuses on providing technical knowledge that is necessary to record and analyze data obtained with each measure. Chapter 6 features a discussion of emerging psychophysiological measures that have tremendous potential value in media psychophysiology research but have yet to be extensively used in published experiments. Measures discussed in this chapter include the startle eye-blink response—a measure that is showing particular promise in indexing the motivational value of media content—and fMRI—a particularly exciting psychophysiological measure that directly records highly localized activity in the human brain. Our discussion of these emerging measures includes a consideration of their potential value as well as general operational details.

The last three chapters of this book cover a range of important topics. Chapter 7 addresses the importance of conducting media psychology research using a combination of psychophysiological as well as self-report and behavioral measures. This chapter opens with a discussion of the specific role of psychophysiological measures in advancing knowledge of how the brain processes media and outlines how distinct types of measures only capture a part of the ultimate mental experience of consuming and being influenced by media content. Chapter 7 concludes with a review of specific measures that are particularly useful to combine with psychophysiological measures in media psychophysiology research. Chapter 8 is a "how-to" guide to setting up and running a media psychophysiology lab. This chapter was particularly informed by our 15 years of both mistakes and accomplishments in setting up labs and conducting media psychophysiology research. We discuss considerations in finding a lab space, ordering equipment, training, as well as conducting experiments. This could actually be the first chapter you want to read if you are either in the process of setting up or currently running a media psychophysiology lab. Chapter 9 concludes this book with a consideration of important contributions to knowledge experiments utilizing psychophysiological measures have already made to media psychology research as well as our thoughts about the exciting future of media psychophysiology research.

A distinct feature of this book that we hope readers will find particularly interesting is that throughout several chapters we have included brief reviews of research that has utilized psychophysiological measures to study how the brain processes media. Ideally this will not only help you better understand these measures but spark ideas for ways that psychophysiological measures might be used to advance your own work and general understanding of media psychology research. We consider it a privilege to be part of the community of scholars engaged in media psychophysiology research and offer this book as a tool that will hopefully help our colleagues both present and future in this endeavor.

ACKNOWLEDGMENTS FOR ROBERT F. POTTER

This book has been a *long* time in the making. And looking back, before it was even a consideration, there were people who were preparing me to write it. As Annie Lang mentions in the Foreword, when we first met I was a confused graduate student not finding particular intellectual satisfaction in cultural studies courses I was taking. I guess she was the first person to push me toward writing this book when—on what I remember as being only our second meeting together—she asked me "Do you want to help me unpack my new lab equipment, it just arrived today?" Annie, I thank you for unleashing a fascination for psychophysiological enquiry that gets bigger with each passing day.

Another person who prepared me to write it was my first departmental Chair, Loy Singleton in the Telecommunications and Film Department at the University of Alabama. Loy was steadfast in his belief that the time of junior faculty should be protected so they could nurture and build research momentum, something so easy to lose during the transition from student to faculty. Because of him—and one other person—I was able to set up my first psychophysiology lab.

That other person was Ed Cook of the Department of Psychology at the University of Alabama at Birmingham. In Chapter 8 I encourage young media psychophysiologists to contact those longstanding in the field for input and assistance. I do so based entirely on the warm reception Ed gave me when I called him and said "I can't get this stuff to work right, can you help?" He came to Tuscaloosa and worked with me to put the final pieces of my lab puzzle together for little more than a burrito lunch at Pepitos, the local Mexican restaurant. Thanks Ed.

Walter Gantz also helped launch this project. As my Chair at Indiana University, Walt appointed me the Director of the Institute for Communication Research (ICR) and allowed my colleagues and me to design an ideal collaborative social scientific laboratory. I thank him for that opportunity and for the encouragement during the final stages of the writing process.

The bulk of the initial writing took place during my sabbatical year at the Interactive Television Research Institute in Perth, Australia. Thanks to my ITRI colleagues—Duane Varan, Steve Bellman, Jenny Robinson, and Shiree Treleaven-Hassard—for a wonderful opportunity to get away from home and devote myself to the project.

That initial writing had to be edited, and I thank the students of T602 from the Fall of 2010 who provided valuable comments and insight.

Sharon Mayell is the Lab Manager at the ICR and Reed Nelson is my department's Fiscal Officer. Both do an unbelievable job keeping the facility running smoothly, allowing me time to tinker in the lab, explore ideas, and learn the things I tried to share in this book.

And finally immense thanks to Linda Bathgate, our extraordinary editor and my occasional bowling partner. This book exists because of your encouragement, patience, and sense of humor.

ACKNOWLEDGMENTS FOR PAUL D. BOLLS

Writing a book like this is a humbling experience. My mind helped produce this work that we hope serves to inspire and promote the use of psychophysiological measures within media research to study a topic I am very passionate about, the media/mind interaction. However, as I worked to produce this volume I became keenly aware of how much I owe to a great scientist, mentor, friend, and my "academic mom" Annie Lang. Annie took me under her wing as a wide-eyed student in a "janitor closet" lab at Washington State and through two labs at two different universities molded me into a productive member of this community of scholars. There are numerous members of the community of scholars who have inspired, prodded, and provided other forms of support that have contributed to the completion of this book. I want to specifically thank my co-directors of the PRIME Lab, Glenn Leshner and Kevin Wise, for their friendship and for bearing the brunt of keeping a lab running while I worked on "the book!" I also want to thank Esther Thorson and Margaret Duffy for helping create an encouraging intellectual work environment where I could complete this project. It is also critical that I thank the students who inspire my work in the PRIME Lab. Your intellectual curiosity helps fuel my passion for this field of research. I need to specifically thank PRIME Lab students, Petya Eckler, Jessica Freeman, Jana Hainey, Anastasia Kononova, Jaime Williams, and Nathan Winters who posed for pictures. Elisa Day shot some of the pictures in this book and Saleem Alhabash helped produce figures. Throughout this endeavor I have been blessed with support from students who at times seemed more excited about the completion of this book than even me. I hope you all know that more than just being my students, you are my friends. Finally, a huge debt of gratitude is owed to Linda Bathgate at Routledge. It is impossible for me to even imagine completing this book without your significant help. You knew exactly when to "cheerlead" and when to "coach" us through FINALLY finishing this book!

1

PSYCHOPHYSIOLOGY IN THE CONTEXT OF MEDIA PROCESSES AND EFFECTS RESEARCH

The general task of a social scientist is to ask questions about how human beings act within a complex world. For most of you reading this book your specific interests focus on how human beings interact with mediated messages—communications coming from television sets, computer monitors, mobile media devices, radios, game consoles, and the like. Social scientists explore these interactions in a variety of ways. Some take a fine-grained and systematic look at what is contained in the content of media messages using a method called content analysis. Others conduct surveys, using a wide range of instruments (phone interviews, mail surveys, website questionnaires) to assess people's attitudes toward media-related issues. Most of this book, however, will focus on a third common technique used by social scientists: the laboratory experiment. If you have taken even the most basic high school science class you are somewhat familiar with the steps of experimental research. In a controlled environment a small number of variables are isolated and precisely varied in order to measure the effects of the manipulations on outcome variables of interest. There are fine books available to guide you in the general practice of experimental design (Babbie, 2010; Kirk, 1994). The overarching goal of *this* book is to show how **psychophysiological measures**—indices of bodily responses reflecting variation in psychological states—are used in experiments conducted by researchers interested in discovering how the brain processes mediated messages. By the time you are finished you will have a working understanding of what psychophysiological indices validly measure and be able to read the ever-increasing body of work being published in the area, some of which will be reviewed throughout this book.

But in order to understand how psychophysiological research methods are used in the modern media psychology lab, it's helpful to first take a general look at the history of social scientific research in media processes and effects. As you'll see, the measurement of bodily responses to media messages makes two brief appearances in the early part of that history, quickly retreating each time. The first appearance is actually only a single study, a module of the iconic **Payne Fund Studies**. Following that, the application of physiological measures disappears from media research for almost three decades due to the rapid and almost complete swing of the psychological discipline toward the behaviorist approach. The second appearance of research that included the observation of physiological responses to media occurs late within that behaviorist tradition, but even then only generates a handful of published studies before again being abandoned. With the luxury of hindsight, this seems to be primarily a result of prevailing, but mistaken, thoughts at that time concerning how different human physiological systems respond to arousing situations. The belief that all physiological indices should increase in response to arousing situations resulted in unpredicted and—at least at the time—inexplicable results. Once again, physiological measures virtually disappear from the media psychology researcher's toolkit for several decades.

Not until media researchers fully embraced the theoretical underpinnings of *psychophysiology*—as opposed to just viewing physiological responses as more and different media effects one could measure—were they able to successfully utilize indices like heart rate, skin conductance and brain wave patterns as indicators of psychological states that vary in meaningful ways during the processing of mediated messages.

A brief history of media effects research

Early research—the impact of film content

With the development and widespread distribution of each medium comes public concern over the effects of exposure to its content. Of particular focus is the impact of seemingly salacious materials on children. With electronic media, this reaction was first seen in the early 1920s as the number of movie theaters in cities and towns across the country rapidly increased. Interested in the impact of the new phenomenon, individual researchers from sociology and psychology conducted meticulous studies primarily focusing on the effects of movie houses on specific municipalities. Reverend J. J. Phelan, for example, published *Motion pictures as a phase of commercial amusement in Toledo Ohio* in 1919, claiming to "gather all available data and allow the reader to make his own interpretation" (p. 11) concerning the impact of film on society. The conclusions drawn in publications like this, however, did not derive from experimentation or careful observation. Instead they seem to have sprung from common understanding of the day concerning human cognition; namely that psychological mechanisms of thought, knowledge, attitude formation, and behavior were uniform across individuals

(Sparks, 2002). As a result, Phelan and others crusading for governmental censorship of the motion picture industry believed that film content had very powerful effects. Under this powerful-effects view, it was, to use Phelan's own imagistic language, as if the attitudes, knowledge, and beliefs contained in a motion picture were applied directly to the psyches of each audience member like they were being poured into the brain by a ladle!

This powerful-effects view resulted in Phelan giving a list of "specific dangers" to children who frequented movie theaters. Things like: an incapacity of sustained studying of school materials, the awaking of morbid curiosity, the development of an abnormal imagination, and even "false delineation of what constitutes true Americanism" (p. 112) all awaited any child who watched too many movies.

Although the research done during this time has largely been associated with a **Hypodermic Needle Theory** of media effects, an examination of individual works show more caution and reticence among researchers of the time (Wartella & Reeves, 1985). For example, although William Healy, a prominent scholar in the field of juvenile delinquency, warned that movies—and perhaps even more so, the darkness of the movie theaters themselves—led to increased sexual activity among youth, he also believed that the susceptibility to such effects was highly variable across individuals (Jowett, Jarvie, & Fuller, 1996).

In the early 1930s came the publication of a series of eight volumes under the title "Motion pictures and youth." Today, students of media history are more familiar with them as The Payne Fund Studies, an interesting fact given that members of the private, philanthropic Payne Fund eventually attempted to distance the use of the fund's name from the publications (Jowett et al., 1996). The reason for their lack of enthusiasm was the fervent political nature of the project's leader Reverend William Harrison Short. Short's intention was to use a series of social scientific research studies to gather enough damning evidence of the effects of motion pictures on youth that demands of governmental censorship would take hold. He believed that the best way to gather this evidence was by enlisting the leading researchers across several fields to design experiments using the highest standards of scientific rigor. In the end, it was likely the scientists' objectivity and precision—which they placed above their own possible personal disdain for movie content—that ultimately led to results which made it hard to suggest strong, uniform effects resulted from movie exposure (Jowett et al., 1996).

Given the focus of this book, it is interesting that one of the 11 Payne Fund Studies relied heavily on the measurement of physiological reactions to movie content. **Wendell S. Dysinger**, a graduate student at Iowa State University, and his professor **Christian A. Ruckmick** were two members of the Payne Fund Study team whose goal was to "discover the emotional effects produced by various types of incidents in motion pictures on children and adults" (Dysinger

& Ruckmick, 1933, p. 3). They did so by designing a series of laboratory and field studies where subjects between the ages of six and 50 watched popular films while dipping two fingers into a box about the size of a small loaf of bread. The box contained liquid electrode allowing skin resistance readings to be taken off their fingers. Pulse rate data were also recorded using a leather arm strap. Even by today's standards, the extent of the Dysinger and Ruckmick data collection task is impressive. Not only did they record physiological data from 89 people across six age categories in the controlled environment of their research labs, but they negotiated to bring their equipment into the back three rows of local movie theaters, allowing them to collect additional data from 61 subjects in a more naturalistic setting.

In contrast to the declarations made by the likes of Phelan, the results of Dysinger and Ruckmick did not show uniform emotional reactions to film. Instead there were interesting variations across the different age categories. For example, skin resistance reactions to scenes from the "erotic" movie *The Feast of Ishtar* showed more arousal among the 16-year-old subjects than any other age group. Now remember, this was in the 1930s when erotic scenes consisted of kissing and groping that would likely be considered mild by today's standards. But still, Dysinger and Ruckmick found fewer reactions to them in the older movie viewers compared to 16-year-olds. Furthermore, even *within* the 16-year-old age group there were substantial differences; some responded with very high levels of skin resistance and some had barely any resistance at all indicative of large arousal reactions. This led to the conclusion that the impact of film "is a matter of individual mental lives and must be regulated or at least judged according to the individual psychophysiological organism . . . of his peculiar mental and physical constitution" (Dysinger & Ruckmick, 1933, p. 115).

Behaviorism's strong influence

As we will see later in this chapter, Dysinger & Ruckmick interpreted their results in accord with several of the theoretical precepts of modern psychophysiology, recognizing the importance of both external and internal *contexts* in being able to predict how individuals will react to a media message. However, this contextual way of thinking was overshadowed in the 1930s by the growing momentum of a major scientific paradigm: **behaviorism** and **classical conditioning**. In the early 1920s, Russian scientist **Ivan Pavlov** demonstrated how organisms could be conditioned to expect certain outcomes following a signal input (Samoilov, 2007). He did this first by repeatedly giving dogs food following a standard signal—such as a ticking metronome or the ringing of an electronic buzzer—and then measuring the activity in their salivary glands in response to the food presentation (Pavlov, 1927). After multiple conditioning trials, the dogs began to associate the signal with the onset of good things to eat. Eventually Pavlov's data showed the

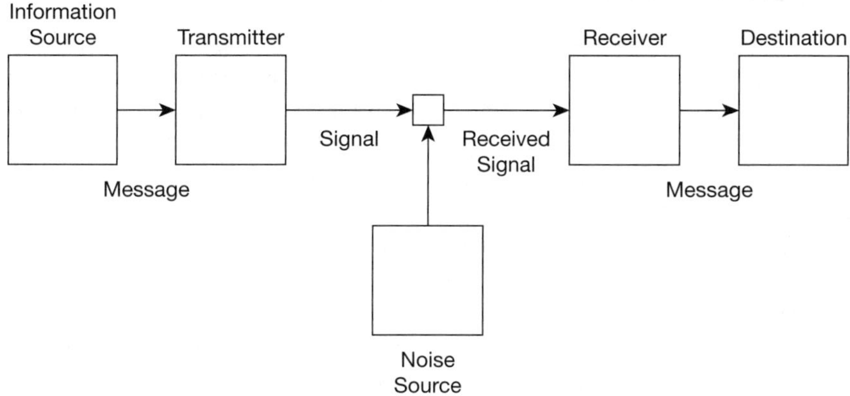

FIGURE 1.1 The Shannon-Weaver model of communications, circa 1949.

dogs beginning to salivate in response to the signal alone, whether food was given or not. This pairing of a stimulus (the buzzer) with an identifiable response (increased saliva in the dogs' mouths) became a guiding metaphor for much of the work done in psychology for the next several decades—an approach known generally as *behaviorism.*

One of the most famous and influential scientists associated with behaviorism—**B. F. Skinner**—believed that the only things necessary for explaining the behavior of any organism—including humans—was a description of the important elements of the external environment and an understanding of the functional connections between them and the behavior of interest (Smith, 1996). According to Skinner and other strict behaviorists, it was not only unnecessary but also somewhat foolish to develop theories about what was going on inside the brain of the animal since we could not possibly measure with any accuracy something that we could not directly observe (Smith, 1996). So, to return to the Pavlovian metaphor, the task of most experimental psychology conducted from the 1930s to 1950s became essentially one of matching an external stimulus to observable responses.

Communication researchers and theorists during this time reflected behaviorist approaches in their work, primarily because many scholars migrating to the field had been trained—and therefore highly influenced by—psychologists immersed in the paradigm (Paisley, 1984). The pattern of the **Stimulus-Response Model**, for example, is apparent in the classic definition of communication from Lasswell (1927/1971): "Who says What to Whom and with What Effect." Later, the **model** proposed in Shannon and Weaver's (1949) *Mathematical theory of communications* (see Figure 1.1) still conceptualized communicative acts in a manner just slightly more elaborated than Pavlov's description of salivating dogs responding to signals 20 years previously.

Early behaviorist communication research

Of course, with communication research in its infancy, using a behaviorist model to establish predictable responses from well-explicated causal stimuli was important and necessary work. Many notable relationships were identified during the early years of the field. Consider the research conducted by Hadley Cantril who explored the massive panic caused by the radio performance of H. G. Wells' *War of the Worlds* on CBS's "Mercury Theater of the Air." The broadcast, which occurred on October 30, 1938, contained multiple on-air reminders that the show was merely a dramatic performance. Nevertheless, all over North America people believed they were hearing a live broadcast of an interplanetary invasion by Martians intent on destroying the Earth! The extent of the panic was so great that Cantril and his colleagues at Princeton University's Office of Radio Research seized upon the opportunity to conduct the first investigation of wide scale public behaviors triggered by a media event (Lowery & DeFleur, 1995). What Cantril hoped to do was take the behavioral responses—which ranged from sorority sisters huddled around radios saying their tearful goodbyes to frantic calls to police stations and attempted suicides—and work backwards to identify the environmental conditions which had served as stimuli. To do so, the researchers conducted a wide-ranging study utilizing personal interviews, surveys, and content analysis of over 12,000 print pieces describing the broadcast and people's reactions to it.

According to Lowery & DeFleur (1995), the researchers from the Office of Radio Research identified four different categories of responses to the radio play:

1. Those who listened to the *War of the Worlds* but decided the reports sounded too much like science fiction storytelling and therefore did not panic.
2. Those who compared what they were hearing in the broadcast to external information, such as a published radio schedule, determined the reports were fictional and did not panic.
3. People who obtained other external information but yet still panicked because they believed the broadcast was true.
4. Those who panicked from the onset of the broadcast and therefore were uninterested in checking what they heard against internal or external searches of further information.

Even though Cantril (1940) believed strict behaviorists would not be comfortable with his conclusions due to the absence of a repetitive conditioning element (but after all, how many times does an alien invasion of the planet repeat itself!), the influence of a behaviorist approach in these categories is hard to dispute. They provide descriptions of the *external* or *environmental* conditions on that October night and explain how they may have influenced a person to act in one of these four ways. These descriptions were either of key elements of the media messages (i.e., the dramatic excellence of the performance itself, the interruption of music programming to present "news" updates about the invasion, etc.), or the societal temperament in general (i.e., the fact that the broadcast occurred so close to Halloween, that war being salient in the minds of many listeners as Hitler's fascist regime gained control in Germany, etc.). However, Cantril did not attempt to describe the processes that took place *within* the individual's cognitive system to arrive at the conclusions they did and exhibit particular behaviors as a consequence.

Another behaviorist researcher, Carl Hovland, advanced the field with a prolific research career spent establishing links between external message attributes and opinion change in message recipients (Hovland, 1957; Hovland, Janis, & Kelly, 1953). Hovland's research interests were greatly influenced by his stint in the US Army during World War II conducting experiments on how film could be used to affect audience opinion change (Lowery & DeFleur, 1995). During the two decades following the war, however, he moved from film to audiotape recordings of individuals making interpersonal arguments. In all he conducted over 50 studies as the director of the Yale Program of Research on Communication and Attitude Change. In his book *Persuasion and communication* (Hovland et al., 1953), for example, one chapter details experiments about the organization of message arguments and the ways in which varying their structure impacted opinion change. Research questions included:

- Should a persuasive message draw an explicit conclusion or should it leave the conclusion implicit and allow the audience to reach it?
- For a message to be maximally persuasive should each side of an argument be presented or only the points in favor of the position being argued for?
- If multiple points are made in an argument, should the message lead with the strongest one or save it for last?

To test these and other questions, Hovland recorded different versions of arguments on issues ranging from international politics to the benefits of higher education. He even included more mundane topics like the usefulness of woodworking as a hobby! In tightly controlled experimental conditions, college students listened to their assigned audiotape and then gave their opinions and attitudes toward the topic. Hovland and his colleagues felt that three things happen when someone changes an opinion:

1. A recommended opinion (the stimulus) is presented.
2. Assuming that the subjects have paid attention to and understood the message, the audience responds or reacts. That is, they think about their initial opinions and also about the recommended opinion.
3. The subjects will change their attitudes if incentives (rewards) for making a new response are greater that (*sic*) those for making the old response (Lowery & DeFleur, 1995, pp. 169–170).

Once again, there was not much work designed to investigate the specifics of the second condition—the one having to do with cognitive processes like attention and comprehension (cf. Cohen, 1957). It was, indeed, *assumed* that "attention" occurred and that "thinking" took place. The mechanisms or processes involved in such internal states were just not explored by behaviorist researchers in the 1950s.

Albert Bandura is another communication researcher closely associated with behaviorism. Bandura developed a model of how people learn through observation which he initially called **social learning theory** (Sparks, 2002). Social learning theory maintained that if a person observes behaviors being performed by a physically- or socially-attractive model—*and* if those behaviors are rewarded—then the observer is likely to behave in similar ways in future situations as long as they physically can and are motivated to do so.

Bandura was primarily interested in how people learned aggressive behaviors and much of his early experiments had school-aged subjects watch modeling stimuli consisting of media messages showing adults acting in an aggressive manner. For example, in one study Bandura and his colleagues (Bandura, Ross, & Ross, 1963) tested whether watching aggressive behaviors in a film resulted in different levels of post-viewing aggressive behaviors in research subjects than watching the same behaviors in cartoon or real-life versions of the same acts. The experimental procedure for this study was similar to many done by Bandura. First, a child subject came to the lab individually and was randomly assigned to a treatment group; they were either selected to see the live-, film-, or cartoon-version of the aggressive behavior or they were assigned to a control group and exposed to no aggressive behaviors at all. When the experiment began, the experimenter brought the subject and another adult into a testing room. The other adult was actually also one of the experimenters—a **confederate** acting as the modeling agent. Both the child and the modeling agent were seated at a table on which there were arts and crafts supplies. The experimenter showed them both how to use the supplies to make creations. After a short time, the experimenter then escorted the confederate to a table on the other side of the room. This table was covered with small toys, a small mallet, and an inflated plastic Bobo doll toy. The confederate was told, loud enough so that the child subject could hear them, that they could now only play on that side of the room. The experimenter then left the two of them—at their separate tables—alone in the room.

As a planned part of the experimental manipulation, the confederate first began playing with toys but after a short while began yelling at the Bobo doll and acting aggressively toward it—sitting on it, punching it multiple times in the nose, hitting it on the head with a mallet, throwing it up in the air and kicking it around the room—for about 10 minutes. Subjects in the film version of the experiment did not share the room with the confederate, but instead were shown a movie of an adult acting in this same aggressive way on a color TV set placed close to the arts and crafts table. Those in the cartoon version also watched the same TV set, but the film was actually a live-action production of *Herman the Cat*, a show made especially for the experiment where "the female model costumed as a black cat similar to the many cartoon cats" appeared walking across the floor "covered with artificial grass and the walls forming the backdrop were warm, bright-colored trees, birds, and butterflies creating a fantasyland setting" (Bandura et al., 1963, p. 5). But, as you might expect, Herman the Cat also eventually beat the heck out of the Bobo doll!

After the modeling session, the child subject was led to another small room that contained a number of attractive toys and told that they could play with them. But, shortly after they became engaged with these toys, the experimenter returned and said that those toys were too nice for the subject to play with. Instead, they would have to go into yet another room and play with toys there. The goal of this step, of course, was to instigate frustration in the child. In the next room the child subject found equal numbers of nonaggressive toys like crayons and paper, cars and trucks, dolls, and plastic farm animals. There was also an assortment of aggressive toys, too. Most importantly an identical Bobo doll, a mallet and peg board, two dart guns, and a tether ball with a face drawn on it and hanging from the ceiling. The child then spent 20 minutes in this room while experimenters observed and coded their behaviors while sitting behind a one-way window.

Bandura's findings were exactly the type that you could imagine William Harrison Short had hoped to find during the Payne Fund Studies:

> Indeed, the available data suggests that, of the three experimental conditions, exposure to humans on film portraying aggression was the most influential in eliciting and shaping aggressive behavior. Subjects in this condition, in relation to the control subjects, exhibited more total aggression, more imitative aggression, and more partially imitative behavior, such as sitting on the Bobo doll and mallet aggression, and they engaged in significantly more aggressive gunplay. In addition, they performed significantly more aggressive gunplay than subjects who were exposed to the real-life aggressive models.
>
> (Bandura et al., 1963, p. 7).

Similar to Hovland's theory of persuasion, Bandura's social learning theory proposed four necessary conditions if modeled behaviors were later to be imitated by a targeted individual: attention, retention, reproduction, and motivation. In other words, if learning of the modeled behaviors was going to occur, one must ensure that behavioral details are first selected from the vast array of information in the target's environment at any one time and symbolically encoded into their cognitive system. If the students in the Bobo doll experiments had, instead of watching the model, been so focused on their arts and crafts, no learning of aggressive behavior could have occurred because none had been attended to in the first place. But, paying attention to the behavior is not enough. Instead, said Bandura, the details of the modeled behavior must be retained in long-term memory and be accessible during appropriate situations. Furthermore, the target individual must be physically capable of reproducing the effect and have strong incentives to do so.

Bandura's research has focused primarily on investigating the impact of different variables on these four necessary conditions for social learning. With the inclusion of the concept *personal agency* (Bandura, 2006), social learning theory has transformed to social cognitive theory (Bandura, 2009). However, in the late 1950s and early 1960s, like the work of Hovland and Cantril before him, Bandura focused almost entirely on external circumstances in a noticeably behaviorist way. In fact, this focus away from closely investigating internal cognitive processes lasted well into the 1970s. Noted communications researcher Wilbur Schramm—in his edited volume entitled *The process and effects of mass communication*—stated that although much of communication took place inside our brain, researchers were forced to view that as impenetrable:

> Most of the communication process is in the "black box" of the central nervous system, the contents of which we understand only vaguely. When we describe communication, we are therefore dealing with analogies and gross functions, and the test of any model [of communications] is whether it enables us to make predictions—not whether it is a true copy of what happens in the black box, a matter of which we cannot now speak with any great confidence.
>
> (Schramm, 1971, pp. 24–25)

Opening the black box—the information processing approach

It is generally accepted that three primary goals of social scientific investigation are prediction, explanation, and understanding (Babbie, 2010; Sparks, 2002). Scientists predict (we often say "hypothesize") what will happen when we bring different variables together. We see this exemplified in the extreme with the Stimulus–Response model of behaviorist work. But beyond that, most scientists also have a strong desire to know *why* things happen the way they do and to *understand* the particular sequence of events that have to transpire in order to obtain a particular effect (Sparks, 2002). Because behaviorism did such a poor job of satisfying these two aspects of the scientific undertaking, the luster of the paradigm began fading by the 1960s. Many psychologists began to believe like linguist Noam Chomsky, "defining psychology as the science of behavior was like defining physics as the science of meter reading" (attributed to Chomsky by Miller, 2003).

What was needed in order to better understand human psychology was a willingness to pry open the "black box" of the mind. Scientists felt that in order to predict and fully explain human behavior they needed to not only identify which environmental stimuli caused predictable effects but also design methods and test hypotheses concerning the specific mental processes and mechanisms behind these S-R connections. Picking from a wide array of disciplines—not only psychology but also philosophy, linguistics, computer science, communication science and anthropology—some social scientists began moving their work in a direction which eventually became known as the *information processing approach*. In their book *Cognitive psychology and information processing: An introduction* Roy Lachman, Janet Lachman, and Earl Butterfield provide a thorough description of how each of these fields contributed to the development of information processing as a discipline in its own right (Lachman et al., 1979). They also provide a discussion of the assumptive principles held by those who began to peek inside the black box. Because many of these principles are also held by media psychology researchers who use psychophysiological methods it is important to summarize them for you here:

1. *Humans have innate capacities.* Behaviorists felt that all of human knowledge and behavior was due to conditioned learning. In contrast, those using an information processing approach believe that humans also have inherited tendencies passed on through generations via the genetic mechanisms of natural selection. There are genetics associated with external and aesthetic traits, of course: height, hair and eye color, skin pigmentation, etc. There are also innate genetic tendencies for certain diseases. The information-processing scientist, however, is more interested in the impact of innate *cognitive* abilities that have evolved in all human beings to a varying extent. And, as we will see, the fact that these abilities were selected for down through millennia when almost everything human beings encountered was real and present, certainly impacts the ways in which we interact today with things mediated through a TV or computer screen—in other words, with things *not* real and *not* present (Reeves & Nass, 1996). But, that's getting a little bit ahead of ourselves. For now, it is important to realize that a key assumption held by those using an information-processing approach is that "part of the job of explaining human cognition is to identify how innate capacities and the results of experience combine to produce human performance" (Lachman et al., 1979, p. 118).
2. *Humans are active information seekers.* Again in stark contrast to the behaviorist approach, which viewed humans as passively waiting to react as environmental stimuli acted upon them, the information processing approach "views people as hungry for information, as constantly scanning their environment in search of relevant developments" (Lachman et al., 1979, p. 118). What causes unpredictability in human behavior, of course, is that human beings are not only motivated by observable external conditions but also by internal motivations that are often unseen and therefore unrecognized by the scientific observer.

3. *Knowledge is stored in the brain.* Humans (and other living organisms) interact with the environment through sensory organs. When reading this book, light is reflected off the page and hits your eyeball. When listening to music through headphones connected to an MP3 player, ears collect vibrations of air occurring at various frequencies. But what happens to these instances of light and sound energy after they enter into the human organism? How are they transferred into the cognitive system? Somehow the different light and shadow patterns reflected from the page become recognized as letters, words, and sentences containing meaning. The varied vibrations get turned into a recognition and appreciation of the musical notes from a favorite song. But if we were to slice open your brain while reading and listening to music we would not, of course, be flooded with waves of light and sound. Those using an information processing approach believe that the human brain first transfers these various energies into some sort of representations of reality. There are debates over what form these representations may take. Some—including Lachman et al. in the late 1970s—believe that knowledge is represented as a series of formal symbolic propositions which the brain then manipulates (Newell, 1990). Others believe that viewing cognition as strict symbol manipulation is too limiting and instead feel that knowledge is represented as a distributed network of neurons that become activated at certain times (Churchland & Sejnowski, 1992). Regardless, the fact that some sort of representation is necessary in a cognitive system is an undisputed assumption.

4. *The Brain is a knowledge manipulator.* Since Lachman et al. (1979) believed that knowledge was stored in the brain in a symbolic manner, they stated this assumption as "*The Brain is a Symbol Manipulator*" and that only a "few relatively basic symbolic computational operations, such as encoding, comparing, locating, storing, and the like, may ultimately account for human intelligence and the capacity to create knowledge, novelty, and perhaps expectations about the future" (Lachman et al., 1979 pp. 114–115). Although the computational operations may be few, evolution has fine-tuned the human cognitive system into one that is very rapid, efficient, and precise in its ability to employ them. Of course, if one takes the distributed network approach, the brain has evolved to rapidly make associations between a series of neurons located across the brain (Clark, 1997; Thelen, 1995). Regardless of how you think knowledge is represented in our brains, the assumption that evolution has fine-tuned the brain into a very rapid processor of that knowledge is central to information processing and to psychophysiology.

5. *Human beings are systems.* Social scientists using an information processing approach view the human organism as a **dynamic system**. The concept of a dynamic system is one that we will return to in more detail when discussing specific assumptions of the *psychophysiological* approach. For now, the

definition provided by Miller (1973) will suffice: "A system is a set of interacting units with relationships among them" (p. 68). Information processing conceptualizes any single behavior (or thought . . . or emotion . . . or memory) as the result of a whole multitude of interactions amongst and between components of different systems within and outside of the individual. Consider again the task of reading the words on this page. But, this time, let's be more specific and think about what is going on as you read and understand a single word, say:

BALL

Your eyes represent an access point to a complex *visual system* where light energy is transduced into bioelectrical energy at the cellular level (Kandel, Schwartz, & Jessell, 2000). Then it is transmitted along a string of neurons—a *neural system*—connecting your optic nerve to a very specific location in the brain known as the visual cortex. To decipher the squiggly lines on the page as the word "BALL" (as opposed to say GXPZ, or even other squiggly lines like ‖⊢◇▣) requires more interaction within another system—this time among brain cells in the visual cortex. Interestingly, investigation of this particular system by cognitive neuroscientists (James, James, Jobard, Wong, & Gauthier, 2005) shows that even though vision is involved in both tasks, different identifiable parts of the visual cortex are activated when processing a word unit ("BALL") compared to processing individual letters appearing alone ("B"). Why? Different tasks necessitate the interaction of different units . . . the involvement of different systems. As we think more closely about reading the word "BALL" off the page, we recognize even more systems that are involved with this simple task. After recognizing "BALL" as a word unit, you likely create a mental image of a ball, for example. What units interact to constitute this process? Why might some readers imagine a baseball, others a football, and still others a rugby ball? What systems are at work as you recall the time when you and a group of friends played volleyball at the beach last summer? Or as you experience mixed emotions; remembering the happiness of that day while also realizing you haven't seen those friends for a long time? Meaning-making, exemplar generation, personal memory, emotion . . . they all are viewed by scientists using an information-processing approach as the outcomes of systems interacting with each other. Recognize how this is a magnitude greater in complexity than the traditional behaviorist view of the world from the 1950s, where action resulted from a connection between two nodes—stimulus and response. To one viewing the world from an information-processing stand-point, this increase in complexity seems appropriate. For although science strives for the simplest explanation of a single phenomenon (a concept known as **parsimony**), we are also after as thorough and complete an explanation as can be teased apart. The notion of the brain as an unknowable "black box" will not be enough! One of the tasks for the information-processing psychologist, then, is to develop models that generate testable hypotheses about how a particular system behaves and interacts with others. A model, in the scientific sense, is an attempt to break down larger experiences into their composite parts (Shoemaker, Tankard, & Lasorsa, 2004), which brings us to the sixth principle underlying those using an information-processing approach.

6. *Systems are divisible and take time to complete.* As the example with the word "BALL" illustrated, an information-processing researcher often begins the task of understanding a cognitive phenomenon by breaking it down into a list of steps—or subprocesses—necessary to realize an end state. Each of these subprocesses can then be explored individually along with, of course, the ways they interact as a system. A further important component within the information-processing paradigm, however, is the idea that each of these subprocesses takes time (Posner, 1978). To contrast information processing with behaviorism again, the importance of time elapsing was never recognized by behaviorists "[b]ecause they were uninterested in internal events, it stands to reason that they would not think of speed as an index of occurrence of events inside the head" (Lachman et al., 1979, p. 119). However, as we will see in Chapter 7, **Secondary Task Reaction Time** (STRT) measures have become instrumental in understanding many of the subprocesses that make up encoding of mediated information. Psychophysiological recording also relies heavily on the concept of time. In fact, just like the STRT measure, time is sometimes exactly what a psychophysiologist records. One way of quantifying cardiac activity, for example, is by counting the number of milliseconds (1/1000th of a second) between peaks in the waveform created by the electrical signals generated by the heart. As we'll learn in Chapter 4, this waveform is called an *electrocardiogram* and the time between peaks is the *inter-beat interval*. In other instances, time can be used to identify meaningful psychophysiological responses. For example, suppose you wonder if the appearance of a close-up video image of a police officer firing their pistol in a cop episodic drama, and the accompanying sound, increases viewer arousal. You could answer this question by measuring skin conductance activity off the hands of viewers as they watched the cop show to see if it increased in response to the firing of the pistol. But, what duration of time will you use to determine whether an increase in skin conductance was *in response* to the pistol as opposed to something else? How long does an evoked skin conductance response take to manifest itself? Defining this will have an impact on the conclusions you draw. We'll discuss the answers to these questions further in Chapter 5 but remember that cognitive processes take time, and just how long they do take is an important consideration in developing theories of media psychology.

7. *Science should work on issues that are applicable to everyday life.* It may seem unnecessary to even state this principle in a book for *media* psychology researchers—after all, people all over the world interact with some form of mediated communication on a regular basis. But three decades after Lachman et al. (1979) it is still worth mentioning this standard for those new to the field—as well as a reminder for those of us who have been at it for some time. A guiding principle *from the very beginning* of the information-processing tradition of enquiry was the desire to understand how the brain worked while processing everyday events. There are two ways this principle can be applied in modern research. The first is to remember that fruitfulness is secondary to naturalness. In academic circles, the term *fruitfulness* means the ability of one's research area to generate future studies and publications. However, generating studies and publishing academic articles that test slight variations among independent variables should not be the *raison d'être* of the media psychology researcher if those variations are not ones meaningfully encountered in everyday life. This guideline can be easily forgotten, particularly with increasingly powerful computer technology that allows us to easily make the smallest of experimental variations to our media stimuli. Add to this the fact that—as we hope to demonstrate in the pages that follow—collecting and analyzing psychophysiological data is also becoming easier all the time, and it becomes all the more tempting to conduct study after study just because you can. Remember the goal is to understand and explain cognition and emotion associated with the everyday phenomenon of media processing, not just to complete another study and obtain statistically significant results.

   While the rapid advancement of computer hardware and software makes it difficult to abide by this principle in one sense, it can also make it easier in another. When researchers first began using psychophysiological measures to explore the processing of media, the equipment was large and bulky, the protocols intrusive and unnatural. Inherent in this seventh principle is a desire, when possible, to explore how media are processed in everyday life *outside* of the laboratory. As we will see in Chapter 6, with new ambulatory psychophysiological measurement devices this is becoming increasingly more possible, less intrusive to the participant, and less expensive for the researcher.

The second debut of physiology in media research

By the early 1960s it became clear that the discipline of psychology was making a dramatic shift, abandoning the doctrine of behaviorism in favor of these principles of information processing (Miller, 2003). The communication discipline did not rapidly follow suit. In fact, 20 years after psychologists began taking up the information systems approach, **Steven Chaffee** (1980) criticized the field by explaining that it had been stuck for too long in what he referred to as "the two-variable model." He described it using recognizably behaviorist language in an essay originally published in the book *Communication research—a half-century appraisal*:

> The two-variable model consists of a measure or manipulation of variation in exposure to media content (independent variable) and an observation of change in some aspect of thought or behavior (dependent variable) that is empirically linked in a systematic statistical fashion to the independent variable.
>
> (pp. 88–89)

Interestingly, it is in these studies from the 1970s, employing the "two-variable model," where we see the second appearance of physiological indices employed by communication researchers (Donnerstein & Barrett, 1978; Donnerstein & Hallam, 1978; Zillmann, 1971). However, these studies did little more than use the measures to demonstrate Stimulus-Response linkages between media variables and physiological changes. **Dolf Zillmann** (1971), for example, used physiological measures in a pretest to identify movie stimuli for later use in a test of **Excitation-Transfer Theory**. In the pretest, 12 male subjects watched segments of six films while their skin temperature, heart rate and blood pressure were measured. The six film clips were "selected on intuitive grounds" as examples of three conditions: Neutral, Aggressive, and Erotic (Zillmann, 1971, p. 423). However, when the physiological data were analyzed and interpreted for each of the films, with an eye toward selection of the final three for use in the Excitation-Transfer experiment,

> [t]he choice of the three most appropriate experimental films was clearly determined by the results obtained . . . [w]ith the exception that a negligibly greater drop in skin temperature was produced by [the chosen aggressive film] than by [the chosen erotic film], the differences between all physiological indices of excitation are in the proper direction. The differentiation in the critical indices of mean blood pressure and sympathetic activation was highly significant. *The three eliminated films either had major deficiencies or were not advantageous.*
>
> (Zillmann, 1971, pp. 426–427, emphasis added)

The priority in this particular pretest was to identify film clips that elevated physiological arousal so they could later be used to test the effect of transferring residual arousal to another task—the lynchpin of the excitation transfer approach. Certainly for that, Zillmann's interpretation served a purpose. But it is difficult to read that excerpt without recognizing the behaviorists' influence—the films selected on intuitive grounds were supposed to elicit specific physiological responses in a classic S-R manner. Those that were thought to be arousing should increase all measures above those that were not. Those that did not follow the expected patterns were eliminated as "not advantageous," or were explained in a caveat—the erotic film had shown greater arousal effects than the aggressive film in all measures *except* skin temperature (which goes down during high sympathetic nervous system arousal).

Zillmann and his students similarly used physiological measures to confirm that specific experimental conditions generated arousal either in pretest situations (Zillmann & Bryant, 1974; Zillmann, Mody, & Cantor, 1974) or as dependent variables in main experiments (Cantor, Zillmann, & Einsiedel, 1978; Zillmann, Hoyt, & Day, 1974). In these studies, like with Zillmann (1971), the focus was on finding an "effect" of certain stimuli (different types of media stimuli, negative provocation by a research confederate, etc.) on physiological systems—primarily the arousal system (Lang, Potter, & Bolls, 2009). These studies then attempted to show that such arousal activation influenced subsequent behaviors, such as presumably delivering electric shocks to a provoking confederate.

Sometimes during this "second wave" of physiological measurement in media research physiological dependent variables did not act as expected *and* subsequent behaviors did not cleanly match. **Edward Donnerstein**, for example, explored the influence of an anger manipulation and the subsequent viewing of an erotic film on the aggressive responses of male subjects toward either a male or female research confederate (Donnerstein & Barrett, 1978). The study used physiological variables to index arousal levels at various points during the experimental procedure. Subjects first came to the lab and met a confederate posing as another subject. The actual subject was told that the nature of the research was to determine the effect of stress on learning and physiological response. They were always "randomly" selected by the primary researcher to do the first cognitive task, prior to which their blood pressure was recorded. The cognitive task was to spend five minutes writing an essay about a specific current event. The subject was told that essay would then be judged by the other participant (the confederate), who would communicate an assessment about the essay's quality by administering up to 10 short (half-second) electric shocks to the subject as well as providing a written critique. The feedback was, of course, predetermined to be either harsh (receiving nine shocks) or mild (receiving one shock) to manipulate the subject's level of anger. Following the shocks and the reading of a written evaluation of the essay, the subject's blood pressure was taken again.

Then it was the confederate's turn to perform a task, which the actual subject was told was to learn a list of nonsense word pairs. While the confederate was "learning" them, the subject was told to watch a film to pass the time and was randomly assigned to view either an excerpt of a nature film or a black-and-white erotic film. The subject's blood pressure was again recorded after viewing the film.

Finally, the subject was given a list of nonsense words to administer to the confederate who was supposed to respond with the correct matched pair. If correct, the subject could award the confederate any number of points—redeemable for money at the completion of the study. If incorrect, the subject was told to administer an electric shock to the confederate at a level of intensity and duration they thought appropriate. The primary researcher told the subject whether the confederate's answer was correct or incorrect. The number of incorrect responses was also predetermined, of course.

Results were more complicated than the authors had expected. Mean blood pressure and systolic blood pressure were used as indices of physiological arousal in the male subjects. Both measures increased in angered subjects after they saw the erotic film—as Donnerstein hypothesized. But unexpectedly, this physiological response occurred *only in subjects who were paired with female confederates*. Those who interacted with male confederates showed a *decrease* in mean and systolic blood pressure immediately following the erotic film. Further baffling was that the angered subjects behaved less aggressively (e.g., gave shorter and less intense shocks) than those who had shown less physiological arousal—a finding completely contradictory to the expectations of the Excitation-Transfer Theory being employed (Donnerstein & Barrett, 1978).

So, in the decade of the 1970s, communication researchers who had tried to include physiological measures in their methodological toolbox found themselves faced with perplexing issues. To begin with, when compared to the paper-and-pencil measures often used in the discipline to collect self-report data, physiological measures seemed both expensive and daunting (Gale & Smith, 1980). Furthermore, there were many known methodological and design problems associated with blood pressure (Stern, Ray & Davis, 1980), the primary measure being employed by communications researchers at the time (Cantor, Zillmann, & Einsiedel, 1978; Donnerstein & Barrett, 1978; Donnerstein & Hallam, 1978; Zillmann & Bryant, 1974; Zillmann, Hoyt, & Day, 1974; Zillmann, Mody, & Cantor, 1974). This expense and aggravation was coupled with the even more bothersome fact that the results being obtained did not conform to the predictions of S-R behaviorism—neither those where the arousing media variables were the stimulus and recorded physiological activity the response *nor* those when physiological arousal was conceptualized as the stimulus and the subsequent behavior (as predicted by Excitation-Transfer Theory) the response. So, just as they had 40 years earlier, physiological measures were placed back onto the shelf by media psychology researchers and not taken down again for some time.

The third time's a charm: psychophysiological approaches to media

Not nearly as much time passed before physiological measures were again employed in the media lab . . . but it was still more than a decade after Chaffee (1980) had encouraged the field to move beyond two-variable studies and begin embracing the exploration of "psychological *processes* that intervene between media exposure and its effects" (p. 89, emphasis added) that they received widespread attention. It came in the form of another overview of the discipline, this one a two-issue special collection of essays in the *Journal of Communication* designed to be "a collective reconnaissance of communication scholarship and its future" (Levy & Gurevitch, 1993, p. 4). One of the essays, by Seth Geiger and John Newhagen, claimed that the information-processing view was still largely ignored by the field:

> Inquiry in individual-level mass media effects has been limited by conceptualizing the human processor as an impenetrable "black box" with unknowable processes taking place between message reception and the traditional outcomes of learning, attitudes, or behaviors. Instead, we see these component processes as both important outcomes and predictors in their own right. In short, the perennial black box of mass media effects can be better illuminated by examining the black box of human information processing that goes on within it.
>
> (Geiger & Newhagen, 1993, p. 42)

Still, they went on to review recent publications in which media scholars were beginning to develop models of how the human cognitive system processes media by harnessing tools developed by psychologists over the three decades since behaviorism's initial wane. For example, some work focused on a central principle in information processing, that cognition takes time (Posner, 1978), and measured either secondary task reaction time (STRT) (Geiger & Reeves, 1993; Reeves, Newhagen, Maibach, Basil, & Kurz, 1991) or response latency (Newhagen & Reeves, 1992)—which quantifies the amount of time it takes a person to respond to questions about a previously seen media message (Cameron & Frieske, 1994). The common researcher across many of these studies, **Byron Reeves**, was also a key figure in the re-introduction of physiological measures to media psychology. As we will see, his studies using brain waves (EEG) were the first to truly bring a *psychophysiological* perspective to media psychology.

There is a key concept in psychophysiology known as the **orienting response** (OR) which is a momentary increase in attention to what's going on in the environment—we will spend more time on the OR in Chapter 4. But, for now, one of the ways that an OR can be identified physiologically is with a momentary change in the bioelectrical signals emitted by your brain. So, if electrodes were put on your scalp and the signal amplified about 20,000 times, the very small electrical signals your brain was generating could be seen on a computer screen. Actually, what would be seen is a very complex waveform . . . a very messy squiggly line. This waveform is actually the summation of many different waveforms oscillating at particular frequencies. Waveforms oscillating at two distinct frequency ranges are of interest when it comes to attention: they are arbitrarily named **alpha waves** and **beta waves**. When you experience an orienting response and momentarily pay more attention to what is in your environment, the waves oscillating in the beta range increase in amplitude and those oscillating in the alpha range decrease. Knowing this, Reeves and his colleagues (Reeves, Thorson, Rothschild, McDonald, Hirsch, & Goldstein, 1985) were interested in using EEG measures to determine which aspects of media caused ORs in viewers. They recorded EEG from 26 right-handed females while they watched two 30-minute sitcoms containing commercials. Another group of 57 women watched the same two sitcoms without having their physiology data recorded but instead completing only memory tests after the programs. The first sitcom was included as part of the procedure to essentially allow the physiology subjects to become used to having four EEG sensors attached to specific locations on the top of their head, plus two others on their earlobes to act as comparison locations (see Chapter 4).

Reeves et al. (1985) placed nine advertisements in the sitcoms across three commercial breaks. They collected the brain wave signals 128 times each second and then extracted the portions of the complex waveform that were in the alpha frequency range of 8–13 Hz. To analyze the data they began by graphing the strength of the alpha waves each half-second for each commercial, averaged across the 26 subjects. Then, they looked extremely closely at the ads themselves, a half-second at a time. For each 500ms they coded whether there was movement of actors or objects on the screen and if the camera cut between two different shots. This fine-grained inspection of both the media stimuli and the physiological response was different from other work at the time that looked at brain waves during ad processing but averaged the physiological measure across much longer time periods (Appel, Weinstein, & Weinstein, 1979; Weinstein, Appel, & Weinstein, 1980; Weinstein, Drozdenko, & Weinstein, 1984). By looking across such a small time window Reeves et al. (1985) were able to conclude that "attention *reacts* to the stimulus. Rapid alpha drops and habituation are likely involuntary reactions to visual stimuli, although the magnitude of drop and the length of recovery may be variable and related to interest in content" (Reeves et al., 1985, p. 252, emphasis in original).

Annie Lang, a student of Reeves at the University of Wisconsin, determined that the same visual structural features Reeves et al. (1985) had shown caused alpha blocking also elicited the predicted pattern of cardiac deceleration associated with the orienting response (Lang, 1990). The impact of Lang demonstrating that heart rate can be used as a physiological correlate with the allocation of cognitive resources to the processing of media cannot be overstated. The comparative ease with which heart rate could be collected, coupled with the related lack of invasiveness experienced by the subject, has led to numerous studies which vary aspects of the television message and use heart rate to determine the resulting impact on cognition. Another early study (Lang, Geiger, Strickwerda, & Sumner, 1993) used cardiac deceleration to investigate whether people pay more attention to a television message during the few seconds following a change of the picture on the screen—which they called, at the time, a "cut." They showed 12 different segments of television to 58 college students. They also recorded the heart rates of a subset of them, synchronizing that with the television presentation. The results of the physiological analyses show that, indeed, on average a person's heart rate slows down following a cut. Furthermore, they showed that there is no difference in the extent of deceleration depending on whether the cut was between two related images (i.e., a cut from one camera shot to another within the same scene) or two unrelated ones (i.e., a cut from a shot of a car in a commercial to a shot of a news anchor at a desk). But, interestingly, there were differences between related and unrelated cuts in other information-processing dependent measures that A. Lang et al. (1993) collected. For example, subjects were not only faster to respond to STRT tones that occurred in the audio track shortly after related cuts compared to unrelated ones but their memory for the content was better as well.

Now, if the pattern surrounding the use of physiology by media scholars was to repeat itself yet again, the publication of this handful of studies would have been the end of the line for another decade or so. But, the third time was the charm! Lang published an edited book a short time later entitled *Measuring psychological responses to media* (Lang, 1994b). Two of the chapters in it focused directly on the proper measurement and interpretation of bodily responses to mediated messages (Hopkins & Fletcher, 1994; Lang, 1994c) while three others discussed physiological measures as examples of larger topics such as experimental design (Reeves & Geiger, 1994), data analysis (Watt, 1994), and setting up a laboratory space (Lang, 1994a). More importantly for the continued utilization of physiology within the field was the book's framing of "explanations of how specific psychological measures could be used to assess the mental processing of mediated messages" (Lang, Bradley, Chung, & Lee, 2003, p. 651). With the widespread distribution of Lang's methods book, and more importantly the theoretical stance it took, the separation from the behaviorist tradition in the field of media psychology moved toward completion. This has been demonstrated by a noteworthy increase in the number of journal articles in the field utilizing the information processing approach in the decade following its publication (Lang et al., 2003). Lane and Harrington (2009) express disappointment in the fact that less than 5 percent of those publications utilize psychophysiological measures. While their point is well taken—*future* media research should strongly consider the added insights psychophysiology can provide to their research endeavors (that's the reasoning behind this book, after all!)—it is also possible to view the field since 1993 in a more optimistic light. Placing the number of studies employing physiological measures within the entire arch of communications research presents a quite encouraging picture. As you have seen during this brief history of mass communication research, there are very few examples of physiology being measured between the years 1910 and 1990. However, Figure 1.2 shows the number of publications in major communication journals between 1995 and 2009 utilizing psychophysiological measures. The increase is obvious, as is the fact that more and more investigators across the world are setting up media research labs containing physiological measurement equipment. Why the change? What has happened to create an environment where physiological measures are accepted as useful?

The primary difference is a separation from viewing bodily measures as *responses* in the classic behaviorist sense. Instead, media researchers are increasingly operating under what has been called the S-I-R paradigm, where the middle letter stands for the importance of psychological processes which *Intervene* between the external world of the stimulus and the observable response (Donchin, 1979; Donchin & Israel, 1980; Porges, Ackles, & Truax, 1983). In other words, the data obtained when measuring bioelectrical signals from various bodily systems in today's media laboratory are interpreted using the basic assumptions of *psycho*physiology . . . assumptions which make up the first topic of Chapter 2.

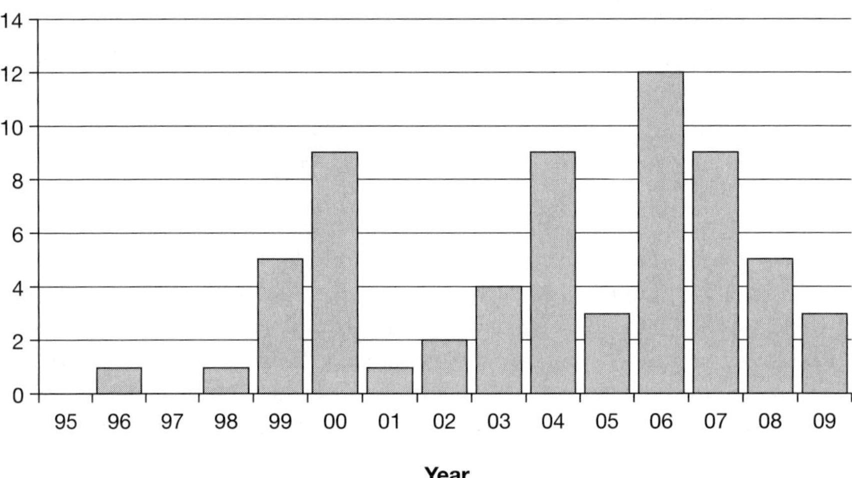

FIGURE 1.2 Number of peer-reviewed journal articles using or substantially mentioning psychophysiological measures published in *Communication Research, Human Communication Research, Journal of Advertising, Journal of Broadcasting & Electronic Media, Journal of Communication,* and *Media Psychology.*

2

PSYCHOPHYSIOLOGY

Theoretical assumptions and a history of the field

In Chapter 1 the use of measures of bodily responses as dependent variables in response to media stimuli were traced across six decades. We saw that physiological indices were not valued for a vast majority of this time span, largely due to the strong influence of behaviorism as a theoretical approach in psychology. It wasn't until the early 1990s, when media psychology researchers began to conceptualize the audience/medium interaction from an information-processing standpoint rather than an S-R behaviorist one, that the quantification of physiological measures during message processing started to be interpreted in ways that made sense—in ways that prevented them from being abandoned and instead used to develop substantial theories of media psychology.

Eventually, physiological measures stopped being viewed as response variables and instead became seen as correlates with psychological phenomena—be they states or traits—in media audiences. In other words, those who were most successful in utilizing physiological variables in the media psychology laboratory were those who abided by the basic assumptions of psychophysiology.

Basic assumptions of psychophysiology

While most psychophysiologists also ascribe to the theoretical underpinnings of information-processing, and therefore agree with the list of principles presented earlier from Lachman, Lachman, and Butterfield, there are several other assumptions which a psychophysiologist ascribes to. These relate specifically to how and why the brain—as the central location of information processing—interacts with other peripheral parts of the body in order to receive information, deliver information, function, and survive. These assumptions are presented briefly here and those who want more extensive treatment are encouraged to read the excellent introductory chapter of the *Handbook of psychophysiology* (2007a) by **John Cacioppo**, **Louis Tassinary**, and **Gary Berntson**.

1. The brain is embodied

As we have already stressed, the psychophysiological approach does not believe that the brain is essentially a "black box" that can't be understood. But this assumption goes farther than merely encouraging us to strive for such understanding. It provides a starting point for *how* to conceptualize the brain— as a human organ connected to all the other organs through a system of afferent and efferent neurological, chemical, and muscular connections. The *embodied cognition* view does not accept the mind-body problem as posed by **Rene Descartes**, who argued that the only thing that can be known with certainty is the existence of the mind—that the body and other physical things could be merely illusionary. Instead, psychophysiologists believe that "cognition depends on the kinds of experiences that come from having a body with particular perceptual and motor capacities that are inseparably linked and that together form the matrix within which reasoning, memory, emotion, language, and all other aspects of life are meshed" (Thelen, Schöner, Scheier, & Smith, 2001, p. 1).

2. The work of the brain and the body happens over time

Bodily and cognitive processes are dynamic, which means that they occur over time. Recognition of the importance of time is key for the psychophysiologist. It impacts experimental design, the selection or creation of stimuli, data collection and analysis and the eventual interpretation and presentation of findings. As we have said elsewhere, dynamic "systems increase and decrease in an analog, not a digital, fashion. Therefore, thinking leads to changes which occur over the course of milliseconds or seconds, whose impacts on the biological and physiological systems grow and wane with the vagaries of thought" (Lang, Potter, & Bolls, 2009, p. 186).

3. The subtractive method applies to analyzing physiological systems

The importance of time as an influence in psychophysiological research allows us to introduce a philosophical and operational approach to psychological research known as the **subtractive method**. The subtractive method is attributed to the Dutch ophthalmologist **Franciscus Donders** (1868/1969) who was fascinated by the experiments conducted by **Hermann von Helmholtz**. Helmholtz applied electrical stimulation to the motor nerves of both animals and humans, and measured how long it took for the stimulation to create muscle contraction. Donders built on Helmholtz's work by designing experiments comparing the time it took human subjects to respond to slight electrical stimulation occurring at different places on the body. So, for example, Donders might apply a slight jolt to the skin on the head, and on the ear and also just under the eye—measuring how long it took the subject to recognize the irritant and respond with a brush of their hand to remove the stimulation. Results showed that it took subjects longer to respond to stimulation the further the point of contact was from the brain itself. In other words, people took longer to brush away the stimulation on the skin at the ear or the eye than for the top of the head. Donders argued that included in his duration measurements were not only the amount of time it took for the muscles to register the stimulation and respond, but also the time it took to complete a cognitive process of evaluating the stimulation as something they wanted to stop with a flick of their hand. But, how could the duration associated with cognitive processes be teased out? The subtractive method was the solution. Donders assumed that if you compared the duration it took to complete one task with the duration it took to complete that same task *plus* a cognitive event, the difference would provide the time required for cognition.

So, in one of Donders's earliest experiments subjects were placed in one of two conditions. In both conditions subjects had an electrode placed on each foot and would receive stimulation to one of them or the other. The subject's task was to raise the hand on the side matching the stimulated foot. The manipulation was, however, that in one condition subjects were told which foot would be stimulated and in the other they were not told, but instead had to figure it out. Those who had to complete the cognitive task of figuring out which foot had been stimulated took longer to raise their hands than those who knew where the stimulation would come from and just had to wait for it and respond when it came. By subtracting the two reaction times, Donders calculated the duration of the mental process. Here we see the nature of the subtractive method.

What does that have to do with psychophysiology? Well, the subtractive approach can be expanded beyond the measurement of time and, as explained by Cacioppo, Tassinary, and Berntson (2007b), psychophysiological measures can be particularly powerful when employed within the subtractive experimental paradigm. Not only can differences in physiological reactions be used to confirm presumed differences in conceptual constructs, but if the proper measures are chosen the nature of what is known about their psychological significance can also inform us about the type of cognitive process being utilized by each. For example, suppose you want to make a claim that psychologically news stories containing visuals showing the victims of violent crime are conceptually different from stories about crime that don't contain such images. Designing a physiological experiment could help you to test that claim; you could plan to show subjects several news stories focusing on violent crime and have half of them contain graphic footage of crime consequences and the other half not. You can probably see how this is, essentially, an experiment based on Donders's approach. By measuring physiological variables while subjects watch both types of news stories you can see what occurs when people process the negative images and compare that with what occurs physiologically when we "subtract" those negative images from the news stories. If there is, in fact, a difference in how your test subjects respond, then based on the logic of the subtractive method you have obtained confirmation for your claim that the types of stories are conceptually different.

But, the benefits of the psychophysiological approach are even stronger than this. "With biological measures . . . the psychological significance of specific physiological differences . . . comes both from the theoretical differences between experimental conditions and from the prior scientific literature on the psychological significance of the observed physiological difference" (Cacioppo et al., 2007b, pp. 7–8). So, to continue with our example, suppose that the physiological measures that you included were skin conductance and frown muscle activity. If you found that those were more active during the news stories with violent content than the stories without, you have indeed separated the two types of stories conceptually. However, we know from past literature both within media psychology and from basic physiological research that those two indices are psychological correlates of the activation of aversive ("fight or flight") systems in the human brain. So, by employing the subtractive method with our physiological measures not only have we identified the two types of stories as conceptually different, we have gained insight into the meaning associated with these types of stories by viewers. Thanks to the subtractive method we have illuminated the darkness in the black box just slightly!

4. The body's primary job is to keep itself alive

The majority of the measures described in this book essentially consist of using electrodes placed on the skin's surface to measure the electrical activity of neurons (Stern, Ray, & Quigley, 2001). It is tempting, if you become a psychophysiological researcher exploring media phenomena, to believe that neurons in the heart fire specifically so that electrical activity can provide an index of the amount of cognitive attention someone is paying to a computer game, or that the amount of sweat a person's palm secretes while watching a TV show is only related to the excitement they feel as a result of the primetime crime drama you are showing them. Although we take careful pains to design experiments where these indices can be used as ways of inferring such relationships, it is important to remember that the majority of the work that the body does at any moment in time is related to the tasks of sustaining life. Food needs to be digested. Respiration has to occur. Blood needs to circulate and hormones need to be secreted and absorbed. As Bernard (1878/1974) puts it, "all the vital mechanisms, however varied they may be, have only one object, that of preserving constant the conditions of life in the internal environment" (p. 121). Easy to say, but hard to untangle when what you are really interested in is the data relating to the processing of media messages—information which lies buried within this activity keeping the organism alive.

The way psychophysiologists have thought about this internal bodily activity has changed over the last 150 years. Bernard was the first to describe how complex organisms exhibit what he called a "milieu interne." **Walter Bradford Cannon** (1929) went on to interpret this as a fluid matrix both created and controlled by the organism itself in order to respond to internal and external conditions. Such a response was, early on, described as a balance achieved to keep the organism stable and prevent it from being destroyed, dissolved, or disintegrated. Cannon (1929) called this balance homeostasis and defined it as follows:

> The highly developed living being is an open system having many relations to its surroundings—in the respiratory and alimentary tracts and through surface receptors, neuromuscular organs and bony levers. Changes in the surrounding excite reactions in this system, or affect it directly, so that internal disturbances of the system are produced . . . it is the integrated cooperation of a wide range of organs—brain and nerves, heart, lungs, kidneys, spleen—which are promptly brought into action when conditions arise which might alter [the body] . . . The coordinated physiological reactions which maintain most of the steady states in the body are so complex, and are so peculiar to the living organism, that it has been suggested that a specific designation for these states be employed—*homeostasis*.
>
> (Cannon, 1929, p. 400, emphasis in original)

Cannon felt strongly that homeostasis was achieved by opposing activation of the sympathetic and parasympathetic nervous systems (Berntson & Cacioppo, 2007). To understand this, it's time for a very brief tutorial on the anatomy of the human nervous system. But don't worry, we will take it slow and easy for now . . . this is only the first part of Chapter 2, after all.

A **neuron**, or nerve cell, communicates bioelectrical signals throughout the body (see Figure 2.1). Perhaps because there are so many of them (over 100 billion) psychophysiologists and anatomists have found it helpful to think about them by grouping them into several different systems—we told you that systems are a big part of our approach to inquiry. The first grouping is really one of convenience, based on location within the body rather than function. The phrase **Central Nervous System (CNS)** refers to neurons located in the brain and the spinal column while the **Peripheral Nervous System (PNS)**, as you may guess, is made up of neurons traveling from the spinal cord to the body's periphery.

Nerve cells can be described more functionally as those that either contribute to the **sensory system** or to the **motor system**. Remember earlier we mentioned how the eye and ear convert energy into bioelectrical signals which then travel onto the brain? The first step of that journey is through neurons particularly tuned to a specific type of stimulation—say, light or sound. As a whole, these specialized neurons make up the sensory system (Kalat, 2007). Motor neurons, on the other hand, originate in the spinal cord and travel outward toward skeletal muscles, organs, or glands. Motor neurons that control skeletal muscles are called

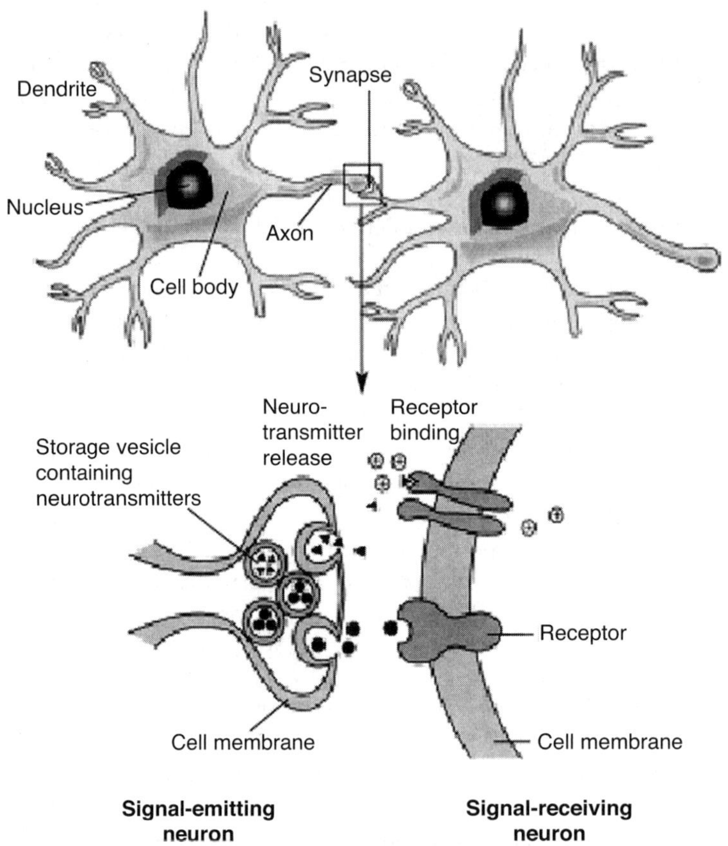

FIGURE 2.1 A basic neuron or nerve cell with discussion of neurotransmitters.

Source: public domain image from Goodlett and Horn, 2001.

somatic nerves (Stern et al., 2001). Those that control organs or glands form what is known as the **Autonomic Nervous System** (ANS).

The ANS is further divided into two branches— the **Sympathetic Nervous System** (SNS) and the **Parasympathetic Nervous System** (PNS). Each sends impulses to organs and glands, prompting them to behave in certain ways. When this happens we say that the gland or organ is being *innervated* by that particular branch of the ANS. As you can see in Figure 2.2, however, most organs and glands in the body can be described as *dually innervated*; that is, they are connected to both the PNS and the SNS which are constantly sending signals to some degree as neither system can ever be thought of as being "off" per se.

The SNS begins with clusters of neurons located on either side of the spinal cord—in a section roughly just below the shoulders to just above the tailbone.

When activated these clusters, known as **ganglia**, pass electrical impulses between each other all along this "thoracolumbar" region. Innervation by the SNS results in preparation for "the four Fs: fight, flight, fright, and sex" (Bear, Conners, & Paradiso 2007, p. 494). This is a crude but effective way of remembering what the SNS does—prepares the organism for activity vital to survival and procreation. So, consider anticipating something that frightens you—an upcoming class assignment where you need to give a five-minute speech, for example. When frightened (or angry, or sexually aroused, etc.), it is the activation of your sympathetic nervous system which results in increased activity in both the heart and lungs and decreased energy expense on digestion (Kalat, 2007).

The Parasympathetic Nervous System (PNS) system is the second branch of the SNS. Neurons that make up the PNS originate in the brain and the lowermost portion of the spinal cord and deliver electrical signals directly to the target organs —bypassing the ganglial chain running along the spine. The parasympathetic system is described in a variety of ways in the literature. Andreassi (2000, p. 67) refers to it as the branch of the ANS devoted to "rest, repair, and enjoyment" (although if the enjoyment level gets *too* high the sympathetic nervous system will certainly become activated!). Kalat (2007) asserts that the "parasympathetic nervous system facilitates vegetative, nonemergency responses by the organs" (p. 85). As Figure 2.2 shows, PNS nerves coming from the lower part of the spine innervate the colon, rectum, bladder, and genitals while those coming from the brain send signals to organs throughout the body—the eye, mucus glands, liver, kidney, and heart all receive parasympathetic signals.

Now with this basic understanding of the parasympathetic and sympathetic systems, Cannon's stance that homeostasis results from the reciprocal activation between the two becomes more clear. In his view, a type of biological give-and-take among the PNS and SNS occurs in response to external situations in order to ensure that the organism survives. Berntson and Cacioppo (2007) point out that the field of psychophysiology has been strongly influenced by the legacy of this conceptualization, even though it is generally no longer recognized as a homeo*static* but more of a homeo*dynamic* process between the SNS, the PNS, the internal world of an individual's cognitions and plans, and the external world of inputs and stressors:

> Moreover, the emphasis on static levels and the fixity implied by the term "homeostasis" does not capture appropriately the variability and dynamic features of visceral control systems. A more appropriate construct is that of homeodynamic regulation, which recognizes that regulatory processes do not reflect simple, rigid, negative feedback mechanisms. Rather regulatory mechanisms are multiple and complex, with lags, limits, and feed-forward components, and may evidence variations in operating characteristics that may themselves be subject to active control.
>
> (p. 463)

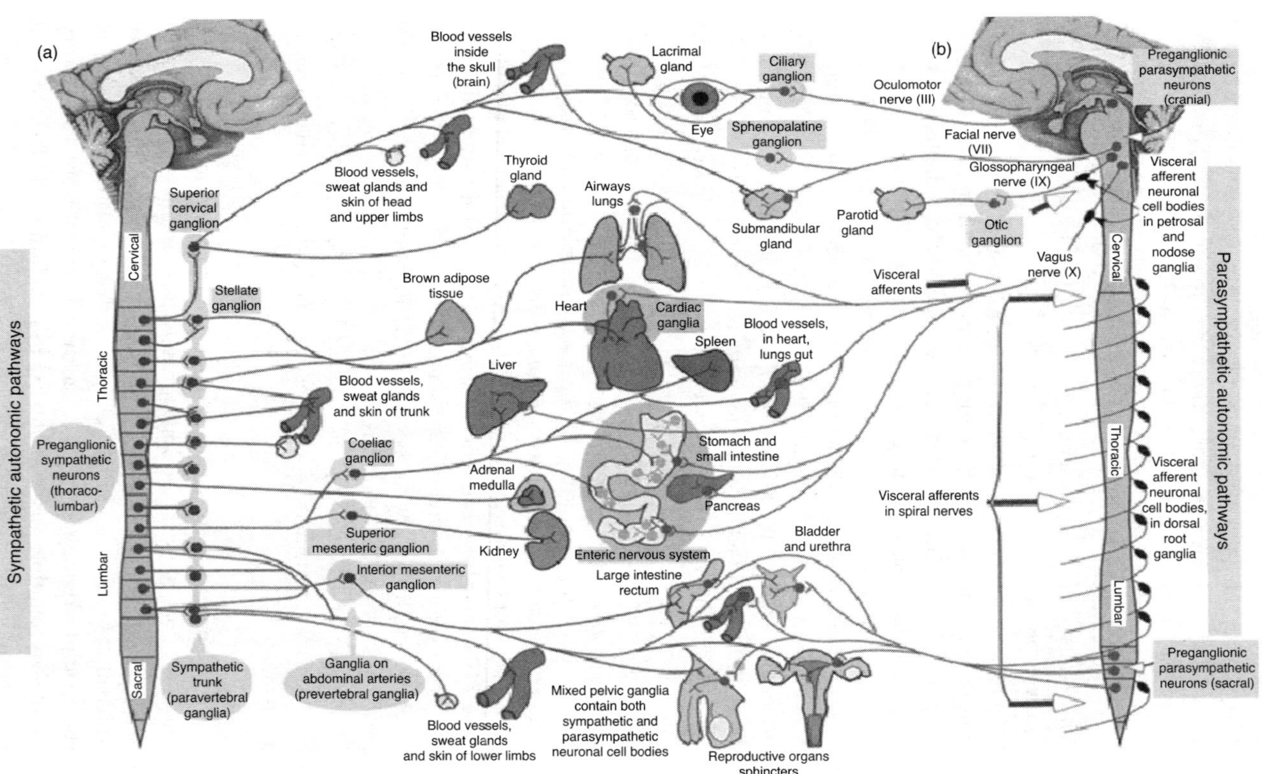

FIGURE 2.2 The sympathetic and parasympathetic divisions of the ANS, showing the dual innervations of most organs.

Source: used with permission from William Blessing and Ian Gibbins, Flinders University SA Australia.

The offshoot of all this homeodynamic interaction keeping your body alive and intact is a lot of bioelectrical activity—all of which is being recorded by the surface electrodes attached to the skin of your research subjects in the media laboratory. Of course, the dynamic interaction between your subject's cognitive system and the media messages you are asking them to process as part of your experiment is in there *as well*. But never forget that it is only a *part* of what is being recorded, and a tiny part at that.

5. Cognitive processes can be inferred from bodily reactions

A psychophysiologist tries to make inferences about cognitive processes by correlating them with observed bodily reactions (Donchin, 1981). The strongest inferences can be made when there is a one-to-one relationship between the two: a single psychological event is associated with one—*and only one*—physiological reaction (Cacioppo et al., 2007b). Unfortunately, this purest form of a one-to-one association is a very rare occurrence for the very reasons we have already discussed: our brains are embodied within a highly interconnected autonomic nervous system. More typically a media psychology researcher will find that the relationships between cognitive processes and physiological responses are more complicated. In one type of instance a single psychological process is associated many physiological occurrences—in other words, a one-to-many relationship is established. So, for example, following the onset of a camera change in a television message a subject's heart rate momentarily decreases *and* their skin conductance increases. Or when processing negative, mud-slinging political ads the startle response to a brief burst of white noise is larger *and* the smile muscle located on the cheek is less activated than during positive ad conditions (Bradley, Angelini, & Lee, 2007). In situations such as this the optimum one-to-one relationship can still be established, and the strong inference from bodily response to cognitive process made, by collapsing the multiple physiological responses into a single **response pattern**—that is, a single set of bodily responses that frequently co-occur.

Things can be particularly tricky with the two other possible relationships between psychological processes and physiological reactions—the many-to-one and the many-to-many. Distilling multiple physiological responses into a single response pattern transforms a many-to-many relationship into one where multiple cognitive processes are associated with one type of bodily response—a many-to-one relationship. Unfortunately establishing this type of relationship doesn't gain us much ground in the area of scientific enquiry since in such a situation there is nothing in the physiological data which allows us to differentiate between multiple psychological states or cognitive processes. As an example, consider an experiment where a media researcher has subjects watch segments from three different types of movies: comedy, suspenseful courtroom dramas, and horror. The physiological measure is frown muscle activity. As expected, the average frown muscle activity is lower during the comedy segments and the researcher draws a logical inference from this one-to-one relation that comedy activates the emotional system associated with good things—the appetitive or approach system—and the frown muscle deactivates as a result (Larsen, Norris, & Cacioppo, 2003). However, when comparing the frown muscle activity during the suspenseful closing argument scenes of courtroom dramas with that of the psychopath killing a victim in horror films they are practically identical in their average increase. Here we have a many-to-one relationship—two types of media content associated with a single physiological occurrence. Although we have every reason to theoretically predict that different emotional and cognitive processes are taking place during the viewing of courtroom dramas and horror films, our physiological data cannot differentiate them.

There are several ways to deal with this. Unfortunately for the poor researcher in our hypothetical situation, many of the solutions should have been considered during the design phase of the study. For example, additional physiological dependent measures would allow for predictions about differences in response patterns during the two types of viewing situations. Also, it is important to remember that the best way to measure emotions is through triangulation of data collected by different methods: physiological, self-report, and behavioral observation (Bradley & Lang, 2000). So, in this case the research subjects could have answered self-reported scale questions after each scene. The researcher could have also made video recordings of the subjects during the experimental session and later coded for the presence of nervous behaviors or posture changes during viewing. Doing so could have allowed for a one-to-one relation to be postulated about frown activity during comedy compared to the two other genres while suspense and horror could be differentiated by the combination of frown muscle activation and discriminating self-reported responses to a fear and anxiety scale and/or the subject's posture in relation to the screen—perhaps most were leaning forward during the dramatic suspense of the courtroom scenes and recoiling during the horror, for example.

Another possibility is that the relationship between both horror and suspense stimuli ("many-") and frown activation ("-to-one") is found only when aggregating across the entirety of the test subjects. If this homogenous group can be divided according to theoretically defensible individual difference factors— say by personality, age, cultural influences, or psychological profile—this may tease out conditions in which horror and suspense *are* differentiated through frown activity in a one-to-one manner for certain psychological types.

Another way of differentiating between many psychological processes which are thought to be theoretically distinct but seem to converge on a single physio- logical outcome is to remember the importance of time as a factor in the process. Because most physiological measures can be collected repeatedly over the entire time course of a media message, collapsing psychophysiological data across time likely obscures important differences between cognitive processes. Looking at bodily response dynamically may be enlightening and allow the researcher to move from a many-to-one classification to a one-to-one. To see how this is the case, consider our hypothetical example again where no difference was found between average frown muscle activation while viewers watched courtroom drama and horror. These findings may have looked like those in Figure 2.3a.

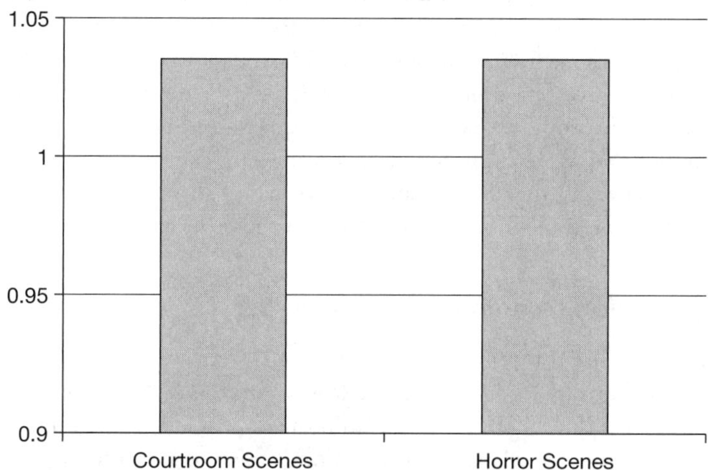

FIGURE 2.3a Average frown muscle activity change scores.

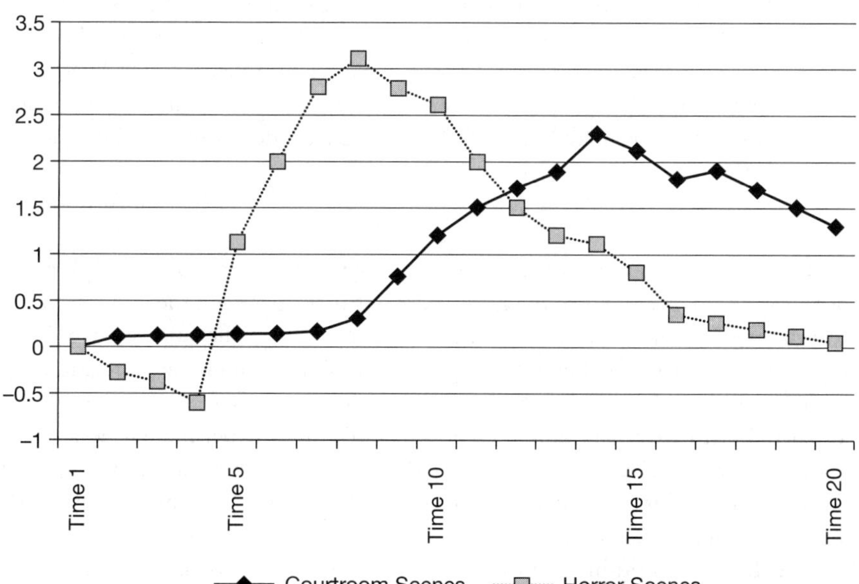

FIGURE 2.3b Frown muscle activity change scores over time.

If the frown muscle activity is not aggregated into a grand mean, however, but analyzed as it evolves over the time course of the messages, differences emerge. In Figure 2.3b we see that these identical means result from very different time series. In general, the horror scenes begin with deactivation of the frown muscle, perhaps suggesting that the subjects were actually enjoying the mystery surrounding the plotlines. But then the increase in negative emotion is quite sudden, early, and large compared to that experienced during the courtroom dramas. In those programs the frown muscle activity follows a slow-building pattern and, although the negative emotion was never as intense in the frown muscle activity during the courtroom scenes, subjects were quite a bit more negative at the end of them than they were at the end of the horror film scenes. Time matters in cognitive processing and therefore it should also matter in your attempts to make inferences from physiological measures back to those processes.

6. Psychophysiological measures are monstrosities

One of us will admit that this phrase is often repeated in the weekly meetings we hold with our lab group . . . likely because it is so fun to say! However, the meaning of the message should not get lost within the dramatic flair one can use to deliver it. So, let's try to explain this assumption by seeing it in the original context in a book entitled *Feeling and emotion* by Gardiner, Metcalf, and Beebe-Center (1937/1970):

> A scientific theory is a description of causal interrelations. Psycho-physiological correlations are not causal. Thus in scientific theories, *psychophysiological correlations are monstrosities*. This does not mean that such correlations have no part in science. They are the instruments by which the psychologist may test his theories. They cannot, however, be a part of his theories.
>
> (p. 385, emphasis added)

This assumption springs from the homeodynamic nature of the relationship between different systems in the human organism *and* between the organism itself and the myriad influences in the external environment. The impact of multiple inputs on the measures themselves makes establishing a single *causal* relationship highly unlikely. And while the researcher tries to control as much variation associated with external context as possible—through experimental design and the setup of the laboratory space itself (Lang et al., 2009)—the most one can expect in the end is a non-causal association between mediated message variables and physiological indices.

The first implication of this is explicitly stated by Gardiner; namely the imprudence of including physiological phenomena as nodes in theoretical models due to the multiple inputs determining the measures and the correlational association between them and the cognitive state of interest. So, for example, in theory development one would not want to include a causal path from people experiencing higher skin conductance levels to a particular outcome. The risk of doing so "is the myriad sources of variance in psychophysiological investigations and the stochastic nature of physiological events and, consequently, the sometimes poor replicability or generalizability of the results" (Cacioppo et al., 2007b, p. 7). Instead, ideally a cognitive or emotional *state*—such as arousal—would be best to include as a causal link when theory building.

Of course, arousal can then be measured physiologically using a large number of indices and analyzed in a number of different ways. And, it's here that the second implication of Gardiner's "monstrosities" quote arises. As time passes technologies get both more precise and sometimes even less expensive. Media psychology researchers will have an increasing array of physiological measures available to them—many of which can be tested for their ability to serve as correlates to cognitive and emotional processes. For example, arousal response to media has been associated with skin conductance (Bolls, Muehling, & Yoon, 2003; Potter, 2009), respiration volume (Gomez, Zimmermann, Guttormsen-Schar, & Danuser, 2005), sympathetic activation of the heart measured via heart-rate variability (Ivarsson, Anderson, Åkerstedt, & Lindblad, 2009), 32-channel EEG arrays (Baumgartner, Valko, Esslen, & Lutz, 2006), levels of testosterone and adrenaline in the urine (Arnetz, Edgren, Levi, & Otto, 1985), and blood flow in the brain (Morris et al., 2009). The development of ever longer lists of associations between physiological measures and cognitive or emotional states may move the field of *measurement* forward, but it does little for progression of psychological theories of communication (Cacioppo et al., 2007b). If developing such theories is the end goal for your scientific pursuits then we urge you to remember that these psychophysiological measures are tools for you to use to identify cognitive and emotional processes and should not be reified. Nor should larger, more complex or more expensive measures be used to identify cognitive processes simply because they are available. Sometimes, a shovel can dig a hole more suited to your purposes than a backhoe.

These are the six basic assumptions of social scientists who use psychophysiological measures in their pursuit of understanding of cognitive and emotional processes. And, although theorizing about the linkage between bodily response and emotion goes back to the teachings of Plato, the field of psychophysiology began with a small group of researchers meeting for the first time in 1950.

Psychophysiology: a field with a long legacy

In the mid-1950s a group of researchers—led by **Albert F. Ax, Chester W. Darrow**, and **R. C. Davis**—would informally gather every year at the American Psychological Association (APA) convention to discuss using physiological measurement to better understand psychological phenomena. In 1959, however, at the convention in Cincinnati, Ohio, the discussions focused on a more formal possibility—organizing an entirely new scholarly society devoted to "the science which concerns those physiological activities which underlie or relate to psychic functions" (Darrow, 1964, p. 4). Although the idea of creating an autonomous organization was not unanimously popular (Edelberg, 1974), in 1960 the Society for Psychophysiological Research (SPR) was created. Darrow served as the first president and the following year the inaugural scientific meeting of SPR was held in New York City (Cacioppo et al., 2007b). The society launched its own journal, *Psychophysiology*, in 1964 with Ax as the first editor. Ax was a natural choice for that role, as he and his wife Beryl had been writing and circulating a mimeographed *Psychophysiology newsletter* since 1955—no small task, as over 800 pages were written during its nine-year run in order to—as Ax put it—"shorten the 'hunting cycle' and thus straighten the erratic path of research in the field" (Fetzner, 1996, p. 135).

Darrow's Presidential Address, entitled "Psychophysiology, yesterday, today and tomorrow," was published in the first issue of *Psychophysiology*. In it he attributed the birth of the field to Darwin's (1872/1965) *The expression of the emotions in man and animals*. Most certainly, when reading almost any page in that work you come across selections which relate bodily activity to cognitive and emotional states. For example:

> We will now turn to the characteristic symptoms of Rage. Under this powerful emotion the action of the heart is much accelerated, or it may be much disturbed. The face reddens, or it becomes purple from the impeded return of the blood, or may turn deadly pale. The respiration is labored, the chest heaves, and the dilated nostrils quiver. The whole body often trembles, the voice is affected. The teeth are clenched or ground together, and the muscular system is commonly stimulated to violent, almost frantic action.
>
> (p. 78)

Of course, Darwin's knowledge about associations between psychological processes and physiology was not only a result of his own observations. He read widely the works of top scholars of his day (Black, 2002) and gave substantial attribution to other physiologists such as Bell (1844), Bernard (1865/1957) and Duchenne (1862/1990). In fact, in *The expression of emotions in man and animals* Darwin included his own line drawings of expressive faces inspired by Duchenne's photographs of subjects smiling as a result of electrical stimulation of muscles as opposed to authentic emotional experience (Black, 2002).

Darwin's case is not unusual. No matter where one claims the history of any discipline "begins," each generation of scientists is indebted to the work of those that preceded it. As a result, when searching for the true beginning of fascinations linking bodily response to cognitive and emotional processes one can go back quite a long way. In the Platonic dialog *Timaeus*, written around 400 BC, the title character tells Socrates a story about the creation of the universe. According to this account, when making human beings the gods put immortal and divine reason and rationality in the head while the mortal passions of pleasure, pain, anger, rashness, fear, and hope were placed in the gut. Concerned that the two would mingle more than necessary and "pollute the divine," reason was separated from the passions by the neck. But compare the above quotation from Darwin with this by Plato:

> The heart, the knot of the veins and the fountain of the blood which races through all the limbs, was set in the place of guard, that when the might of passion was roused by reason making proclamation of any wrong assailing them from without or being perpetrated by the desires within, quickly the whole power of feeling in the body, perceiving these commands and threats, might obey and follow through every turn and alley, and thus allow the principle of the best to have the command in all of them. But the gods, foreknowing that the palpitation of the heart in the expectation of danger and the swelling and excitement of passion was caused by fire, formed and implanted as a supporter to the heart the lung, which was, in the first place, soft and bloodless, and also had within hollows like the pores of a sponge, in order that by receiving the breath and the drink, it might give coolness and the power of respiration and alleviate the heat. Wherefore they cut the air-channels leading to the lung, and placed the lung about the heart as a soft spring, that, when passion was rife within, the heart, beating against a yielding body, might be cooled and suffer less, and might thus become more ready to join with passion in the service of reason.
>
> (Jowett, 2008)

Although there is a greater sophistication in Darwin's piece from the 1800s, the similarities between the two—and between the *Timaeus* and explanations of homeostasis by Cannon in the 1930s for that matter—are striking.

Following Plato, the next key figure in the history of psychophysiology is **Galen of Pergamon** who lived from AD 130–200. Galen was one of the most prolific physiological, philosophical and medical writers of antiquity distilling the work of those who came before him—Plato, Aristotle, and Hippocrates, among others (Boylan, 2007). However, as every generation of scholar is constrained by both the ideas of the past and the social and intellectual milieu in which they live, Galen was also a citizen of the Greek city of Pergamon—a place known for its fantastic 200,000 volume library, a huge altar to Zeus, *and* an intricate series of waterways and aqueducts designed to deliver water throughout the city (Bromehead, 1942). With this technological marvel of interleaved lead pipes central to and vital for the culture, in hindsight we see how sensible it was that Galen and others of the time believed health to be due to a balance of fluids in the body—specifically the four humors of blood, phlegm, black bile, and yellow bile (Boylan, 2007). By dissecting monkeys—human dissection was prohibited in Pergamon at the time—Galen developed a theory where organs existed to generate these humors and veins distributed them through the body based on the principles of hydraulics. Galen's fluid-transportation view of human physiology was almost universally accepted for about 1,500 years (Cacioppo et al., 2007b).

The first time we see Galen's grip on physiological thought begin to loosen is in the 1500s. Interestingly, its undoing came about as the result of work done by **Vesalius** who himself was not only well-versed in Galen's approach but called him "the prince of physicians and preceptor of all" (Saunders & O'Malley, 1950, p. 13). Still, Vesalius was a brilliant young Italian anatomist and a strict empiricist devoted to meshing the inherited views of bodily function with his own direct observations. And, unlike Galen, Vesalius was able to obtain human cadavers for dissection and observation, often stealing them in the dark of night from gibbets or pit graves of plague victims.

After earning his doctorate in medicine at the young age of 23, Vesalius became a Professor of Surgery in Venice where he conducted dissections and lectured to crowds of students (as well as other faculty members) from across Italy. As part of his lecture experience he created large charts displaying line drawings of the anatomy being explored at that particular event. Their popular reception led to the publication of six such drawings—the *Tabulae Sex*—in 1538. Although it is hard to believe given the importance of graphics and figures in most of today's psychophysiological, biological, and anatomical publications, this was a rare occurrence at the time. Still it met with great approval and almost instant plagiarism by other anatomists (Saunders & O'Malley, 1950).

One year later Vesalius entered into a controversy surrounding the common Galenical medical practice of venesection or bloodletting. The translation of the writings of Galen and Hippocrates into both Arabic and Greek had resulted in substantial differences in the specific procedures surrounding the practice—where blood was drained from an ill patient and how much was taken. Up until that time, those who published opinions surrounding the debate relied on a mixture of inherited opinion from past authority and observation of the treatment outcomes of ill patients. However, with the publication of his *Venesection letter* in 1539, Vesalius was the first to provide conclusions informed from direct observation and illustration of the venous system.

> The effect was startling. Thereafter every future participant in the controversy was compelled to appeal to the body which, in turn, led to the discovery of the venous valves . . . Furthermore, Vesalius in devoting so much attention to the venous system was unwittingly exposing one of the weakest aspects of the Galenical anatomy. Thus, it is with this small work that we first perceive the slow and gradual loosening of traditional

authoritative bonds whence eventually emerged the principle that the validity of a hypothesis rests solely on the facts established by observation.

(Saunders & O'Malley, 1950, p. 18)

Viewing the venous system through direct observation was an enlightened approach at the time, and one which—along with challenges the work of Galileo, Bacon, and Newton made to the intellectual and religious authorities at the time—inspired the work of **William Harvey** whose doctoral dissertation completely refuted the "canal" conceptualization of blood distribution in the body (Cacioppo et al., 2007b). The work, *On the motion of the heart and blood in animals* (1628/1998), presented both thought experiments and calculations designed to refute the Galenical idea that blood moved rather haphazardly throughout the body, traveling in both directions through both arteries and veins. Harvey's calculations were based on observations of the amount of blood present in the left ventricle of cadavers during dissection. Multiplying that by conservative approximations of the percentage of the total volume the ventricle expelled by a single beat and estimates of how many beats the heart made in 30 minutes, Harvey showed that the total volume of blood moved in just half an hour—even by these conservative calculations—far exceeded the amount of blood contained in the whole human body (Massey, 1995). The resulting conclusion, of course, was that the veins and arteries actually formed a *circulating* system with blood flowing in specific directions throughout the body—arteries away from the heart into the body, veins returning to the heart. In Figure 2.4 we see a line drawing of Harvey's which he used to support his theories by asking readers to imagine they applied a tourniquet to the arm of a man after he had been exercising, noticing that below the blockage toward the hand the arteries do not pulse while above the tourniquet "the artery begins to rise higher at each diastole, to throb more violently, and to swell in its vicinity with a kind of tide, as if it strove to break through and overcome the obstacle to its current; the artery here, in short, appears as if it were preternaturally full" (Harvey, 1628/1998).

The next substantial historical development in psychophysiology came in the late 1700s with the work of **Luigi Galvani** on electrical transmission by muscles and nerves (Stern et al., 2001). Until then, bodily movement had been hypothesized as resulting from the movement of fluid through nerves which—*à la* Galen—were conceptualized as a series of pipes throughout the body (Cacioppo et al., 2007b). But in 1781 Galvani observed someone—some say his wife while making a frog-leg dinner—touch a knife to a frog's nerve and noticed the emission of a spark simultaneous with the contraction of the frog's leg. Galvani wondered if muscles resembled capacitors—essentially storing up electrical energy for subsequent discharge and the resultant muscle contraction (Cajavilca, Varon, & Sternbach, 2009). Galvani conducted a number of experiments exploring increases in electrical stimulation on subsequent muscle activity as well as showing that the electrical stimulation could come from environmental electricity such as

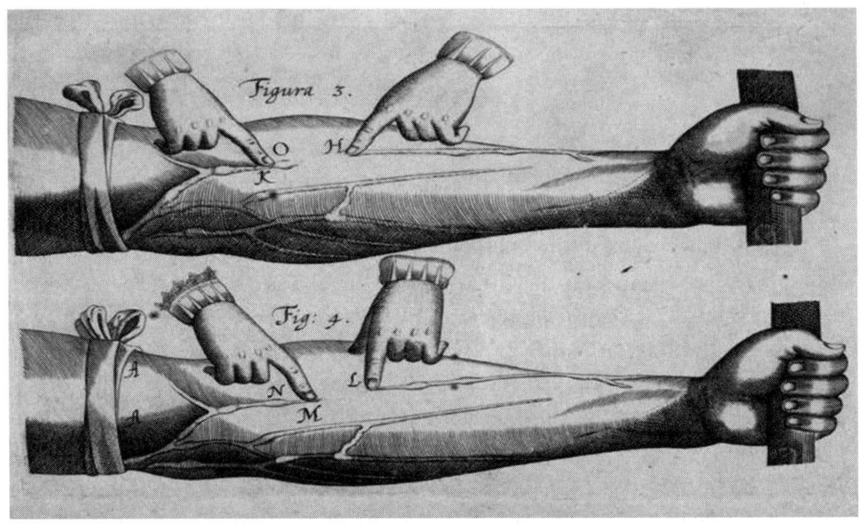

FIGURE 2.4 Harvey's tourniquet thought experiments in the 1600s led to recognition that blood circulated through the body through arteries leading away from the heart and veins moving toward it.

Source: courtesy, The Lilly Library, Indiana University, Bloomington Indiana.

that present in the air during a thunderstorm. During this experimental period, Galvani also showed that absent any external electrical stimulation whatsoever, a frog's muscles could still be made to contract when two different types of metal were brought in contact across them. Although in Galvani's mind this phenomenon strengthened the (correct) view of biological muscle as an electrical capacitor, the direct result of the experiment was a scientific debate that delayed general acceptance of the theory for decades (Cajavilca et al., 2009). **Alessandro Volta**, a physicist from Italy's University of Pavia, thought muscles contracting after pieces of two different metals were connected across them was a function of the electrical properties of the *metals*—with the contraction a mere artifact— and not due to the conduction of electricity originating in the muscle cells themselves. The tensions between Galvani and Volta started a robust series of experiments and counter-experiments—with Galvani showing, for example, that the electrical circuit could be closed and the muscle made to contract by connecting a wet piece of paper to the muscle or connecting muscle tissue from even an entirely different frog to the experimental leg. However, Volta's counterpoints to Galvani became more popularly accepted, especially after he was able to demonstrate that bringing silver and zinc into contact with each other resulted in the generation of a small electrical current. In 1800 Volta developed and distributed the first cell battery and his popularity soared. As a result, so did his view that muscles did not generate electrical signals of their own accord.

It wasn't until 1849 that the work of another brilliant young academic, **Emil du Bois-Reymond** at the University of Berlin, was able to show that it was Galvani who in fact had the correct theory (Cacioppo et al., 2007b; Meltzer, 1897). Du Bois-Reymond invented a nerve galvanometer and used it to show that there was indeed electrical current moving across a muscle neuron—transference now known as an **action potential** (Pearce, 2001). Furthermore, du Bois-Reymond and his student Julius Bernstein went on to develop and empirically confirm the physiological model of neurons still used today with negative and positive ions on either side of a semi-permeable membrane of a muscle neuron at rest (Brazier, 1959). This potential energy existing across the membrane—what is now referred to as the *resting potential*—was also shown by Bernstein to be equivalent to the excitation necessary for muscle contractions taking the extremely brief durations that Helmholtz had measured. (You remember Helmholtz, we talked about him in connection to Donders and the subtractive method.)

With the acceptance that human cells were capable of producing electrical current within the body, efforts began to develop instrumentation for measuring it. The first such device was the capillary electrometer in the late 1870s (Burch & DePasquale, 1964). This device used a tube filled with mercury, the shape of which would change based upon electrical current. By shining high intensity light on the shape one could record the changes in contour in real time, thereby capturing a representation of the changes in electricity emitted at the body surface. This technique was first used to measure the electrical activity of a frog's beating heart in 1880s and then by placing electrodes on a human in 1887 (Stern et al., 2001). The invention of the string galvanometer by Einthoven in 1904 made the recording of the ECG more practical because it no longer required the high intensity light source or the unstable mercury (Burch & DePasquale, 1964; Andreassi, 2000). However, as can be seen in Figure 2.5, the methodology was

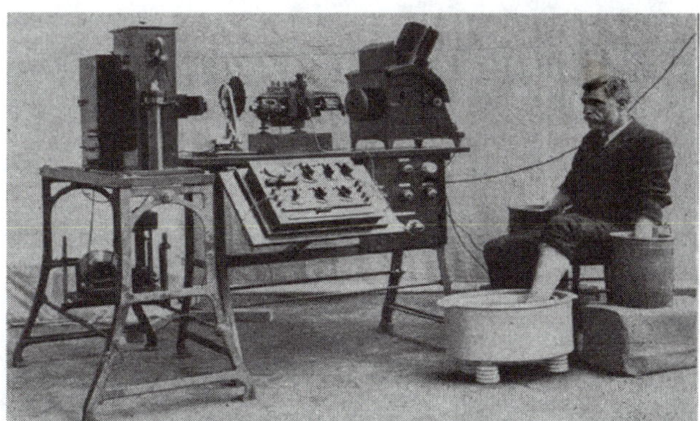

FIGURE 2.5 An early Einthoven string galvanometer manufactured by the Cambridge Company

Source: reproduced from *British Medical Journal*, S.L. Barron, 1, 720, 1950 with permission from BMJ Publishing Group Ltd.).

still not a piece of cake. As we will see in Chapter 4, a lot of progress has been made in lessening the intrusiveness of recording heart rate.

The general trajectory toward more simple yet accurate recording devices is, of course, also true for all other psychophysiological techniques. However, we would not be where we are today were it not for pioneering measurement work that began in the late 1800s and early 1900s. Particularly applicable for the measurements we'll be focusing on in subsequent chapters are the measurement of sweat secreted on the skin to indicate sympathetic nervous system activation which was first done by Féré (1888), the use of the oscilloscope to measure facial muscular activity by Jacobson (1927) and the first measurement of brain activity at the scalp surface using EEG by Berger (1929).

Benefits and drawbacks of psychophysiology

Even though we have come a long way in making measurement of bodily responses less intrusive than Einthoven's string galvanometer, Figure 2.6 reminds us that in today's media psychophysiology lab there are still multiple electrodes attached directly to a person's body—each with leads dangling from them (see Figure 2.6).

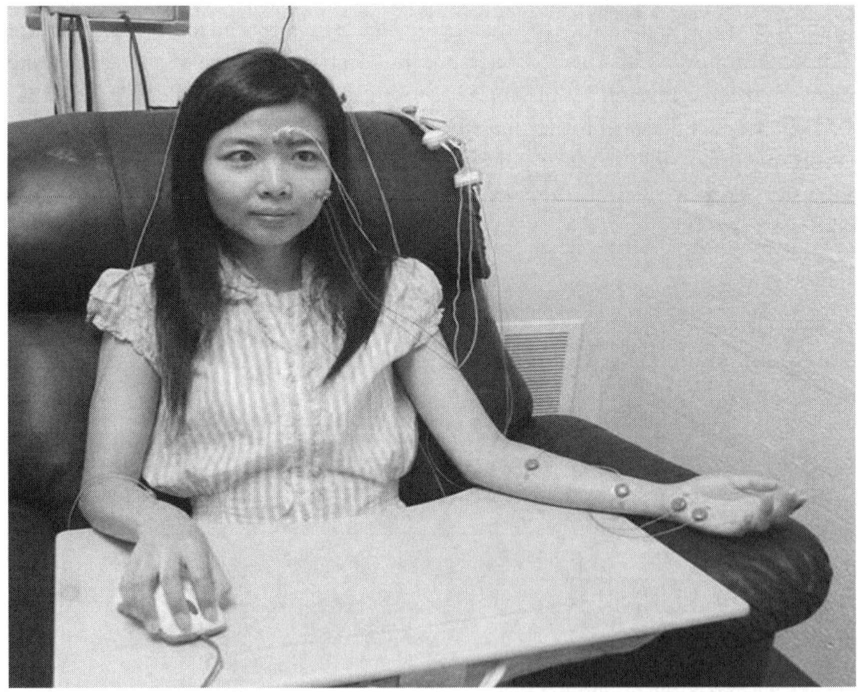

FIGURE 2.6 Participant in a typical physiological recording session in the media psychophysiology lab.

Some of them, in fact, are placed very close to the eye—a very important body part when it comes to watching TV or playing a computer game. So, one lead dangling in your subject's peripheral vision can certainly impact the media experience and the validity of the results. Of course, there is a question about the **ecological validity** of the experimental setting as well.

Ecological validity is the extent to which the experimental situation resembles the real life situation. It's a good bet that no one reading this book regularly watches television, listens to music, or surfs the web in a room by themselves with electrical sensors attached to their bodies. If you do, please seek help. Certainly, the artificiality of the viewing situation is one of the drawbacks to psychophysiological research.

The potential anxiety experienced by the research subject as a result of the measurement procedure is another. Conducting psychophysiological research requires physical contact with the subject—wiping their hands with distilled water, placing weird-seeming sensors filled with gel on the skin and face. This can be very disconcerting to some. Here a researcher's ability to establish rapport with a subject is vital to ease the possible anxiety associated with the situation. And certainly, being as empathetic as possible and trying to see the situation through the eyes of the subject is a good rule of thumb. So, for example, one of us once heard a graduate student tell a subject "I'm not getting a good impedance reading from this electrode so I'm just going to go get a syringe and inject more electrolyte into it." We had a teachable moment with that student later, as the same information could have been communicated to the subject in a much less stressful way by saying something like "I'm not seeing what I should from this sensor, so I'm just going to put more goop in it and see if that helps." Nevertheless, the most soothing demeanor and calm language will not remove the fact that physiological recording is intrusive by its very nature.

A related issue is the slightly elevated level of subject risk associated with psychophysiological measures. These are issues beyond social discomfort or anxiety mentioned above. The researcher places electrodes on the surface of the subject's skin and then plugs them into electrode leads. These leads are then plugged into amplifiers, forming a low impedance connection with the AC current powering the amplifier from the wall outlet. Essentially, due to the adherence of the electrodes, the subject is placed in a completed circuit. Because of this, periodic safety checks are a must in your lab to ensure that the building it is housed in and the equipment it contains remain electrically safe. Specific safety issues are addressed in Chapter 8.

For some, a final drawback associated with psychophysiological data collection techniques may be the care and precision required by the researcher during every data collection session. Several signals that media psychophysiologists are interested in are very small and originate from very specific locations. For example, say you are interested in measuring positive emotion during humorous radio advertise-ments (Bolls, Lang, & Potter, 2001) and therefore want to measure muscle activity using electromyography (EMG). Particularly, you are interested in the *zygomaticus major* muscle group since it is responsible for the upturning of the lips when a smile is formed (Tassinary, Cacioppo, & Vanman, 2007). However, this group is overlapped by the *levator anguli oris* group and extremely close to the *levator labbi superioris* group, both of which are related to the upcurl of the lip during both disgust and anger. In order to obtain the most valid data possible, accurate placement of the electrodes is of the utmost importance. Furthermore, the electrical signals that you are collecting are very small and a lot has to go into making sure they can be accurately measured. This includes things prior to the experiment, like designing the lab space to be electrically quiet. But it also requires diligence during each data collection session by preparing skin surfaces to create the lowest impedance possible in the connection between electrodes and the signal source. This often means thorough preparation of the skin surface, using slight abrasion with special swabs and the application of conductive gel both in the electrode and on the skin itself. In EEG work this can be even more time-consuming as electrodes must be placed in specific locations on the head to correspond to brain areas associated with your research questions and hypotheses. Special EEG caps make this spatial location simpler, but still dead skin from the scalp surface must be removed and hair pushed to the side in order for the electrode to make the low impedance connection necessary. During the experiment, too, physiological signals must be monitored and adjustments made to amplification, for example, in order to ensure that useable data are obtained. So, if you aren't someone who likes to "get your hands dirty," and being involved with attention to detail at all stages of an experiment—design, data collection, and analysis—then psychophysiological research is likely not for you.

However, if you are willing to commit to this level of detail you will find psychophysiological measures beneficial. They allow you to measure multiple bodily responses simultaneously in real time during media consumption. Each response gives you insight into cognitive and emotional processes associated with that particular media context—processes that the subject may not want to, or be able to, tell you about. They are one of the strongest lights we can shine into what used to be considered a black box—the embodied human brain.

So, here is the plan for the rest of the book. In Chapter 3 we provide some necessary vocabulary—the terms and concepts that all psychophysiologists have in their arsenal of understanding. Then, in Chapters 4 and 5 we make what we believe to be an artificial distinction for ease of reading and reference. In Chapter 4 we focus on measures of physiological systems that have been associated with concepts traditionally referred to as *cognitive* such as attention, cognitive processing, cognitive effort, and memory. Specifically we look at how to go about measuring heart rate using the electrocardiogram (ECG) and brainwaves with the electroencephalogram (EEG). In Chapter 5 we do the same for concepts traditionally referred to as *emotional* such as arousal, positivity, negativity, sadness, joy, disgust, and the like. You will learn how to measure specific muscle groups on the face using the electromyograph (EMG) and electrodermal activity (EDA) in the form of skin conductance level and responses.

Chapter 6 discusses new psychophysiological measures that are beginning to appear in the literature as correlates of psychological states during interactions with media messages. Each measure discussed has an established history within the field of psychophysiology, cognitive psychology, or cognitive neuroscience, however they will likely be utilized to a greater extent in media psychology labs in the coming decade.

As mentioned in several places throughout the current chapter, psychophysiological measures work best when used in conjunction with other forms of measurement because each give us insight into different stages of an ongoing cognitive process. Because of this, in Chapter 7 several measures are described which are often coupled with psychophysiological indices in media psychology. Common psychological questionnaires, secondary task reaction times, continuous response self-report measures, thought-listing, and memory measures are all explored.

Chapter 8 is designed to inform you about of the practical issues researchers face in implementing psychophysiological measures in experiments on cognitive and emotional processing of media. Topics include dealing with sources of external signal noise, safety concerns, research design, and analysis approaches.

Finally, Chapter 9 hopefully ties it all together, providing an overview of recent research in major areas of communication research that illustrates how psychophysiological data increase both the practical and societal importance of media psychology research. Chapter 9 also discusses the exciting scientific environment in which media psychology researchers presently work as well as the growth in the use of psychophysiological measures in both academic and proprietary media industry research. We conclude by considering several trends that we see unfolding in the future of media psychophysiology.

So, if you're ready, let's get ready to pry open the black box that is the human cognitive and emotional system using psychophysiological measures and the meaning they provide. We begin in Chapter 3 with the important basics you need to know when it comes to psychophysiological vocabulary, concepts, and equipment.

3
KEY TERMS AND CONCEPTS IN PSYCHOPHYSIOLOGY

Now that you have a sense of the history of psychophysiological measurement, both as a field and as an approach used by media psychology researchers, it is time to introduce some terms and concepts that are central to the approach. This chapter is short but important, designed to familiarize you with key ideas and vocabulary in order to make later chapters easier to follow. It begins with a discussion of basic topics of signal recording and then moves to iconic characteristics of psychophysiological responses in humans. The chapter is not by any means exhaustive in its detail. You are encouraged to consult other excellent psychophysiology textbooks such as Andreassi (2007); Cacioppo, Tassinary, and Berntson (2007a); and Stern, Ray, and Quigley (2001) prior to starting your own work. Furthermore, a chapter by Marshall-Goodell, Tassinary, and Cacioppo (1990) provides wonderful coverage of the bioelectrical principles central to psychophysiological recording.

Tracing the basics of the signal chain from body to computer

Psychophysiological recording focuses primarily on the collection of electrical signals or **biopotentials** at the skin's surface. When measuring skin conductance (see Chapter 5) the electrical signal is actually provided from *outside* the body in the form of a very low voltage originating from the recording equipment itself. The more the skin conducts that voltage the more sweat has been released by activation of the sympathetic nervous system. More common though is the recording of signals that originate as a result of the firing of **action potentials** by muscle or nerve cells deep within the body. An action potential is the all-or-nothing discharge of about 70mV that occurs due to a rapid change in the dispersion of ions across the semi-permeable membrane surrounding the neuron. When the cell is at rest, a larger concentration of negative ions exists inside this membrane compared to outside—this is the **resting potential** first discovered by Bernstein and du Bois-Reymond in the early 1850s as mentioned in the last chapter.

Circumstances arise, however, which cause the semi-permeable membrane to allow positive sodium ions to enter the cell and negative potassium ions to exit. When approximately 25mV worth of charge transfers across the membrane the cell "fires," dispersing the entirety of its 70mV charge. Often this energy release is sufficient to change the polarity of adjacent cells and a propagation of action potentials occur. Still, 70mV is a very small signal, even when it happens multiple times across a large cluster of neurons. And not only is the signal minuscule, but action potentials occur *below* the skin surface while the recording electrode usually sits *upon* it. For this reason the media psychology researcher collecting psychophysiological data needs to do something at most steps of the **signal chain** in order to amplify the bioelectrical signal prior to recording. The concept of the signal chain is a way of envisioning the different steps that the signal takes as it moves from action potential to the symbolic/numeric representation in the recording computer. Thinking in terms of the signal chain will be useful when you must troubleshoot recording errors in your lab . . . when you know you *should* be recording a signal but for some reason are not. Trust us; this will happen more often than you expect. To encourage you to use the metaphor of the signal chain when thinking about your psychophysiology lab, each major link is discussed below.

Electrodes and leads

Electrodes are small round cups with flat bottom surfaces covered by a metallic substance designed to conduct the bioelectrical signal. The metal is most often silver/silver-chloride (referred to using the elemental abbreviation Ag/AgCl) but other conductive metals such as gold and platinum are also used. Most of the measures used in modern psychophysiology laboratories are taken using **bipolar recording** techniques. In bipolar recording the electrical signals are compared across two active sites. In practice this means that two electrodes are needed for every measure: two for heart rate, two for each facial muscle group recorded, etc. Often, a third electrode acts as a ground to identify and eliminate electrical signals identical across the two electrodes in the bipolar pairing. Using a ground electrode affects the risk to the subject and you should refer to the specific instructions for your recording devices concerning electrical grounding. There are two important general rules across all labs, however. The first is that you should *only use one ground electrode on a subject at a time*. The second is that *a subject should be connected to a ground electrode prior to connecting other electrodes*.

Electrodes come in different sizes and are referred to according to the diameter of their recording surface. Two common sizes are 4mm and 8mm (Figure 3.1) and you should always use identical sizes for any individual bipolar measure. Because the biopotentials being recorded are so small, the largest possible surface area is desirable. However, where you are trying to place the electrode sometimes makes the use of the larger 8mm ones impractical. In the media research lab this is particularly the case when measuring facial EMG since larger electrodes may occlude vision or be too heavy for the adhesive collar to support when placing the electrode perpendicular to the floor on the surface of the face.

To boost the signal strength, electrodes are filled with an **electrolyte gel**. Disposable electrodes are often built into an adhesive collar and come pre-gelled by the manufacturer (see Figure 3.2). It is still useful to keep electrolyte gel on hand, even if you decide to use pre-gelled electrodes. We have found that adding a very small amount of electrolyte gel to in essence "freshen" the gelled surface of pre-gelled electrodes results in better signal quality. The collar of the disposable electrode is placed on the skin of the subject and an **electrode lead** snapped

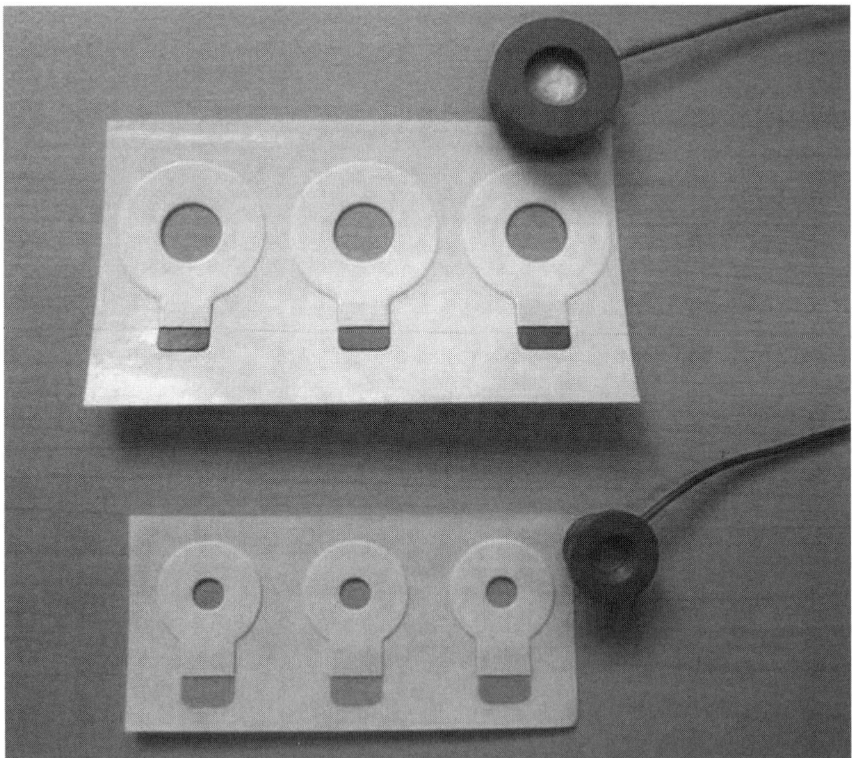

FIGURE 3.1 Standard-sized electrodes have an 8mm recording surface. Mini-electrodes, often used for facial EMG recording, have a 4mm recording surface. These are reusable electrodes that the researcher must fill with gel and attach to the subject using adhesive collars.

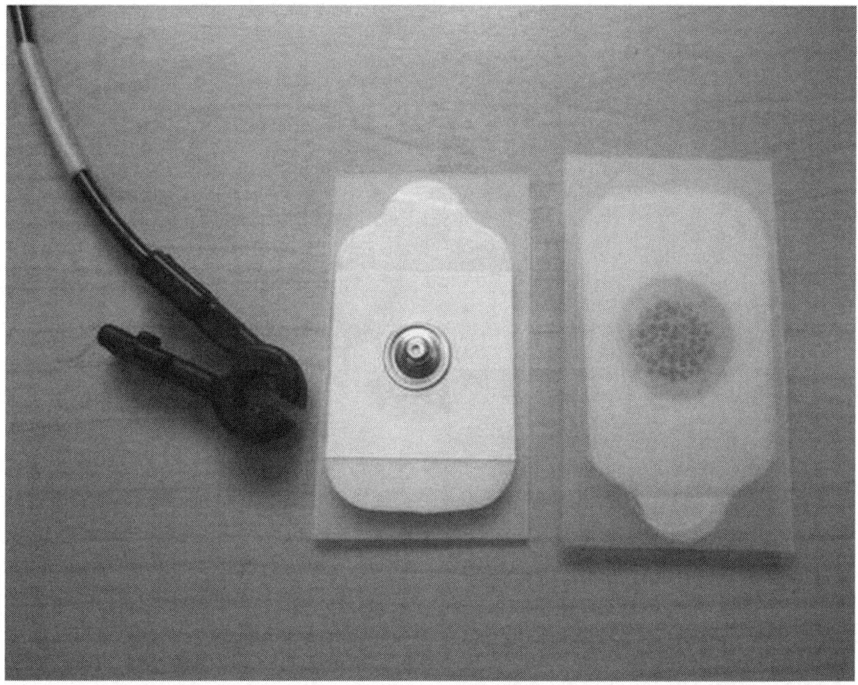

FIGURE 3.2 Disposable electrodes are intended for a single use. They are usually
purchased within an adhesive collar and pre-gelled with electrolyte.
The electrode lead, on the left, snaps onto the metal button on
the non–adhesive side.

onto it. After the experiment the lead is unsnapped from the collar/electrode,
which is then discarded.

Reusable electrodes, on the other hand, require adhesive collars to be attached
to them and must be filled with gel by the researcher prior to adhering them to
the subject (see Figure 3.3). Surgical hydration syringes can be filled with
electrolyte and used to inject it into the empty reservoir of the electrode. When
filling reusable electrodes you should be careful not to scrape the Ag/AgCl surface
of the cup with the syringe tip. You should also do all you can to minimize the
number of bubbles in the gel. Due to the nature of bipolar recording if one of
the electrodes has a smaller recording surface area than the other due to bubbles,
the resulting measurement may be invalid.

We have found the following electrode-prep steps effective at lessening the
bubbles in electrolyte gel. First, fill the electrodes about 10 minutes before the
experimental subject arrives, injecting slightly more gel than the cups can hold.
Use a toothpick to gently remove any large bubbles that initially occur. Then,
set the electrodes on a flat surface allowing the gel to settle and giving small bubbles
time to work to the surface. Just prior to applying the electrode to the subject

take the toothpick and run it along the flat surface of the adhesive collar to remove excess gel. Finally, when removing the non-adhesive backing just prior to application, give the reservoir a final visual inspection to make sure no bubbles have developed (Figure 3.3).

As the first links in the signal chain, the electrode and electrode lead are good initial places to investigate if you can't observe an electrical signal from the subject. For those using reusable electrodes, be sure to thoroughly clean the electrodes after each use. When cleaning reusable electrodes, be careful of the solder point where the lead attaches and try to prevent excess abrasion of the Ag/AgCl surface.

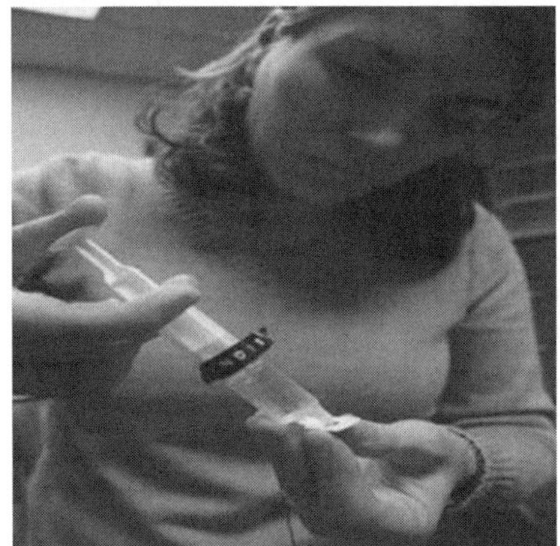
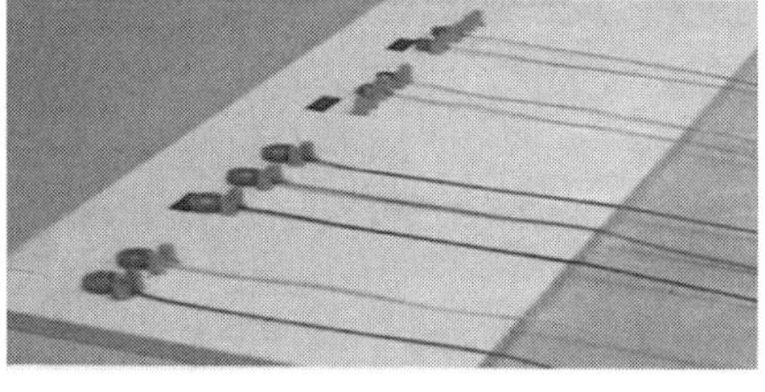
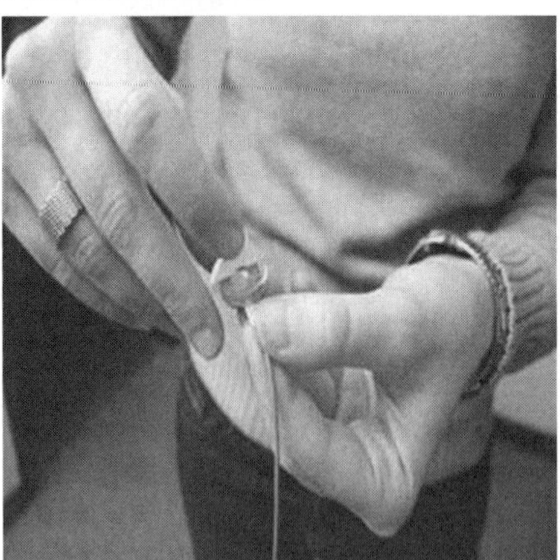

FIGURE 3.3 Preventing bubbles in the electrolyte gel is an important step when reusable electrodes are used in the lab. A successful technique is to overfill the electrodes initially and then allow the gel to settle for several minutes prior to adhering them to the subject. Note in the bottom picture that the location where the lead is permanently connected to the reusable electrode is very delicate and should be handled gently.

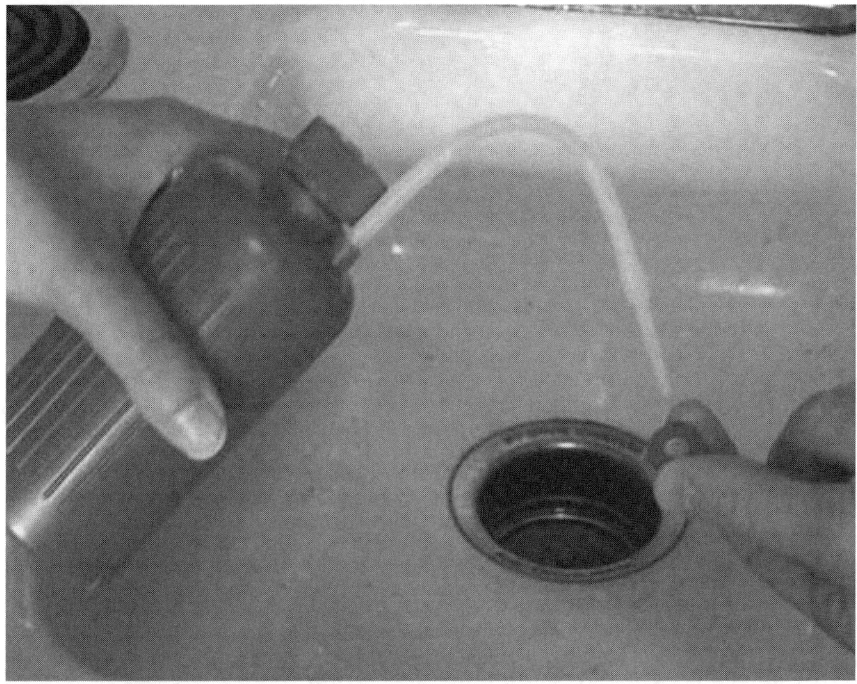

FIGURE 3.4 A thin stream of warm water from a surgical squeeze bottle can easily remove gel from the electrode without risk of abrading or removing the Ag/AgCl on the recording surface.

Some researchers remove the gel using small cotton swabs. An even less abrasive option is to use a Water-Pik® or surgical squeeze bottle to deliver a thin stream of warm water into the cup and blast-wash the used gel out (see Figure 3.4).

After removing the gel, rinse the electrode with distilled water to wash away mineral deposits and let it dry completely before using it again.

Other things to consider about electrodes and leads if you are not receiving an expected signal: if you are using disposable electrodes was the gel still semi-fluid or have the electrodes been sitting in a storage cabinet for so long that the gel has dried out and become viscous? Do you have a good connection between the removable electrode lead and the snap connector on the electrode? If your lab has reusable electrodes, perhaps the delicate soldering point where the electrode lead joins the electrode has been damaged. Another possibility is that you have filled the electrode with the wrong gel; we'll learn in Chapter 5 that there are two different kinds used with reusable electrodes and the one you choose depends on the measure being recorded by that sensor.

A related issue surrounding electrodes is the **impedance** of the signal coming out of them. Impedance is essentially the amount of resistance that the bioelectrical

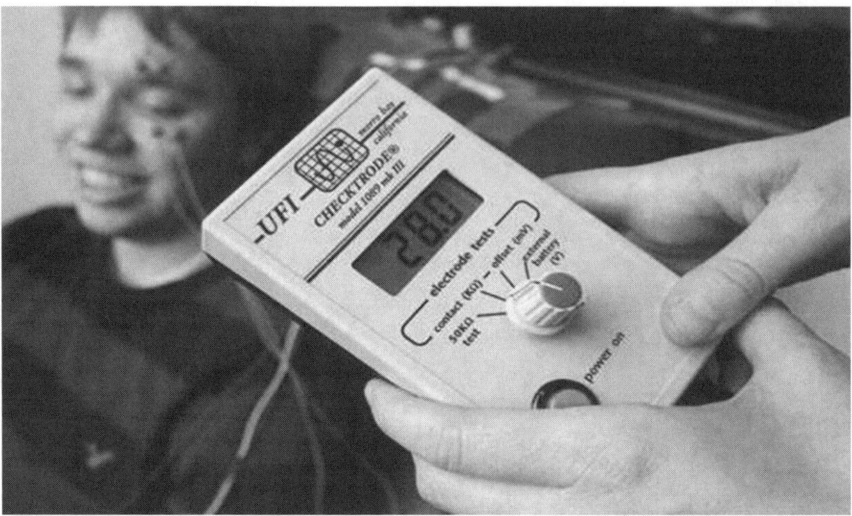

FIGURE 3.5 Impedance meter used to check electrical impedance across a bipolar set of electrodes.

signal encounters as it travels from the skin surface, through the electrolyte gel, and passes out of the electrode lead. High impedance levels result in greater susceptibility of the signal to influences by subject movement (called **movement artifact**) and extraneous oscillations of AC current in the lab itself from things like wall outlets and TV monitors. The use of an impedance meter is recommended (see Figure 3.5), with optimal readings varying based upon the particular signal being recorded *and* the input impedance level of the next link in the signal chain: the **bioamplifier** (Marshall-Goodell et al., 1990). For example, Tassinary, Cacioppo, and Vanman (2007) recommend cleaning and gently abrading the skin surface prior to facial EMG recording to bring impedance levels to between 5 and 10 k⏐. Newer EEG bioamplifiers, however, have higher input impedances which allow higher impedance at the electrode site (Pizzagalli, 2007). This is good if you happen to be recording at 19, or 64, or 256 locations on the scalp since it decreases the time required to bring the impedances of all those channels to a low level.

Photoplethysmographs

Electrodes are a specific type of **transducer**. A transducer converts one form of energy into another. So, in the case of electrodes biopotential energy is transferred into an electrical signal that can then be amplified by the bioamplifier. Although most of the chapters that follow will refer to physiological recording using electrodes, some published research in media psychophysiology employs another type of transducer: the **photoplethysmograph** or PPG (Anttonen, Surakka, & Koivuluoma, 2009; Detenber, Simons, & Bennett, 1998; Lim & Reeves, 2009). The PPG uses a light emitting diode to illuminate the skin of either the finger or the earlobe (see Figure 3.6). By measuring the light reflected back to a photo-sensor on the device, the amount of light absorbed by blood passing that location is measured to quantify the trace of the blood pulse allowing heart rate to be calculated. The fact that a single point of contact can provide the measurement is a benefit to using PPG as opposed to the two or three electrodes required to measure heart rate. However, realize that PPG does not

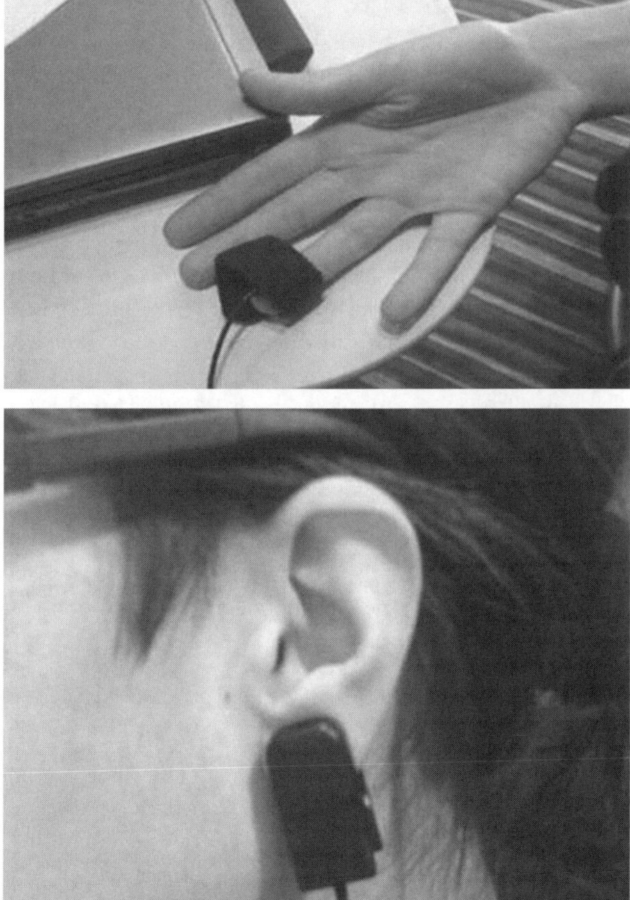

FIGURE 3.6 A photoplethysmograph is a single-point transducer that uses reflected light to detect the volume of blood flow. Common points of contact are the finger or the earlobe.

directly measure the electrical signal generated from the cardiac muscles but instead estimates the time between heartbeats based upon milliseconds between the maximum pulse of blood at the periphery. This IBI estimation is then used to calculate heart rate in a way which confounds the dual innervation of the heart *and* vasculature constriction by the parasympathetic and sympathetic nervous systems. Therefore, if you are interested in eventually using the milliseconds between heartbeats to determine the combined contribution of both autonomic systems using heart–rate variability analysis (see Chapter 6) then using a PPG is not advised.

Electrode cables and bioamplifiers

In some recording systems the PPG or the two electrodes used for a particular bipolar measurement plug into an **electrode cable**, which in turn connects to the bioamplifier at a single point. Other systems allow for each lead to plug directly into the bioamplifier (see Figure 3.7).

A bioamplifier, as you might expect, is designed to amplify the signal to a point where it can be recorded by a computer. It is helpful to think of a bioamplifier as a volume knob allowing you to "turn up" the signal being received from the electrodes. Older bioamps often allow continuous increases in volume similar to how you would turn up the sound of your car stereo. Newer bio-amplifiers, however, tend to use step-functions in the amplification or *gain*. For example, the bioamplifier in Figure 3.8 has five gain settings the researcher can use to boost the signal received from the electrode leads by 100, 1,000 (1K), 5,000, 10,000, or 50,000 times. The gain setting is determined according to the initial voltage of the signal being collected and the parameters of the software program being used to record it. However, if you trying to find a missing signal the first place to check on a bioamplifier are the connections where the electrode leads or cables go into the unit and the gain settings. You need to make sure the signal is getting in and that it is being amplified sufficiently for you to record it.

Filtering

Sometimes you are only interested in physiological signals that oscillate within a particular frequency band. Signals at all other frequencies are then, in essence, noise and the researcher may want to eliminate them. This is done using filtering. Off-line filtering is where the entire physiological signal—"noise and all"—is amplified and recorded by a computer during the experimental session. Filtering is then done after the data collection is completed—it's done "off-line"—using computer software which removes the unwanted frequencies. Therefore, when off-line filtering is done a **bandpass filter** is not a part of the signal chain. However, as you can see on the right side of Figure 3.8, there are times when

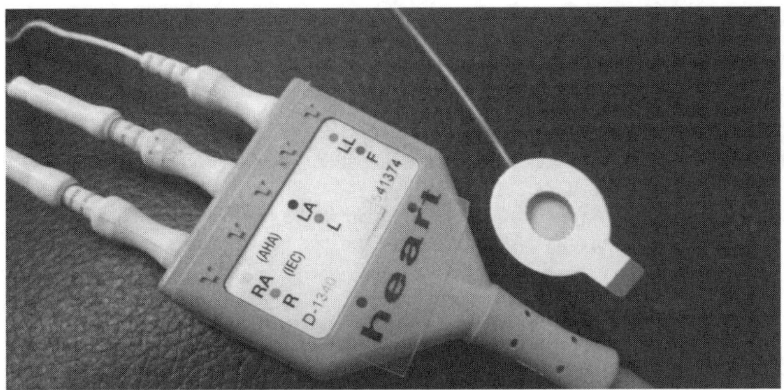

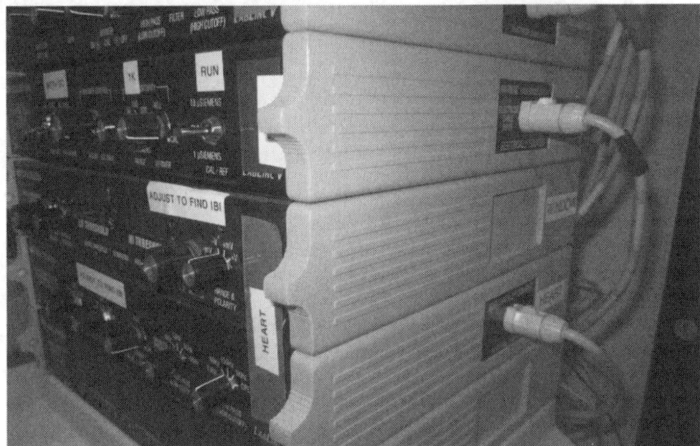

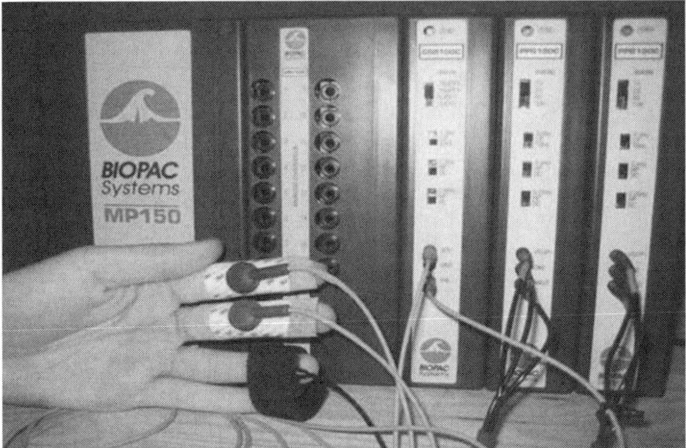

FIGURE 3.7 Top: an electrode cable with the two leads of bipolar electrodes and a ground electrode plugged in. Middle: the electrode cable is then led through a pass-through in the wall and plugged into the bioamplifier. Bottom: a system that does not use an electrode cable but instead allows the leads to be plugged into the bioamplifier directly.

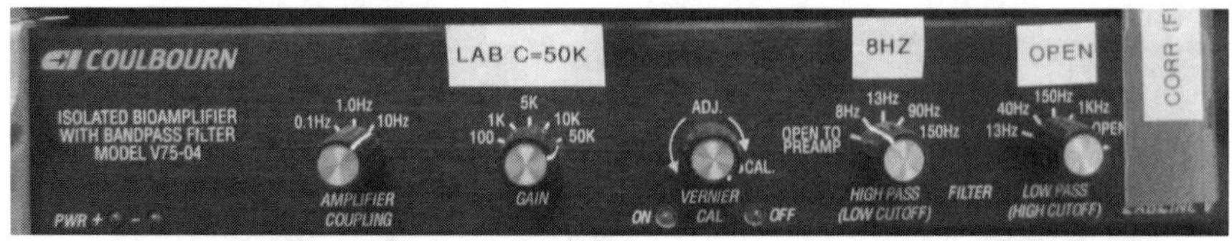

FIGURE 3.8 An example of a bioamplifier with gain set to boost the signal 50,000
times. High- and low-pass filters are located on the right.

filters are part of the bioamplifier and therefore become a link in the signal chain.
When they do you are filtering "online."

There are two major categories of online filters that may be a part of the
bioamplifier: a high-pass and a low-pass filter (Stern et al., 2001). They are named
according to the type of signal that they let *pass* and continue on in the signal
chain. So, a **high-pass filter** allows the researcher to set a frequency point above
which the signal will pass and below which all signals are attenuated. A **low-
pass filter** is set such that all frequencies *below* the setting will pass but those
above are attenuated. In Figure 3.8 you see the high-pass filter is set to 8 Hz
(signals oscillating at a frequency of eight-times-per-second) and the low-pass filter
is set to "Open" (i.e., there is no high frequency cut-off point for the low-pass
filter). This means the bioamplifier *accepts* all frequencies coming in from the
electrode cable but its filters are set to only let those *pass* if they are above 8 Hz.
If you are filtering online, an important link in the signal chain is to make sure
the filters are set to allow the desired frequencies to pass through to the next part
of the chain: the AD/DA board.

AD/DA boards

The final important link in the signal chain of most labs is the AD/DA board.
AD/DA is an abbreviation for Analog-to-Digital/Digital-to-Analog. An AD/DA
board is necessary because of differences between computers and living organisms.
Bioelectrical signals produced by living organisms are continuous. Your heart,
for example, is always generating voltage at some level which is collected by ECG
electrodes and delivered to the bioamplifier. Computers, however, are unable to
accept continuous signals because they work with discrete values. So, in order
to get a representation of the continuous signal into the storage computer we
must chop the signal up into a series of discrete voltage values. This process is
called **sampling** and it occurs in most labs at such a rapid rate—anywhere from
20–1,000 times per second—that the resulting sequence of discrete (digital)
sampled values closely resembles the continuous waveform emitted by the living
organism it is representing. The AD/DA board is the piece of equipment that
takes these samples from the output from the bioamplifier and inputs the discrete
values to the storage computer.

Most AD/DA boards consist of two important parts. There is an interface box which allows for both digital and analog input and output channels. Researchers use these in a variety of ways to communicate between stimulus presentation computers, physiological data collection computers and bioamplifiers. The second part is the interface card which is installed in the card slot of the data collection computer. AD/DA boards are sold as integrated parts of data collection systems or as stand-alone components that all bioamplifiers must be connected to if the signals from them are to be sampled and recorded. If you are not particularly savvy with computer hardware, or do not have access to a technician who is, you should probably consider using the integrated AD/DA approach since they will be set to interface with all your bioamplifiers by the manufacturer. More details concerning the selection of bioamplifiers and AD/DA boards are provided in Chapter 8.

For now, however, an important thing to check in the signal chain of your lab is that your AD/DA board is accepting signals from the particular bioamplifiers in the appropriate channels. For example, when collecting psychophysiological data you will be using a software program of some sort to interface between the AD/DA card in the computer and the AD/DA interface box. The software will have some way for you to tell it which of the channels in the AD/DA board will be dedicated to each measure. So, let's say you have identified analog channel 1 as the place where data from your subject's corrugator (frown) muscle activity will be collected. This will only be successful if, in fact, you have wired the output from the corrugator bioamplifier to enter the AD/DA board through analog channel 1. If you have accidentally plugged the output from the bioamplifier into another analog input channel the signal chain will be broken. Then even though your subject is frowning, the electrodes are filled with bubble-free gel, and the leads are intact and plugged into the proper bioamp, no signal will be reaching the AD/DA board in the place that the data collection computer will be expecting it. The result . . . no recorded signal.

One final consideration associated with AD/DA boards is how often each measure should be sampled during data collection. More frequent sampling increases the amount of computer storage space required per subject. And, although computer storage capacity gets larger and cheaper with each passing month, the total size of computer memory required per subject can quickly increase if you are sampling from many different channels. For instance, if you are recording a subject's heart rate, skin conductance, and four different sets of facial muscles while they watch 60 minutes of television and sample each channel 1,000-times-per-second (1,000 Hz) that amounts to over 21 million samples per subject! So, you may decide to vary the sampling rate, setting it only as high as each measure requires. If you do, it is important to realize that being too frugal in your sampling may result in **aliasing**—a phenomenon where the shape of the waveform resulting from sampled values looks nothing like the true biological waveform being represented. In this way, properly setting the sampling rate can be considered the final important link in the signal chain. A rule of thumb to avoid aliasing is known as the **Nyquist function**. According to the Nyquist function, a sampling rate set to twice the frequency of the phenomenon of interest will reproduce the original continuous waveform with the optimum degree of precision necessary to represent it. For instance, we know that the waveforms of meaning comprising the EEG recording oscillate between one and 60 times every second (1–60 Hz, Pizzagalli, 2007). So, sampling in EEG must be at least 120 Hz—although most researchers recommend even greater sampling rates than that for EEG, normally around at least 250 Hz. Similarly, if we know that most of the ECG signal for measuring heart rate occurs in the range of 13–40 Hz then a sampling rate of 80 Hz (80 samples per second) will yield an extremely accurate representation of the original continuous ECG signal for subsequent analysis.

Psychophysiological signal vocabulary

Now you have a brief understanding of the different links in the signal chain. In the chapters that follow we will spend time focusing on specific issues surrounding individual types of electrode placement and amplification corresponding to particular measures. But first, a few more pieces of vocabulary are worth presenting. This section introduces some common terms surrounding psychophysiological signals themselves.

Tonic and phasic responses

Two common terms refer to the duration over which the researcher is interested in exploring a psychophysiological response. **Tonic responses** are those occurring over comparatively long periods of time, often not in response to any particular event but rather to an experimental condition. Wise, Bolls, Myers, and Sternadori (2009), for example, designed a within-subjects experiment where subjects read news stories on a simulated news website. A primary independent variable was the way the news story was written: either in typical "inverted pyramid" style or in a chronological narrative style. After reading the story for as long as they wanted, the subjects were to click onscreen to play a 60-second video clip concerning the news story. Wise et al. (2009) hypothesized that processing the video clips after reading the inverted pyramid stories would require more cognitive effort than clips viewed after reading narrative stories. As we will discuss further in Chapter 4, they operationalized cognitive effort as deceleration in heart rate. Their analysis—the results of which can be seen in Figure 3.9—consisted of collapsing results across the eight stories on each of the two levels of the story-style factor and comparing the physiological responses across the entire 60-second time period. This is an example of a tonic analysis.

The second type of response is the **phasic response** which occurs across a comparatively brief time window and is usually in reaction to a specific stimulus

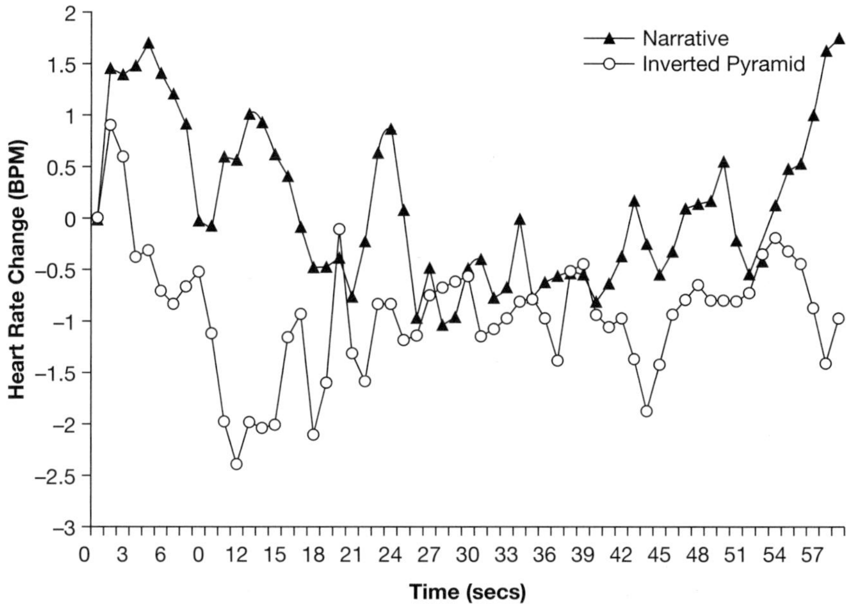

FIGURE 3.9 An example of a tonic analysis of cardiac data where heart rate activity for eight Narrative stories and eight Inverted Pyramid stories were averaged and presented across the 60-second duration. This analytic approach allows a comparison across a relatively long time-frame and is not concerned with specific evoked responses (source: figure reprinted from Wise et al., 2009, with permission from Taylor & Francis Ltd.).

feature. For example, Potter, Lang, & Bolls (2008) were interested in which auditory structural features resulted in orienting responses which they operationalized as brief decelerations in heart rate for the six seconds following the feature onset. In an experimental setting they collected heart rate data from subjects while they listened to a simulated radio broadcast in which auditory structural features had been identified. Then they calculated the average heart rate activity in the 10-second time window immediately following the onset of each feature. An example of a phasic result from that study is shown in Figure 3.10.

Change scores

A closer look at Figures 3.9 and 3.10 reveals that even though both represent cardiac decelerations over one-second increments, there is a difference in how that change is represented on the Y-axis of each graph. In Figure 3.10 the units are beats-per-minute (e.g., 72.6) while in Figure 3.9 they are **change scores**. A change score is calculated by subtracting a uniform baseline value of the

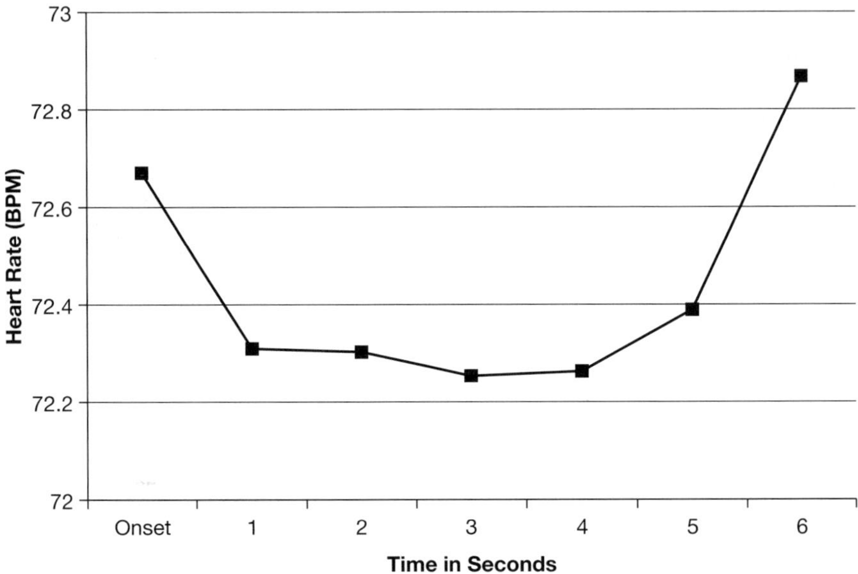

FIGURE 3.10 An example of a phasic analysis of cardiac data. The heart rate activity for all subjects was averaged in response to the onset of audio structural features and then the brief, evoked response was analyzed in the subsequent six seconds.

Source: used by permission from Potter, Lang, & Bolls, 2008, © 2008 Hogrefe & Huber Publishers www.hogrefe.com.

physiological measure from the value of the measure at each subsequent point in time. The baseline value is usually measured prior to stimulus onset when subjects are instructed to relax and wait for the beginning of the next message. In Wise et al. (2009), for example, their change scores were calculated "by taking participants' heart rate during each second of the video and subtracting the average heart rate during the 5 seconds immediately prior to video onset (baseline)" (p. 541). The use of change scores is very important when conducting experiments using a between-subject design because it helps to neutralize any between-group variance due to individual differences in physiological state or reactance; variance which, by design, is not present in within-subject designs as we will see in Chapter 8.

Habituation and sensitization

Another concept that any psychophysiologist should comprehend is that of **habituation**. Stern et al. (2001) define habituation as "the reduction of responding that occurs to the repeated presentation of the same stimulus" (p. 55). In other words, if the same media phenomenon is presented over and over the emotional or cognitive processes resulting from it may diminish with each subsequent exposure. This is likely to be reflected in the associated psychophysiological response patterns. For example, consider the experiment by Bruggemann and Barry (2002) where they showed 29 males and 29 females the same two video clips, in sequence, a total of 10 times. The clips were both about a minute long and one was from the television comedy *Mr. Bean*, the other was a violent scene from the film *Reservoir Dogs* (you know the one . . . where the man gets his ear cut off!). The skin conductance activity was recorded while the subjects watched the two clips in sequence, separated each of the 10 times by a self-report rating period. In Figure 3.11 you see that the mean skin conductance level during the two clips increased initially in the first trial, but then habituated over time.

Interestingly, Bruggeman and Barry found a greater initial increase in skin conductance for the violent film clip compared to the comedy for those who had scored high on a self-reported psychoticism scale (HP) compared to those who scored low on the scale (LP). However, the HP subjects habituated to the violent scene quite quickly, while the LP subjects actually showed a greater difference between mean skin conductance during the two types of films during the second and third trial than the first (see Figure 3.12). This is an example of **sensitization**, when the size of a psychophysiological response increases with repeated presentations of the same stimulus.

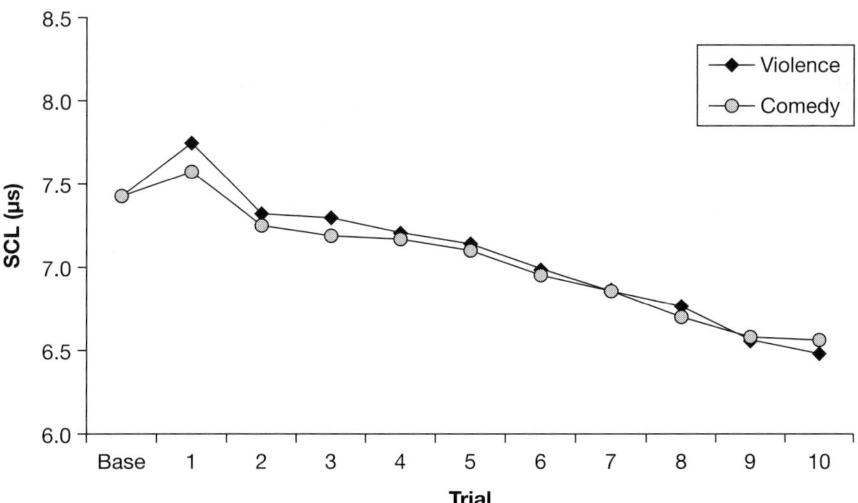

FIGURE 3.11 An example of habituation of skin conductance level after 10 presentations of the same violent or comedic video clip

Source: figure reprinted from Bruggemann & Barry, 2002, with permission from Elsevier.

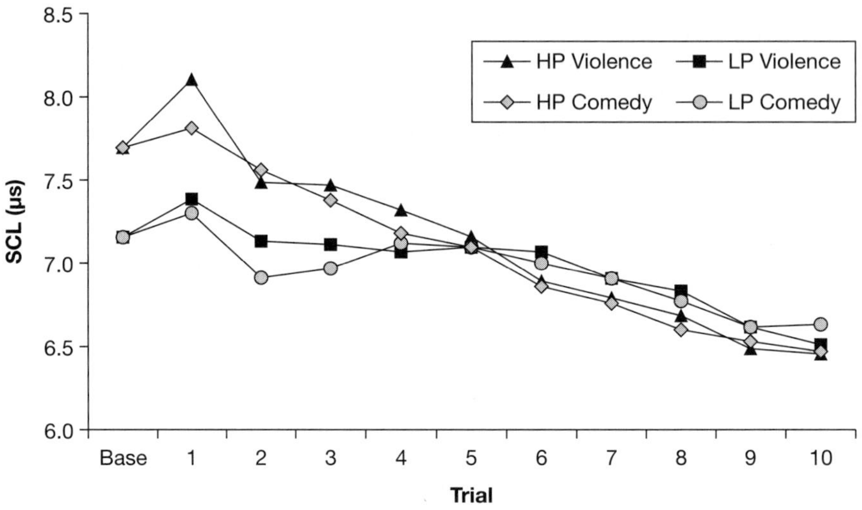

FIGURE 3.12 Example of habituation and sensitization

Source: figure reprinted from Bruggemann & Barry, 2002, with permission from Elsevier.

Summary

So, now you have a basic understanding of the general hardware used to measure psychophysiological signals. Plus, you have the conceptual model of *the signal chain* to help you generally follow a variety of signals from the subject's body to the data collection computer. And finally you know some general ways media psychology researchers look at psychophysiological signals when it comes to analysis—using change scores or whole values and looking for either tonic or phasic changes.

Now, it's time for you to move from the general to the specific. In the next two chapters we look at how these basics have been applied to help us open the black box of human processing while exploring the cognitive responses (Chapter 4) and the emotional responses (Chapter 5) to media.

4

PSYCHOPHYSIOLOGICAL MEASURES OF COGNITIVE PROCESSING OF MEDIA

Both this chapter and Chapter 5 focus on specific psychophysiological measures that can be used in studying cognitive and emotional processing of media respectively. The previous chapters of this book reviewed the history of psychophysiological research, foundational concepts and biological processes, as well as basic technical details that apply to psychophysiological measures in general. We move forward now by discussing theoretical, conceptual, and operational details involved in the current use of several specific psychophysiological measures commonly used in research conducted by media psychology researchers. Media psychology researchers investigate the mental processes that underlie the highly complex conscious experience of media consumption as well as the subtle, and not so subtle, way media content may influence individuals. The proper application of psychophysiological measures in this area requires solid theoretical understanding of relationships between specific cognitive and emotional processes evoked during media use on the one hand, and physiological activity on the other. We therefore begin this chapter, as well as the next, with a general theoretical consideration of mental processes involved in cognition and emotion engaged through media use and then move to discussing details involved in the application of the specific measures covered. It is worth noting, before we proceed, that our theoretical discussion of mental processes engaged by media exposure will be limited to more recent theorizing about cognition, emotion, and media that we apply in our own work. You ultimately may want to pursue a more historical discussion of these concepts as your interest in them grows.

Methodological developments—allowing more direct and detailed observation of human cognition—combined with subsequent theoretical advances have led to greater understanding than ever before of the mental processes engaged during media exposure. Such advances are the very lifeblood of media psychology research (and science in general, actually). We believe that the application of psycho-physiological measures to the study of cognitive and emotional processing of media has arguably been one of the greatest methodological advances our field has seen. As mentioned in Chapter 1, one of the benefits of psychophysiological measures is their ability to index mental processes as they occur in real time. They can thereby provide insight into processes engaged by the act of consuming media—both highly conscious and relatively unconscious processes. Yet despite the fact that psychophysiological measures enable media psychology researchers to observe dynamic mental processes unfolding in real time during media exposure, the ultimate value of this methodological advancement hinges on the degree to which the data obtained continue to spark subsequent theoretical thinking that provides useful knowledge of the rich and complex experience of media consumption. This requires a constant focus on understanding the nature of the human brain and how it processes mediated messages.

The act of consuming media—in all of its wide variety of formats and content—engages a host of mental processes that ultimately yield our conscious experience of being entertained or informed by media. It is these mental processes that lay the foundation for any previously documented effect of media on individuals. In Chapter 1 we discussed how prying open the black box of human cognition and emotion and systematically studying dynamic mental processes engaged by media exposure has moved the field of communication from one of research focused on shallow descriptions of static media effects to a field where researchers attempt to develop rich, insightful theoretical explanations of the interaction between the human mind and media. Scholars who study media psychology must remain focused on understanding the host of mental processes engaged by a wide variety of media content delivered over constantly changing technological platforms. It is important for media psychology researchers—if we are to continue to contribute to a scientific understanding of the influence media has on individuals—to also continue conceptualizing this wide variety of content delivered in new and different ways in a manner grounded in the theoretically-relevant mental processes rather than media industry conventions. It could be easy, given the warp speed at which media technology changes, for researchers to get caught up in the excitement of new media technology and regress to studying static "new effects" rather than systematically investigating how specific features of new media engage cognitive and emotional processes manifested in an embodied mind. This is, in essence, a challenge to researchers to maintain an appropriate focus on the "processor" of media—a mind that is embodied in the human brain—that mentally processes content in predictable and functional ways.

In order to maintain an appropriate focus on understanding the "processor" of media, researchers need to be dedicated to adopting an ever-evolving theoretical perspective on the nature of human cognition and emotion as well as maintaining the methodological expertise to study how the mind processes media. Scholars in the psychological sciences are continuing to increase knowledge of how mental processes are instantiated in an embodied mind and it is this body of knowledge media psychology researchers must stay abreast of in order to remain on solid conceptual and operational footing when using specific psychophysiological measures to study how the mind processes media.

The mental processes embodied in the human brain that psychophysiological measures index involve a dynamic interaction between human cognition and emotion. Thus, before diving into a detailed theoretical and operational discussion of specific psychophysiological measures of cognitive and emotional processing of media we need to briefly review the nature of the connection between emotion and cognition. The interaction of emotion and cognition has important theoretical and methodological implications for using data obtained through psychophysiological measures to understand cognitive and emotional processes engaged during media use. Neuropsychologists are revealing just how interdependent cognition and emotion are for enabling individuals to effectively negotiate life in complex social environments (Damasio, 1994). Mediated messages—as a form of complex social stimuli—seem likely to trigger extensive interactions between cognition and emotion in the minds of individuals consuming media. These interactions are discussed at a slightly more detailed level in this chapter on psychophysiological measures of cognitive processing in order to lay the foundation for a more general treatment of this issue in Chapter 5.

Media use—in the form of everything from highly immersive games to more traditional news and entertainment programming—can easily transport us beyond our relatively narrow "real world." It exposes us to characters, places, and events that we are unlikely to directly experience and which are significantly more mentally engaging than our real life experiences. This point is quite obvious to anyone who studies media—probably as well as most people who consume it—but media scholars have not always demonstrated a similar awareness of how consuming media that transports us beyond direct, unmediated sensory experience likely ignites complex interactions between cognitive and emotional/motivational mental processes.

One theoretical perspective includes explicit awareness of how cognition and emotion interact in the processing of mediated messages, and is therefore more consistent with how the brain is actually structured to process information. The theoretical approach places emphasis on the features of media which are salient to a human brain rather than traditional media-related features. Lang, Potter, and Bolls (2009), for example, recently suggested that the foundation of a strong conceptual definition of "mediated message" must include mention of a stream of sensory information that varies in motivational/emotional significance. This reflects a theoretical perspective in information processing known as **motivated attention** which claims that the amount of attention paid to any stimulus in our environment is modulated by the emotional/motivational significance of perceived information (Lang, Bradley, & Cuthbert, 1997). This theoretical perspective has recently been applied to motivated cognitive processing of mediated messages (Bradley, 2007b; Lang, 2009). Given that media present wide and varying cues signaling motivational/emotional significance, it makes sense for media psychology scholars to embrace a motivated attention theoretical framework.

A motivated attention perspective has some interesting implications for research and theory surrounding the media and mind interaction. This is because the evolution of the modern brain to attend to and preferentially process information with motivational significance happened over millennia—during times when the details that seemed to be relevant to us as biological beings (be it food or predators or mates) were actually there in our immediate environment. Today, with HDTV sets, 3D movies, highly immersive video games and the like, our brains are hard wired to respond to things of motivational relevance *as if they were really there* when in the modern world they may merely be a compilation of pixels (Reeves & Nass, 1996).

Another implication of adopting the motivated attention approach for media psychology research is that it makes it impossible to study cognitive or emotional processes engaged during media use in isolation. All theories of how the mind processes media need to include interacting cognitive and emotional processes. Further, on a purely methodological level, when using psychophysiological measures to study mental processes engaged during media use you must keep in mind that any data collected as an operationalization of cognitive processes will be simultaneously impacted by emotional processes and vice versa. For example, research on how individuals process fear appeals and disgusting visual images in televised anti-smoking messages indicated that variation in heart rate—often employed as a psychophysiological measure of cognitive processing—was accompanied by meaningful variation in facial EMG—the measurement of muscle activity associated with emotional response (Leshner & Bolls, 2005). Operational details of these two measures are thoroughly covered in the appropriate sections of this chapter (heart rate) and the next (facial EMG). For now, however, the important point is that results like those obtained by Leshner and Bolls illustrate how the interactions between cognitive and emotional processes are reflected in psychophysiological data.

Adopting this theoretical perspective also calls for careful consideration of how the interplay between media content and media structure impact motivated attention. Just as emotion and cognition are intertwined, so too are the content and structure of a media message when it comes to the impact of that message on the human brain. You've heard the old saying "It's not just what you say; it's how you say it." Research has found that to be true when it comes to your brain processing media. Remember how concerned the members of The Payne Fund Studies were about the impact of "salacious" topic matter in films like *The Feast of Ishtar*? And how Lang and her colleagues found that people paid momentarily more attention to TV during both related and unrelated cuts? Well, it turns out both these things interact to influence motivated attention as a media message unfolds dynamically over time (Lang, Bolls, Potter, & Kawahara, 1999). The importance of the impact structural features (e.g., cuts, camera angle, etc.) have on the limited capacity human cognitive system, in fact, has led Lang to move beyond her previous rough conceptualization of structural complexity (e.g., "related and unrelated cuts") and develop a more intricate quantification system for the load placed on the cognitive system by structural changes in a message (Lang, Park, Sanders-Jackson, Wilson, & Wang, 2007).

The embodied, motivated attention theoretical framework we apply in our own research into cognitive and emotional processing of media proposes that there are no purely cold cognitive processes or purely hot emotional processes. The cognitive processes of allocating mental effort to selecting information in our environment to pay attention to, think about, and remember are fueled by our motivations and emotions (Berntson & Cacioppo, 2008; Lang & Bradley, 2008). Conversely, it is arguably not possible to have emotional processes engaged unless emotionally meaningful stimuli—which by definition can only be meaningful based on stored information retrieved from long-term memory—are cognitively attended to. This extensive and dynamic interaction between cognitive and emotional processes is anatomically embodied in a human brain that consists of extensive neuronal connections between areas believed to be highly involved in cognitive processing *and* areas thought to be the center of emotional responding (Tucker, Derryberry, & Luu, 2000). These interconnected areas of the brain are engaged during media exposure in patterns of cognitive/emotional processing that vary according to the sensory properties, motivational significance, and structural features of media content.

An embodied, motivated attention framework provides what we believe is the strongest theoretical rationale to use psychophysiological measures to index cognitive and emotional processes engaged during media exposure. It also serves as a general framework for understanding the interaction between cognition and emotion. It is important, however, to still recognize that cognition and emotion involve distinct, separable, mental processes, which is why we can talk about separate psychophysiological measures for each (Cacioppo, Gardner, & Berntson, 1999). Put more specifically, the mental processes of attending to and remembering information contained in the media you consume—cognitive processing of that media—interact with but are distinct from mental processes involved in your deriving emotional meaning from that media. We recognize that these are distinct mental processes with specific related psychophysiological measures by covering the related, unique conceptual and operational details of psychophysiological measures of cognitive processing and psychophysiological measures of emotional processing in separate chapters. The next chapter explores emotion while the remainder of this chapter focuses on psychophysiological measures of cognitive processes. In it a conceptual foundation for studying cognitive processing of media is presented and two exciting psychophysiological measures of cognitive processing —heart rate and EEG—are described.

Conceptualizing cognitive processing of mediated content

Cognitive processing of mediated content broadly refers to the mental act of attending to and remembering information presented through some form of medium. Scholarly research on understanding cognitive processes engaged during media use is epistemologically rooted in cognitive psychology—a shift in psychology away from radical behaviorism to a cognitive approach centered on understanding how humans acquire and use knowledge and information (Bryant & Rockwell, 1991). Early on, researchers interested in cognitive processing of media content specifically focused on investigating attention, particularly attention paid to television, with much of the research being conducted on children (e.g., Anderson & Burns, 1991).

Researchers who conducted the early work on how individuals pay attention to television—consistent with how attention is conceptualized in cognitive psychology—viewed it as consisting of separable cognitive processes related to the selection of information from one's environment and processes related to effort or depth of processing (Anderson & Burns, 1991).

The last two decades of the twentieth century saw a tremendous amount of research on how individuals pay attention to television. Some of the earliest work in this area was conducted on children's viewing of *Sesame Street* and how different production features of that educational series captured and held attention—as measured by the extent to which children looked at the TV screen and later remembered information from it (Anderson & Levin, 1976). One of the fundamental questions this research attempted to answer was whether attention was primarily driven by conscious, strategic choices of individual viewers or was more automatically captured by content and formal production features (e.g., Alwitt, Anderson, Lorch, & Levin, 1980; Huston & Wright, 1983; Lang, 1990). Scholars also probed the nature of **attentional inertia**, a phenomenon in which it was shown that the longer an audience member continues viewing a segment of television content the more likely they are to keep paying attention to it and become less easily distracted away from the screen (Anderson & Lorch, 1983; Choi & Anderson, 1991).

The early work investigating how individuals pay attention to television laid a foundation for developing an in-depth theoretical view of how the human brain cognitively processes media content. Models developed in the 1980s were fairly sophisticated, reflecting the operation of both unconscious and conscious mental processes and various forms of memory (e.g., Anderson & Bryant, 1983; Thorson, 1989). However, a majority of the research on which these models were based relied on behavioral and self-report measures incapable of revealing the subtlety involved in cognitively processing media content. As a result, they glossed over many of the intricate, dynamic processes involved—processes that psychophysiological measures now enable us to explore.

In the current age, when media researchers can readily use psychophysiological measures to study the extensive and intricate work performed by the brain during exposure to mediated content, it is imperative that researchers have a detailed conceptual and operational understanding of the nature of mental activity. Here we present two conceptual and operational considerations that are particularly relevant to researchers wishing to use psychophysiological measures to study cognitive processing of media content. First, on a conceptual level, realize that the conscious experience of consuming media—created by the working brain—emerges from specific dynamic subprocesses. These subprocesses can be described as perceiving, taking in, making sense of, and remembering relevant aspects of the media content being consumed. Second, on an operational level, the work performed by the brain during media exposure is fueled by observable biological activity that underlies psychophysiological measures of cognitive processes. These two considerations taken together mean that utilizing psychophysiological measures to study cognitive processing of media involves mapping observable biological activity within a physiological system to subprocesses involved in mentally processing media content. Fortunately, the connections between patterns of physiological activity and many cognitive processes have been well established and media researchers can concentrate on learning how to validly and reliably use psychophysiological measures to study cognitive processing of media.

Rigorous, valid measurement of cognitive processes engaged during media exposure requires a careful, nuanced conceptualization of the distinctions between "attention" and "memory." An individual might pay attention to media content and fail to have highly detailed or accurate memory for information presented (Bolls, Lang, & Potter, 2001). Second, memory cannot be adequately described as a singular broad concept. Memory consists of mental processes related to recognition, recall, and retrieval (Zechmeister & Nyberg, 1982). While containing some theoretical and practical value, taken broadly, the concepts of attention and memory gloss over important processes involved in the cognitive processing of mediated messages. For instance, if a researcher simply measures "attention" paid to a mediated message, more micro-level mental processes that produce human attention may be overlooked. Here, the term *micro* certainly does not imply less importance. It is these underlying mental processes that are the nuts and bolts of cognitive processing and therefore are what researchers need to observe if they are truly going to increase knowledge of how different forms of media content are cognitively processed. Variation in these micro-processes underlying human attention has the possibility to alter any observed effects of "paying attention" to a message.

Research we have conducted on imagery in radio advertisements illustrates the importance of studying specific cognitive processes that underlie attention and memory (Bolls, 2002, 2007; Bolls & Potter, 1998). Previous research has shown that individuals report paying more attention to high versus low imagery radio ads and high-imagery ads are more memorable (MacInnis & Price, 1987).

However, through the use of psychophysiological measures of cognitive processing and more detailed tests of message recognition we discovered that most of the cognitive effort invested in processing a high-imagery ad may be dedicated to retrieval—a specific process underlying memory that involves the activation of neuronal networks representing stored memories at the expense of encoding— a specific process underlying attention (Bolls, 2007; Bolls & Lang, 2003).

Psychophysiological measures have been used to observe the operation of dynamic subprocesses that underlie cognitive processing of mediated messages (see Lang et al., 2009 for a recent review). It is also clear psychophysiological measures of cognitive processing of media content hold the most promise for revealing the dynamic functioning of mental processes across time. Early in the history of cognitive processing of media research such insight was recognized as critical for the development of theoretical models that include description of mental processes—evoked by messages—leading to specific patterns of activation that represent memory (Bryant & Rockwell, 1991). Experiments in which psychophysiological measures of cognitive processing of media are used to gain insight into how the mind processes media must be grounded in a theoretical model capable of generating testable hypotheses concerning how an embodied human mind processes motivationally relevant sensory information. Thus, here we review the theoretical model that underlies a substantial amount of research in which psychophysiological measures have been used to study cognitive (and emotional/motivational) processing of media content.

The limited capacity model of motivated, mediated, message processing

Annie Lang and colleagues have conducted numerous experiments over the past two decades developing a model of cognitive processing of media that has recently been called the Limited Capacity Model of Motivated, Mediated, Message Processing, abbreviated **LC4MP** (Lang, 2009). Many of the premises of LC4MP are similar to those covered in Chapters 1 and 2. The foundational principle of the model is that individuals are limited-capacity information processors. The notion of limited cognitive capacity is not only a premise of the LC4MP but has also been incorporated into theories advanced by some of the most respected psychologists during the earliest published experiments on human attention and memory (Wickens, 1984). Put into the practical context of cognitive processing of mediated messages, limited capacity simply means that the human cognitive system does not have the capacity to thoroughly process all the bits of information contained in a media message. According to the LC4MP, information contained in a mediated message gets transformed into a dynamic memory representation that changes across time through three subprocesses: Encoding, Storage, and Retrieval. These three subprocesses are performed in parallel during exposure to media content.

Here is how these components work together—and although the process must be discussed in a linear manner, remember that all these sub-processes are going on simultaneously in parallel as the message is processed. It is also important to remember that memory is a process—not a place that exists in the human brain. **Encoding** involves the selection of incoming information from the message for further processing—resulting in a short-term, working memory pattern of neuronal activation that represents the selected information. At the same time, cognitive resources are also allocated to **retrieval**—resulting in the activation of neuronal memory networks that represent previously encountered information and knowledge. Concurrent encoding and retrieval results in a unified pattern of neuronal activation that forms a memory representation of a mediated message an individual can actually make sense of. Along with encoding and retrieval, a portion of the information contained in a mediated message that was encoded is linked with information that was activated during retrieval through the memory process of storage. **Storage** results in a memory representation that consists of a new pattern of neuronal organization that could be activated through retrieval at a later time. The simultaneous and parallel nature of these subprocesses means that storage is occurring while additional information from the continuous stream of media content being consumed is encoded and details contained in stored memory representations are retrieved, etc.

A specific example may help clarify the nature of encoding, storage, and retrieval as cognitive subprocesses engaged during media use. Imagine that you are viewing your favorite primetime televised drama. At any moment during this episode there is a multitude of information that could be selected to form your continuous, temporary memory representation of this program during encoding. This information ranges from a physical characteristic of any object shown on screen, to action and dialogue contained in the storyline. For instance, an advertiser with an in-program product placement might want you to encode and ultimately store the fact that the main character in the program drives a Ford Mustang. Chances are, however, your primary motive for viewing this program is to escape into an entertaining narrative so you will likely allocate most your cognitive resources to encoding information directly relevant to the storyline such as ongoing dialogue between the characters. Encoding this dialogue is made meaningful by the simultaneous activation of previously stored knowledge through the subprocess of retrieval. At a minimum, retrieval must result in a pattern of activation representative of your knowledge of the language the characters are speaking. The pattern of activation brought on by retrieval could also represent stored information about the characters and program based on exposure to that evening's storyline or previous episodes of the program as well as details about how this genre of program generally proceeds—sitcoms follow different patterns than action drama, for example. It is important to note that the simultaneous performance of encoding, retrieval, and storage during cognitive processing of a mediated message forms patterns of activation that underlie a conscious mental representation of information reflecting actual bits of information in a message to varying degrees. Further, as an individual allocates more resources to retrieval during a media message, a smaller proportion of the limited resources are left to engage in detailed encoding of the message. Likewise, as more cognitive resources are allocated to encoding detailed information contained in the continuous stream of media content being consumed, there are fewer cognitive resources left to engage in retrieval and storage to the degree needed to thoroughly form a detailed memory representation that can easily be activated at a later time.

An additional premise of LC4MP is that cognitive resources are allocated to media messages in the form of both **controlled processing** and **automatic processing** (Lang, 2009). This premise represents the resolution of one of the foundational questions of the field: whether attention is primarily consciously and voluntarily allocated to media or done so more automatically and unconsciously due to features of the stimulus. The answer is both. The degree to which cognitive resources are allocated to encoding, retrieval, and storage is determined through processes that range from being more or less automatic to consciously controlled (Lang, Potter, & Bolls, 1999; Schneider, Dumais, & Shiffrin, 1984).

An individual's interests and goals for media use underlie the controlled allocation of cognitive resources to processing a message (Lang, 2009). A clear example of this involves the goal of information seeking. Our personal interest in obtaining information that aids survival is one reason why individuals might consciously allocate more cognitive resources to encoding negative news such as stories of crime, violence, and disasters (Shoemaker, 1996). Research utilizing psychophysiological measures of controlled allocation of cognitive resources to encoding news stories has indeed indicated that the presence of graphic, negative content in news stories increases cognitive resources allocated to encoding (Lang, Newhagen, & Reeves, 1996). A mechanism through which resources are automatically allocated to encoding media content is the **orienting response** (Lang, 1990). The orienting response has been termed the "what is it" response and results in a temporary increase in cognitive resources allocated to encoding novel or signal stimuli we encounter in our environment (Graham, 1979; Graham & Clifton, 1966; Sokolov, 1963). Several features of mediated messages have been found to evoke orienting responses in attentive individuals. These features include, as mentioned already, related and unrelated cuts in TV (Lang, 1990; Lang, Geiger, Strickwerda, & Sumner, 1993). But orienting has also been found to occur in response to sound effects and voice changes in audio (Potter, 2000; Potter, Lang, & Bolls, 2008), and animation on web pages (Diao & Sundar, 2004; Lang et al., 2002).

Cognitive resources allocated to processing media messages on a conscious, voluntary basis results in cognitive processing that is more tonic, or enduring across time. Cognitive resources allocated to processing media messages on a less conscious, automatic basis results in cognitive processing that is representative of a phasic, or temporary, response to specific stimuli or features within content (see Chapter 3). It is important to note that controlled and automatic allocation of cognitive resources during media exposure dynamically co-occur while an individual processes information. The automatic, phasic allocation of cognitive resources occurs against a background of ongoing controlled, tonic allocation of resources.

Given a fundamental understanding of the human brain and a solid theoretical framework for the application of psychophysiological measures of cognitive processing to studying mental processing of media, we are ready to consider conceptual and operational details of specific psychophysiological measures. The next sections of this chapter are aimed at giving you a strong understanding of two psychophysiological measures that can be used to study cognitive processing of mediated messages. First we will discuss cardiac activity and then measurement of the electrical signal underlying brain activity through the use of the electroencephalograph (EEG). Cardiac activity is more commonly observed in experiments on cognitive processing of media than EEG. This is likely due to the fact that the expense and technical expertise required to collect and analyze brain wave activity makes heart rate a much more accessible measure for most media researchers. Thus, we will discuss cardiac activity more extensively than EEG, although both measures have the potential to provide exciting insight into cognitive processing of mediated messages.

Cardiac activity: a physiological measure of cognitive processing

What can the heart tell us about thinking? This question is not only interesting but also the title of a chapter in the book edited by Annie Lang entitled *Measuring psychological responses to media* (Lang, 1994c). Implied in the title of the chapter is the assumption that cardiac activity—as reflected by increases and decreases in heart rate—is a valid physiological indicator of cognitive processing. As mentioned in Chapter 1, Lang's book coincided with the third, most sustained, and currently ongoing appearance of physiological research methods in the media laboratory. The chapter by Lang was the first publication to provide an in-depth discussion of the use of heart rate as a psychophysiological indicator of cognitive resources allocated to processing media content. Lang distilled conceptual and operational details of this measure in a way that helped researchers think more clearly about using heart rate to draw inferences about how individuals cognitively process media.

Our discussion of heart rate will hopefully serve to similarly strengthen theoretical and operational thinking while including adequate technical detail to enable interested readers to use this measure in their own research. Modern media psychology research can undoubtedly continue to be strengthened by the use of heart rate to provide insight into how individuals allocate their limited cognitive resources to processing mediated messages. Researchers working in the first decade of the twenty-first century have used heart rate to measure variations in cognitive resource allocation due to features of media content like written style of Internet news stories (Wise, Bolls, Myers, & Sternadori, 2009), size of photographs (Codispoti & De Cesarei, 2007), number of radio advertisements in a commercial break (Potter, 2009), animation of Internet advertising (Chung, 2007; Diao & Sundar, 2004), televised graphics (Fox et al., 2004; Thorson & Lang, 1992), and imagery evocation by radio advertisements (Bolls, 2002). In our discussion of heart rate as a psychophysiological measure of cognitive processing we cover the psychological meaning of changes in heart rate—grounded in the anatomy and physiology of cardiac activity—as well as the equipment required to measure and analyze heart rate.

Psychological meaning of heart rate

The connection between cardiac activity and cognitive processing may not be intuitive at first consideration. You are likely more accustomed to associating your heart with your emotions rather than with how much mental effort you invest in processing information on your favorite website when you surf the Internet. Colloquial references to "feelings of the heart" abound and *emotional* states undeniably have profound physical consequences including changes in heart rate. Like most organs, the heart is dually innervated by the sympathetic and parasympathetic branches of the nervous system—a biological aspect of cardiac activity we will be discussing later on. Practically, this means that the speed at which your heart is beating at any moment in time is based on a combination of bio-impulses from both systems. Generally speaking, sympathetic nervous system activation has been associated with arousal while variation in parasympathetic nervous system activity is believed to reflect variation in cognitive resources allocated to perceptual processing of information in one's environment (Berntson, Cacioppo, & Fieldstone, 1996; Wetzel, Quigley, Morell, Eves, & Backs, 2006). A good rule of thumb is that your sympathetic system—as the "fight or flight system"—tells your heart to beat faster while your parasympathetic system tells your heart to slow down. This means that the sympathetic nervous system contributions to changes in heart rate do reflect the influence of the arousingness or emotionality of a situation. However it is usually the case that increases in sympathetic activation associated with emotional media messages are also accompanied by increases in *interest* and *attention* paid to the message content. This is because, you'll remember, our evolutionarily-old brains do not initially recognize the motivationally-relevant content of arousing media (sex, violence, etc.) as being mediated but instead think it is real and present (Reeves & Nass, 1996). So, when something that is threatening appears on the screen, we are both aroused by it and pay attention to it—just like we would in real life. This dual influence on the heart—with the sympathetically-driven arousal telling it to speed up at the same time that the parasympathetically-driven attention is telling it to slow down—is also likely the reason why cardiac data collected by Zillmann (Cantor, Zillmann, & Bryant, 1975; Zillmann, Mody, & Cantor, 1974) and Donnerstein (Donnerstein & Barrett, 1978; Donnerstein & Hallam, 1978) did not behave in predictable ways in response to pornography. If researchers are not careful it is easy to overlook a potential confound in the study of emotional media content. Emotional media content not only evokes an affective reaction but is also something we pay attention to. Thus, embodied mental processing of emotional media content involves both sympathetic and parasympathetic activation. The best measure of sympathetic activation evoked during media exposure is thought to be skin conductance, which we address in Chapter 5. This is because skin conductance is not dually innervated, but activated only by the sympathetic nervous system.

It has long been an assumption of researchers working under the LC4MP theoretical perspective that media messages—even arousing media messages—are rarely *so* arousing that the sympathetic innervation will completely overcome the deceleration resulting from the parasympathetic innervation of cardiac activity. Nevertheless, it is still true that parasympathetic innervation forces the heart rate down while the lesser influence of the sympathetic system pulls it up. For this reason some researchers have turned to an analysis of heart rate variability (HRV). Ravaja (2004a), for example, strongly recommends that media researchers who use heart rate to index cognitive processing use HRV analysis to tease out and specifically identify the unique contributions of the sympathetic and parasympathetic nervous system to changes in the beats-per-minute representation of heart rate. HRV will be addressed in more detail in Chapter 6. However, we believe there is adequate psychophysiological research establishing a solid connection between changes in heart rate as a beats-per-minute measure and variation in cognitive resource allocation to information processing to have confidence in using it to index cognitive resources allocated to processing mediated messages. As long as adequate control exists in the experimental context and selection of stimuli, heart rate measured in beats-per-minute can be confidently placed in the methodological toolbox of media psychology researchers. This is especially true if it is triangulated with results obtained through other measures.

The connection between heart rate and cognitive resources allocated to encoding information in one's environment dates back to research conducted on attention and orienting in the 1960s demonstrating that cardiac deceleration is reliably evoked with the orienting response (Graham & Clifton, 1966; Lynn, 1966; Sokolov, 1963). Lacey's information intake-rejection hypothesis proposed that cardiac deceleration reflects preparatory processes that aid sensory intake from the environment whereas cardiac acceleration reflects defensive responding or disengagement from processing environmental stimuli indicative of information rejection (Lacey & Lacey, 1974). There are a couple of nuanced theoretical interpretations concerning the exact function that heart rate deceleration serves in encoding information from the environment. One perspective is that cardiac deceleration functionally makes individuals more receptive to potentially meaningful stimuli in the environment, thus improving response effectiveness (Lacey & Lacey, 1980). A slightly different perspective holds that cardiac deceleration acts to actually improve the quality of sensory input resulting from encoding information from one's environment (Graham, 1979). Ultimately it appears that cardiac deceleration observed as individuals allocate more cognitive resources to encoding information from the environment reflects the working of processes which serve to facilitate the intake of potentially meaningful information (De Pascalis, Barry, & Sparita, 1995; Jennings, 1992). The bottom line is that psychophysiological research into the psychological meaning of changes in heart rate when individuals are engaged in information processing of potentially meaningful sensory stimuli—like mediated messages—indicates that cardiac deceleration reflects an increase in cognitive resources allocated to encoding information into working memory while cardiac acceleration reflects a rejection of environmental stimuli in support of other processes involved in responding and adapting to one's environment (Lang, 1994). This conceptualization has proven quite useful to researchers studying media psychology as cardiac deceleration and acceleration have been studied at both a phasic and tonic level (Lang et al., 2009).

Despite the fact that there is a solid body of psychophysiological research to draw upon and conclude that heart rate can be used to index cognitive resources allocated to encoding mediated content, we must still keep in mind that any observed change in heart rate is the result of a complex combination of sympathetic and parasympathetic nervous system activity. The psychological meaning of all psychophysiological responses—including changes in heart rate —is fundamentally rooted in underlying biological processes, which, in this case, have to do with the anatomy and physiology of the human heart. There are excellent texts describing this in great detail (Brownley, Hurwitz, & Schneiderman, 2000). We recommend reading such sources because an extremely detailed description of the cardiac system is beyond the scope of this chapter. Rather, the purpose here is to describe basic characteristics of the human heart that lead to a physiological signal media researchers can use as an indicator of cognitive resources allocated to encoding. It is important to note that psycho-physiologists who examine more complex spatial and temporal characteristics of the cardiac signal must be grounded in a much more detailed knowledge of the cardiovascular system than presented here. The following paragraphs are intended to provide enough information on properties of the human heart so scholars interested in media processes and effects can understand the theoretical connection between cardiac activity and cognitive processing of media.

Basic anatomy and physiology of the cardiac system

The human heart is essentially an electromechanical system. The system consists of a pump (your heart muscle) and a group of channels (your arteries, ventricles, capillaries, and veins) through which blood necessary for cell function is distributed throughout your body and then returned to the heart. Critical to your heart's ability to supply blood to your body is its ability to reliably and consistently contract and expand in a more or less steady, rhythmic manner. Extreme variation in the steady, rhythmic nature of cardiac activity is a symptom of cardiac disease and ultimately can lead to heart failure.

The fact that the heart is designed to accomplish its work in a steady, rhythmic nature has implications for researchers who wish to use variation in cardiac activity as an indicator of cognitive processing of mediated messages. Strong variation in heart rate is typically only evoked through sudden, large changes in physical activity or other forms of extreme stress. Most experiments on cognitive processing of media messages are performed under conditions of relaxation rather than physical activity and media content rarely contains images capable of evoking the high levels of stress that lead to extreme variation in heart rate. In most experiments, the observed variation in cardiac activity due to cognitive processing of mediated messages will be small. The need to observe such small changes makes it all the more important for researchers to understand basic characteristics of the cardiac signal in order to reliably measure responses during exposure to media messages. This also means that estimates of effect size reported in experiments in which the impact of some feature of media on heart rate was analyzed will be small. It is important for all scholars to recognize that this is an instance where small effect sizes do not reduce the practical or theoretical importance of an experiment's results.

Rhythmic contraction of the heart is driven by a coordinated conduction system that leads to excitation and contraction of the **atria** and **ventricles** through electrical depolarization and repolarization of heart cells. Electrical stimulation of the heart begins with an influx of positively charged ions into the interior of the heart. This leads to **depolarization**, a state where cells on the interior of the heart muscle are positively charged relative to cells on the exterior. Depolarization of cells in the **myocardium**—striated muscles located in the walls of the heart—causes the heart to contract. **Repolarization** is the process where interior heart cells become negatively charged relative to the exterior cells. This creates a resting state for the heart muscle. A continuous cycle of depolarization and repolarization of heart cells causes the heart to beat. Thus, cardiac activity is in essence electromechanical activity in that electrical current generated in heart cells leads to the mechanical contraction and relaxation associated with a beating heart.

The cardiac signal consists of both electrical and mechanical events. Mechanical events associated with the beating heart occur simultaneously with electrical changes in the heart. In other words there is specific change in the ongoing electrical signal generated in the myocardium that occurs every time the heart contracts and relaxes. This set of repetitive electrical events, and the accompanying mechanical motion of the cardiac muscle to move blood through the veins and arteries, form what is termed the **cardiac cycle**. The cardiac cycle is initiated by depolarization (contraction) of the atria during which the ventricles are resting. This is followed by ventricular depolarization where the ventricles contract while the atria repolarize. Finally, all chambers of the heart go through a period where they remain in a state of repolarization. The phase of the cardiac cycle where heart muscle contracts is known as *systole* and the phase where heart muscle is relaxed is called *diastole*. One complete cardiac cycle is defined as a full sequence of systole and diastole in the atria and ventricles.

A majority of experiments in which cardiac activity has been used to index cognitive processing of media involves measurement of the ongoing cardiac electrical signal, although pulse rate (a mechanical event) is occasionally measured in media experiments using a photoplethysmograph (Anttonen, Surakka, & Koivuluoma, 2009; Detenber, Simons, & Bennett, 1998). The voltage generated by cardiac activity is strong enough to be reliably recorded off the surface of the skin by placing electrodes on the limbs or trunk of the body to obtain a standard **electrocardiogram** (ECG). Required equipment, electrode placement, and technical considerations involved in recording a standard ECG will be discussed shortly. Prior to that, it is important to understand the properties of the ECG as a waveform.

An ECG represents changes in voltage amplitude that occur during the cardiac cycle. Thus, it depicts cardiac activity as a voltage waveform forming what most readers will likely recognize in Figure 4.1 as a cardiac waveform. This basic waveform consists of three primary waves that together represent one complete cardiac cycle. The primary waves in the ECG are generated at the occurrence of specific electromechanical events in the heart. The P wave is generated during atrial depolarization, the QRS complex in the cardiac waveform represents electrical stimulation of the ventricles, and the T wave occurs while the ventricles are repolarized (Hurst, 1998; Stern et al., 2001). Researchers studying cognitive processing of media are typically most interested in variation in the amount of time between R spikes in the cardiac waveform generated during the QRS complex of the cardiac cycle. This specific portion of the ECG waveform is referred to as the *inter-beat interval*.

Several aspects of cardiac activity have been examined in psychophysiological research but the most common indices used to study information processing are related to variation in heart rate or heart period. Both indices are obtained by measuring the inter-beat interval (IBI). **Heart rate** is the commonly known index expressing cardiac activity at any given instant in terms of the number of beats that would occur in one minute (BPM) at that that level of activity. **Heart period** is expressed as milliseconds between R-spikes in the QRS complex of the cardiac cycle. Heart rate and heart period are reciprocals; researchers can easily convert back and forth between these two psychophysiological metrics by dividing 60,000 by either heart rate or heart period. So, for example, an IBI of 750ms equates to 80 BPM . . . 60,000/750.

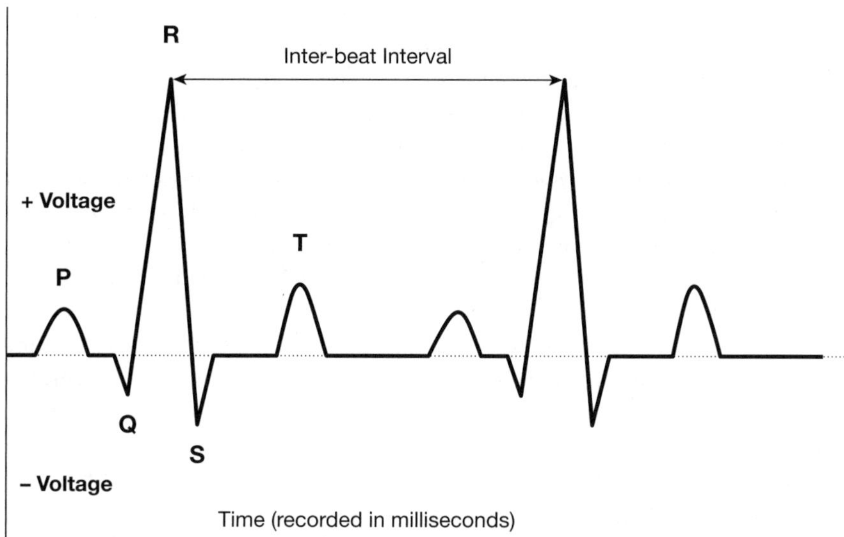

FIGURE 4.1 An idealized cardiac waveform similar to what would be recorded by ECG.

Psychophysiologists have measured heart rate and heart period to study how individuals invest mental effort in performing a wide range of cognitive tasks such as visual attention, mental imagery, mental arithmetic, and language processing (e.g., Berntson et al., 1996; Deschaumes-Molinaro, Dittmar, & Vernet-Maury, 1992; Pfurtscheller, Grabner, Brunner, & Neuper, 2007). The effect of PNS and SNS activation appears to be more linear for heart period than heart rate leading to the suggestion that heart period—milliseconds between R-spikes recorded in the ECG—may be a better metric than heart rate in using cardiac activity as a psychophysiological measure of cognitive processing (Berntson, Cacioppo, & Quigley, 1995). Nevertheless, in our own research—as well as much of the research on cognitive processing of media—heart rate is the most common metric for data analysis. It is highly possible that this was due to heart rate being more intuitive for readers and editors to understand during the resurgence of psychophysiological research in the early 1990s. Now, with an increase in acceptance and understanding of cardiac activity as a measure in general, future researchers may want to consider utilizing the benefits associated with the linearity of heart period when making analysis and reporting decisions.

The validity of heart rate or heart period as measures of cognitive processing is grounded in the biological connection between the autonomic and central branches of the human nervous system and the heart. As discussed in Chapter 2, the theoretical perspective of an embodied brain leads to the belief that mental activities are driven by physiological processes occurring throughout the autonomic and central nervous systems. Thus, mental processes—enacted by the brain in the central nervous system—can be studied by observing their influence on activity of the autonomic nervous system. The autonomic nervous system innervates every major organ in the human body including the heart. Thus, broadly speaking, cognitive processes evoked during exposure to a media message have a top-down influence through the central nervous system on activity of the autonomic nervous system and variation in this nervous system activity changes the speed at which the heart beats. Specific areas of the brain that have been identified as having a possible significant influence on autonomic nervous system activity influencing heart rate include the hypothalamus, amygdala, anterior cingulate cortex, and areas of prefrontal cortex (Berntson, Quigley, & Lozano, 2007). It is interesting to note that particularly the hypothalamus, anterior cingulate cortex, and prefrontal cortex are brain areas that have been specifically identified as playing a significant role in attention and memory (Jansma, Ramsey, de Zwart, van Gelderen, & Duyn, 2007). Cortical and sub-cortical areas of the brain influence autonomic nervous system activity through connections in the brainstem. From this point, there are separate anatomical pathways for para-sympathetic and sympathetic innervation of the heart. Parasympathetic activity flows through the **vagus nerve** to the **sinoatrial (SA) node** located in the upper part of the right atrium of the heart. Sympathetic activity flows through cervical and thoracic ganglia and nerves to the SA node. Figure 4.2 displays these neural pathways between the brain and the heart.

Understanding autonomic influences on heart rate and heart period is critical for an accurate interpretation of changes in these physiological measures recorded during experiments. In review, the autonomic nervous system consists of two independent branches—the sympathetic (SNS) and parasympathetic (PNS) nervous systems. The human heart is innervated by both. Central nervous system activity engaged while an individual cognitively processes a media message could increase or decrease either SNS or PNS activity leading to changes in how fast the heart beats. Increased SNS activity speeds up the heart while decreased activity slows it down. The opposite is true for PNS activation. Increased PNS activity slows down the heart while decreased activity speeds it up.

Early on it was believed that the SNS and PNS were exclusively reciprocally activated with increased activity in one branch leading to a decrease in activity of the other. However, thanks to the work of researchers like Berntson, Cacioppo, and Quigley (1993), we now know that activity in the SNS and PNS can also be coactive, where activity of both branches increases or decreases. The activity can also be decoupled; that is, where change in activity in one branch is accompanied by no change in activity in the other. Thus, regardless of the metric in which cardiac activity is analyzed—heart rate or heart period—media researchers need to be aware that they are using a psychophysiological measure that is under the influence of multiple patterns of autonomic nervous system activity; however, with rigorous theoretical thinking—grounded in an embodied theoretical perspective as well as an understanding of the nature of cardiac

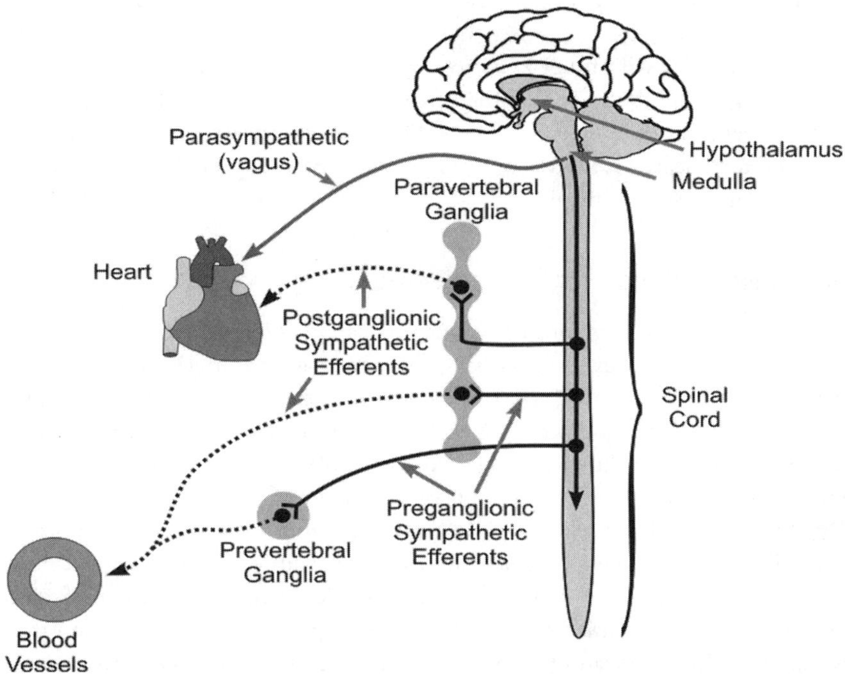

FIGURE 4.2 Neural pathways between the brain and heart through which the sympathetic and parasympathetic branches of the nervous system influence cardiac activity

Source: figure used with permission from R. Klabunde, 2010, www.cvpharmacology.com/vasodilator/ Central-acting.htm.

activity—researchers can interpret both phasic and tonic changes in heart rate or heart period as indicative of changes in cognitive resources during the processing of mediated messages. It is indeed the psychological interpretation of heart rate that has led to this measure yielding significant insights into how the mind cognitively processes mediated messages. The additional knowledge and skills required to validly use heart rate or heart period to index cognitive processing of mediated messages have to do with the operational details of obtaining a reliable ECG from experiment participants.

Recording the ECG in the media research lab

The good news for researchers wishing to set up a lab to study cognitive processing of media messages is that compared to other psychophysiological measures, the equipment necessary to obtain an ECG is relatively inexpensive, easy to set up, and easy to use. As a result you will find equipment necessary for recording ECG in almost every existing media psychophysiology lab. The clear advantage to the beginning researcher is that there is an existing network of colleagues familiar with using ECG to measure cognitive processing of media as well as a significant body of published research utilizing the measure that can be easily referenced (see Lang et al., 2009). This section covers the necessary equipment and technical procedures involved in collecting and using the ECG to study cognitive processing of media.

Equipment and technical procedures for recording the ECG

Recall that the ECG waveform represents changes in voltage amplitude associated with specific electrical events occurring in the atria and ventricles. It is important to note that the ECG is indeed a *representation* of these events. This is because the signal that is actually being measured is the voltage that travels from the heart to the surface of the skin where electrodes are placed. Obviously this signal is not going to be as strong as the electrical signal actually occurring in the heart. The voltage of the R wave in the QRS complex of the cardiac cycle—the portion of the ECG used to measure heart rate—can be as little as 2mV by the time it reaches the surface of the skin where it can be picked up by surface electrodes. This bioelectrical potential is relatively large compared to the voltages of other psychophysiological measures (e.g., the EEG waveform picked up at the surface of the scalp) but still must be significantly amplified in order to generate a recordable and interpretable ECG waveform. The technical challenge in measuring bioelectric potentials like those generated by the heart is to provide a low-impedance, electrochemically stable pathway for the signal to travel from the surface of the skin to a computer where the analog waveform can be displayed and the signal can be sampled and digitized for statistical analysis. Computers and software packages for psychophysiological data collection will be discussed in more detail in Chapter 8. Here—as well as in all discussions of specific psychophysiological measures—the focus is on specialized physiological equipment and procedures for recording the psychophysiological signal of interest.

The ECG is detected using electrodes strategically placed on the surface of the skin to accurately record the signal in a manner that gives the best representation possible of the voltages generated by electrical activity occurring throughout the cardiac cycle. A reliable ECG signal can be produced by placing surface electrodes on the limbs or the trunk of the body. Electrodes can be placed in several configurations, but each must represent a pattern that forms **Einthoven's Triangle** around the heart. Named after the Dutch cardiac physician and Nobel Laureate Willem Einthoven, the inverted triangle can be seen in each of the standard lead placements described below and displayed in Figure 4.3. The ECG is recorded using a three-lead bipolar placement where two recording electrodes are referenced to a third ground electrode. The standard patterns of electrode placement for recording the ECG are as follows:

Lead I: recording electrodes are placed approximately 2 inches below the elbow bend on the left and right arms with a ground reference electrode placed on the left wrist. Polarity is set so that when the electrode placed on the left arm is positively charged relative to the electrode on the right arm there is a positive deflection in the P and R waves in the ECG (refer to Figure 4.1).

Lead II: one recording electrode is placed on the right arm, 2 inches below the elbow bend, and the other is placed just above the left ankle with a ground reference electrode placed on the left wrist. Polarity is set so that a similar ECG pattern as mentioned for the Lead I placement is observed when the electrode placed on the left ankle is positively charged relative to the electrode on the right arm.

Lead III: recording electrodes are placed on the left arm, 2 inches below the elbow bend and just above the left ankle with a ground reference electrode placed on the right wrist. Polarity is set in a manner that is similar to the Lead II placement in that the described ECG pattern should occur when the electrode on the left ankle is positively charged relative to the electrode on the left arm.

Lead I and Lead II placements are recognized as adequate for the purposes of most psychophysiological research. The Lead II placement may result in an R wave that reliably approaches 2mV—a greater voltage than likely obtained with a Lead I placement—which could confer some advantage to this particular electrode placement pattern (Andreassi, 2007). In most of our own research, however, we have successfully utilized a Lead I placement to prevent the increased invasiveness possibly associated with putting electrodes on the subject's leg.

One source of noise that has implications for ECG electrode placement is movement artifact. The electrical activity generated by the movement of muscles located around areas where electrodes are placed can introduce noise into the ECG signal. The easiest way to eliminate this source of noise is to clearly instruct participants to relax and sit as still as possible during exposure to experimental stimuli. This obviously is not always possible, particularly if the experiment involves studying more interactive forms of media consumption such as surfing the web or playing games. One alternative electrode placement that has been recommended for contexts in which movement artifact may be problematic involves placing electrodes along the sternum of the chest (Andreassi, 2007). In the context of media research, however, invasiveness becomes an issue once again. In our own work we have obtained decent results from addressing movement artifact by moving recording electrodes to the left and right sides of the collarbone just below the trapezoid muscles. It is also possible that a Lead III placement utilizing the left arm and left ankle as the recording sites could address some movement artifact problems in studying interactive media such as extensive use of a computer mouse which is typically done using the right hand and arm.

Lead I placement:
Left forearm (+),
Right forearm (-),
Left wrist (ground
reference)

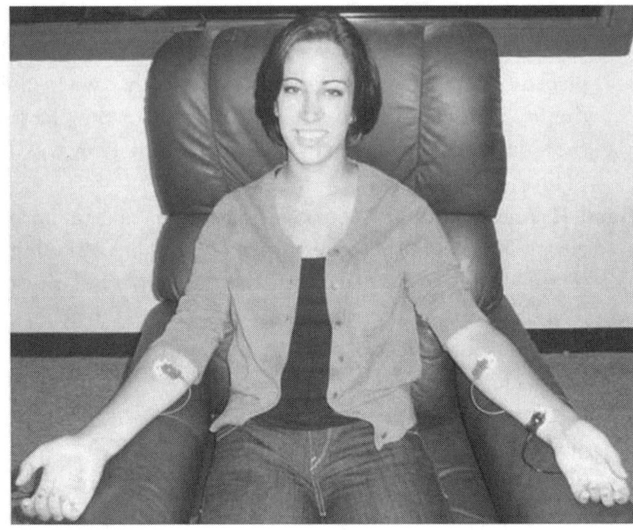

Lead II placement: Left ankle (+),
Right forearm (-), Left wrist
(ground reference)

Lead III placement: Left ankle (+),
Left forearm (-), Right forearm
(ground reference)

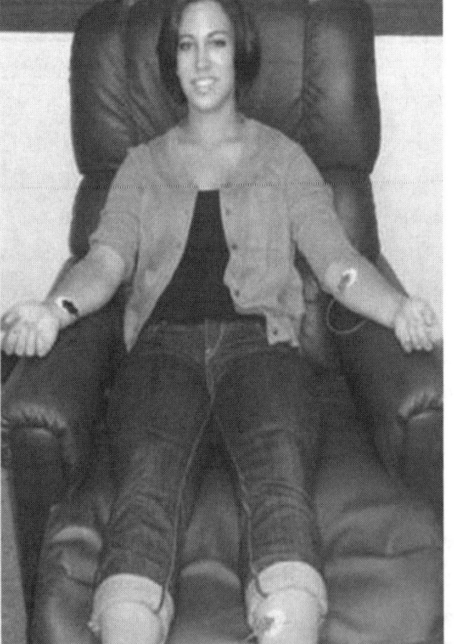

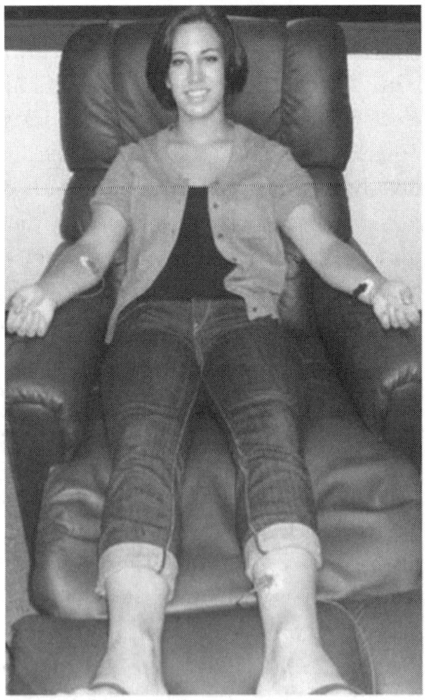

FIGURE 4.3 Standard ECG lead placements. Note how each placement forms an inverted triangle (Einthoven's Triangle).

Regardless of the electrode placement used to record the ECG, a low impedance connection must be made between the recording surface of electrodes and the surface of the skin. In order to minimize electrical impedance, electrodes should be placed on skin surfaces relatively free of hair and that have been gently abraded to remove material such as dead skin cells, dirt, and oil. The voltage recorded in an ECG is large enough that skin prep is significantly less critical for measuring heart rate than other psychophysiological measures. Simply wiping down participants' skin surface with an ordinary paper towel dampened with water or rubbing alcohol should be adequate. Many psychophysiological supply vendors sell alcohol skin prep pads that work extremely well for this purpose. The primary advantage of using specialized skin prep pads is that these pads are convenient to use if an experiment involves the measurement of other psychophysiological signals that require more thorough skin preparation where such pads are almost a must—such as facial EMG. It is extremely important to remember that alcohol-based skin prep pads or paper towels dampened with rubbing alcohol should never be used in prepping skin for the collection of skin conductance—a point we will bring up again in Chapter 5.

The standard electrode for recording an ECG is an 8mm, Ag/AgCl floating electrode. Silver-silver chloride electrodes are the best electrodes because they have been shown to have a low bias potential and have a lower likelihood of becoming polarized to each other, ultimately resulting in a more noise-free signal (Stern et al., 2001). Floating electrodes have an epoxy housing that forms a cup around the recording surface. This means that the most critical component of electrodes, the recording surface, does not make direct contact with the skin; rather, a highly conductive electrode gel is placed in the cup to establish a connection with the skin. Researchers need to make sure that they minimize the presence of air bubbles in the cup of the electrode when filling electrodes with gel due to the resulting increase in impedance and lack of validity resulting from the concept of bipolar measurement, where the signal at one electrode (the one with bubbly gel, say) is compared to the signal at another (bubble-free). Follow the procedures described in Chapter 3 for filling electrodes. Keep in mind that overfilling electrodes can result in them slipping off during a recording session due to electrode gel seeping under the adhesive collars attached to the skin. Again, as mentioned in Chapter 3, some researchers find disposable, pre-gelled electrodes to be preferable. However, if you work in a lab that runs a high number of subjects, this can result in a substantial expense over reusable electrodes. (But then again, a high volume of subjects will mean that if you go the reusable route you'll be filling *a lot* of electrode cups with gel.) You should also recall from Chapter 3 that if you are using pre-gelled electrodes, placing a small amount of fresh electrolyte gel on the pre-gelled surface of the electrode can result in better ECG signal quality.

Electrodes are placed on the prepped skin surfaces in one of the appropriate lead configurations and connected to electrode leads that carry the signal to a bioamplifier. Electrode leads will have three connections labeled positive, negative, and ground. It is important to pay attention to the polarity of these connections when recording an ECG because as mentioned above in our discussion of electrode placement, correctly connecting the positive electrode—usually the one on the left arm or left ankle—yields a correct ECG waveform consisting of a positive deflection of the P and R waves.

A bioamplifier is used to amplify and filter the ECG voltages. The highest voltage in the ECG signal occurs at the generation of the R wave and it is not uncommon for this signal to need to be amplified using a gain setting of 5 or 10K. The objective in amplifying the ECG signal is to obtain a large, clearly distinguishable R wave that can be reliably detected in order to record the inter-beat interval—milliseconds between R waves. Amplifying the ECG signal, however, also amplifies any noise in the signal. Sources of noise include movement artifact, which was already mentioned, as well as other sources of stray voltage that can be present in a lab environment. A common source of electrical noise that can appear in any psychophysiological measure is 60 Hz (U.S.) or 50 Hz (Europe and Australia) interference generated by electrical equipment as well as fluorescent and halogen light bulbs. Details of dealing with sources of ambient electrical noise in the media research lab environment will be discussed in Chapter 8. Here it is just important to note that these frequencies should be filtered out of the ECG signal. Some bioamplifiers will come equipped with **notch filters** that selectively filter out electrical signal in the 50 and 60 Hz range. In recording the ECG it is more useful to filter the signal by using a low pass filter setting on the bioamplifier. Remember that low pass filters attenuate electrical signal occurring above the frequency that is set. The highest frequency that needs to be recorded from the QRS complex in the cardiac cycle in order to reliably record a standard ECG is about 12 Hz; therefore, setting a low pass filter on the bioamplifier in the range of 30–35 Hz minimizes electrical noise in the signal and serves to reduce artifacts due to muscle movements (Stern et al., 2001). The high pass filter on the bioamplifier—a filter that attenuates electrical signal occurring below the frequency that is set—should be set on the lowest frequency possible.

The electrical signal recorded by the bioamplifier generates the analog ECG waveform that can be displayed on a computer monitor. Obtaining a measure of heart rate or heart period from this analog signal requires digitizing the signal and detecting the R wave voltage in order to record the inter-beat interval. This is accomplished through a specialized electrical circuit known as a **Schmitt trigger** which produces a pulse output signal whenever a preset voltage is exceeded. This pulse then enters the physiology data collection computer as a digital input through the AD/DA board. The trigger voltage is set so that it is likely to only be tripped by the voltage of the R wave in the ECG; then a computer clock times the milliseconds between successive output signals of the Schmitt trigger. So, when recording cardiac activity in this manner the ECG waveform itself is actually not stored but rather only the IBI in milliseconds. In place of a Schmitt trigger, some equipment vendors sell what is known as a dual comparator/window discriminator which allows both a low threshold and high threshold voltage to be set to define a voltage range that will result in an output signal being generated.

It should be mentioned that some systems do not utilize a Schmitt trigger or dual comparator at all during data collection. Instead, these systems record the entire ECG waveform by sampling it as an analog signal. Identification of the QRS complex, and the milliseconds between the R waves, is then done offline using a peak-detection algorithm. There are few downsides to this approach, aside from vastly increasing the size of data files associated with each subject.

A recording problem that has been noted with the use of a Schmitt trigger is that the preset voltage may not always occur at the same point in the R wave, which can introduce measurement error in the range of several milliseconds (Jennings et al., 1981). It is imperative that researchers know how the particular equipment they are using to measure heart period generates digital output with the occurrence of the preset voltage. It is recommended that the preset voltage at which output will be triggered corresponds as closely as possible to the peak voltage of R waves in the ECG signal. On a dual comparator/window discriminator this will typically mean setting the low threshold voltage to this peak level making sure the high threshold voltage is set above this point. The first step, therefore, in obtaining a reliable measure of cardiac activity is to exercise the care and attention to detail necessary for obtaining an ECG waveform that is as free of noise as possible. Researchers should examine the ECG waveform and address any recording problems possibly due to electrode placement, amplification, and filtering prior to attempting to adjust the preset voltage for a Schmitt trigger. This procedure improves the likelihood of setting the threshold voltage on a Schmitt trigger at a level that reliably generates output signals at the occurrence of successive R waves and is less susceptible to either missing the occurrence of an R wave or falsely triggering. Heart period recorded by a Schmitt trigger can be converted automatically into heart rate in BPM by sending the output to a cardiotachometer. Both metrics—heart period and heart rate—can of course be submitted to statistical analysis.

Analysis of cardiac activity data

No matter how carefully researchers set a Schmitt trigger to detect R waves to record heart period, there will be some amount of error resulting in recording artificially long or short IBIs. This is a result of either the false positive detection of R waves or missed R waves in the ECG signal. So, for example, if the threshold of a Schmitt trigger is set such that 5,346 milliseconds passes between R waves . . . something is wrong. Either more than five seconds has passed since your research participant's heart has beat or you have missed several R waves. Conversely, if your participant readjusts their sitting position in their chair and moves the electrode leads abruptly then you may have movement artifact that causes the threshold of the Schmitt trigger to be crossed in rapid succession. This may result in a string of "IBIs" in the very brief millisecond range (e.g., 35, 334, 12, 4, 55, 34, 26, etc.). Here it is obvious that your subject's heart did not beat seven times in 500 milliseconds! Thus, the first step in analyzing cardiac activity is cleaning the data by detecting invalid inter-beat intervals and replacing them with a more likely value. Common ways of dealing with invalid inter-beat intervals involve summing the string of unlikely data and dividing the resulting number of milliseconds by a value that results in equal and more likely IBI values. Here it is best to be conservative and rigorous in your decision-making. The best indication of what the IBI values should be during the time segments in question are the IBIs surrounding it. Pay attention to preceding and subsequent IBIs that you are confident are valid, looking for trends of increase or decrease, when determining your replacement estimated values. We have found that it is best to clean heart period data blind to condition and be willing to recode invalid segments as missing data if logical and conservative estimates cannot be determined as replacements of obviously invalid IBIs.

Editing IBIs can easily be done using specialized computer programs for cleaning and editing inter-beat interval data; however, researchers must be aware of the technical details of exactly how these computer software packages clean the data. The best software packages for this purpose will provide a substantial amount of user control that can include setting values in milliseconds to define artificial inter-beat intervals. An acceptable range of valid IBIs would be between 600 and 1,200 ms, therefore you should instruct your cleaning algorithm to identify anything outside of this range. If heart rate directly recorded by a cardiotachometer is going to be analyzed, it is critical to identify outliers in the sampled data that need to be replaced. This might be done using mean replacement or alternatively —since the best predictor of heart rate at time t is heart rate at time t-1—bad data could be replaced with the most recent good value. It is critical to rigorously check the output of any data cleaning and make note of the proportion of inter-beat intervals in a data segment that had to be cleaned or designated as missing data. Data segments in which a significant portion of the collected data had to be cleaned or designated missing should be discarded.

After cleaning the data, researchers must decide whether to conduct a **heart time analysis** or a real time analysis. Analyzing data in heart time involves submitting the IBI values to statistical analysis. Heart period is aperiodic, meaning that the number of beats will vary across exposure to each stimulus message in an experiment as well as between participants. This will be true even if every stimulus in an experiment results in recording periods of equal length. Thus, statistical analysis in heart time is typically performed on a predetermined, theoretically meaningful number of beats so that each IBI is a data point submitted to analysis. The most obvious application for conducting data analysis in heart time rather than real time is in analyzing psychologically meaningful phasic responses such as the orienting response, analysis of which is discussed in more detail below.

A real time analysis of cardiac activity can be conducted on either heart period or heart rate data. This analysis involves submitting data that has been averaged over a chosen unit of time. The choice of the unit of time over which data will be averaged is up to the researcher. The decision of the unit of time, however, should be justified according to the need to capture meaningful variation in cognitive resource allocation given the nature of media being studied. For instance, highly emotional advertisements that often also include a lot of production features such as cuts and edits can often contain very sudden content changes which likely have a meaningful impact on the allocation of cognitive resources to message encoding. In this case, it would be necessary to average data submitted for a real time analysis over shorter time increments, say one second, to capture the expected frequent fluctuations in cognitive response. Cardiac activity averaged across each media stimulus in an experiment can be useful as a global indicator of cognitive resources allocated to processing; however, recall that one of the primary advantages of psychophysiological measures is the ability to observe cognitive and emotional processing across time—capturing momentary fluctuations in responses indicative of variation in cognitive resource allocation occurring within the stimulus messages. If the data analysis is going to be performed on heart period, the inter-beat intervals are simply averaged and then submitted for statistical analysis. If the metric for data analysis is heart rate, the sampled inter-beat intervals will be averaged and then converted into heart rate BPM per unit of time (e.g., BPM per second). Recall that heart period is aperiodic data so in averaging the data across time it is critical to use a weighted average procedure.

Depending upon the hypothesis or research question being pursued, cardiac data can be analyzed at a tonic or phasic level. Analyzing data for tonic activity focuses on looking at longer-term variation in cardiac activity across exposure to media stimuli. Analysis of phasic activity, on the other hand, focuses on examining momentary, temporary changes in cardiac activity evoked by specific events such as the onset of a production or content feature believed to be psychologically meaningful. The most common statistical analysis for both phasic and tonic analyses of cardiac activity collected in experiments on cognitive processing of media has been repeated measures ANOVA.

There are two properties of cardiac activity that have significant implications for statistical analysis. First, heart rate BPM or heart period values collected during a recording session are not uncorrelated which violates the **sphericity assumption** for repeated measures ANOVA. This makes it necessary to adjust the degrees of freedom for analysis by using the Greenhouse-Geisser or Huynh-Feldt corrections to determine statistical significance. Second, heart rate and heart period are substantially affected by the **law of initial values (LIV)** meaning that any change in either of these metrics of cardiac activity resulting from exposure to stimulus messages will be substantially impacted by levels of cardiac activity occurring prior to exposure (Lacey & Lacey, 1962). Although the practical impact of the LIV is complicated and how to best deal with it controversial (Geenen & Van de Vijver, 1993; Stern et al., 2001), a common attempt is to analyze psychophysiological data using **change scores**. This means that analysis of cardiac activity is most appropriately performed on change from baseline activity scores. Thus, a measure of baseline activity must be collected during experiments. Because tonic activity changes over the course of an experimental setting, it is best to measure baseline activity for a period prior to the onset of each stimulus message rather than simply at the beginning of the lab visit. This has the advantage of controlling for carryover effects on cardiac activity from previous messages. There should also be enough time for participants to relax between the end of a stimulus message or the completion of any self-report measures collected between stimulus messages and the recording of baseline activity prior to the next stimulus message—allowing heart rate to return to a more truly resting baseline level. This resting baseline period, however, should not be so long that participants become restless. A resting period of around 20 seconds should be adequate with baseline activity recorded in the five seconds prior to the onset of stimulus messages. Change scores can then be calculated by either averaging the five seconds of baseline activity or using the last second prior to message onset as a baseline measure. Baseline activity is then subtracted from each averaged data point collected during exposure to stimulus messages.

A special case of phasic data analysis worthy of discussion here involves experiments in which researchers explore whether or not specific features of media evoke orienting responses. The orienting response has been termed the "what is it" response and is psychologically meaningful because it reflects a phasic, automatic increase in cognitive resources allocated to encoding stimuli (Lynn, 1966). The identification of features of media that evoke orienting responses has been a tremendously fruitful line of media psychology research shedding insight on some of the most psychologically meaningful features of media that are capable of automatically capturing attention (Diao & Sundar, 2004; Lang, 1990; Lang et al., 2002; Potter, 2000; Potter et al., 2008).

An orienting response analysis can be conducted in either heart time or real time. If the analysis is conducted in heart time the beat occurring just prior to onset of the feature believed to cause the evoked response is used as the baseline measure and change from this beat is calculated for the next 10 beats after onset of the feature. Orienting analyses of features of media that have been conducted in real time use either heart rate or heart period in the second prior to onset of the feature being tested as baseline and calculate change scores from this point over the next six to 10 seconds of data collection. These change score values, graphed over time, constitute what is known as the **cardiac response curve** (CRC). The first step in performing the analysis is to visually inspect the CRCs to see if they follow one of two operationally-defining patterns. As noted by Lang

(1990)—one of the first published studies on orienting to structural features of media—cardiac activity reflecting an orienting response follows either a monophasic or a biphasic pattern. The monophasic pattern resembles a U-shaped pattern for heart rate and an inverted-U pattern for heart period. The biphasic pattern will resemble a sideways S, initially decreasing if the unit of analysis is heart rate and increasing if heart period. If visual inspection of the CRC graphs reveals either of these patterns the researcher proceeds to statistical analysis of the data. This is done through a trend analysis—a special case of ANOVA—looking for either a significant cubic or quadratic trend in the data. If this pattern of cardiac response is observed and statistically significant the researcher concludes that the feature of media being studied has evoked orienting responses in individuals.

Examples of research using heart rate to study cognitive processing of media

Heart rate is one of the earliest and most extensively used psychophysiological indicators of how individuals cognitively process media. The use of this measure has certainly continued in exciting ways in the twenty-first century. Much of the more recent research has examined how features of information presented on the Internet impact cognitive processing. This area of research is psychologically interesting from a media processing perspective because it allows an examination of how user control over the presentation of information impacts cognitive processing. For example, Lang and colleagues studied how user control over the presentation of static and animated Internet banner advertisements impacts orienting responses to these ads (Lang et al., 2002). They found that only animated banner ads evoked orienting responses as evidenced by the phasic cardiac response curves. Further, user control of the ad's onset made no difference in this pattern of results. Diao and Sundar (2004) similarly found that pop-up window ads reliably evoke the cardiac OR.

Heart rate continues to illuminate the black box of cognitive processing of more traditional forms of media as well. Potter (2009) used tonic analysis of heart rate change scores to investigate the impact of clutter in radio commercial breaks on listeners. In a within-subjects experiment listeners were exposed to two simulated radio broadcasts, each containing a five-minute advertising block. In a counter-balanced design, one of the stations played five, 60-second commercials during the block while the other played 10, 30-second commercials. Results showed deceleration in heart rate, suggesting more attention being paid during the commercial breaks containing fewer overall units. In fact, there was an increase of cardiac activity above baseline for the ad breaks containing the 10 shorter ads which could be interpreted as cognitive disengagement.

Our discussion of heart rate and very cursory review of recent media processes and effects research utilizing the measure has hopefully provided insight into how it can be used to provide insight into cognitive processing of mediated messages.

As the media environment continues to evolve with a wider range of content and structural features that could have significant implications for cognitive processing of media delivered over new technological platforms, heart rate will remain an exciting, reliable, and fairly easy to use, psychophysiological measure of cognitive processing. Let's now turn to a discussion of a second specific psychophysiological measure of cognitive processing, the electroencephalogram (EEG).

EEG: a measure of cortical activity underlying cognitive processing of media

The electroencephalogram (EEG) is unique among all the specific psycho-physiological measures discussed in this book. EEG is a direct measure of central nervous system activity evoked by information processing in the brain. The other measures—heart rate, skin conductance, and facial EMG—measure patterns of *peripheral* nervous system activity that researchers then use to draw inferences about cognitive and emotional processes embodied in CNS activity. This makes EEG an exciting psychophysiological measure with tremendous potential to contribute to the development of theoretical models of media processing. The mystique and potential for generating scientific knowledge from being able to, in essence, "read the mind" has intrigued scholars as well as society at large since the EEG was first recorded in humans by Berger in 1929 (Stern et al., 2001).

The EEG involves measuring extremely small biopotentials, in the range of 10^{-6}V, recorded from the surface of the scalp. These signals are generated by neural activity in underlying cortical areas of the brain. Scholars working in cognitive neuroscience have significantly increased knowledge of the functional neuro-anatomy of the major lobes of the brain to a level that allows the development of hypotheses concerning patterns of activation during cognitive processing of sensory stimuli (Sauseng & Klimesch, 2008). The brain is divided anatomically into four regions whose activity can be studied utilizing EEG: the frontal, parietal, temporal, and occipital lobes (see Figure 4.4). The entire human brain is a large-scale mass of interconnected neurons that appear to be arranged in millions of sub-networks all connected by inhibitory and excitatory processes (Varela, Lachaux, Rodriguez, & Martinerie, 2001). It is the summed electrical activity generated across networks of neurons arranged in what has been termed neuronal assemblies that is recorded by the EEG.

The following is a very simplistic explanation of the physiological activity that gives rise to the biopotentials recorded with EEG. So, here comes the second neuroanatomy lesson of the book. This one will only be slightly more intense than our discussion of neurons in Chapter 2. Biopotentials, including those in the brain, are generated at the occurrence of action potentials within neurons. Neurons consist of a cell body, axon, and dendrites. The action potential generated in the cell body

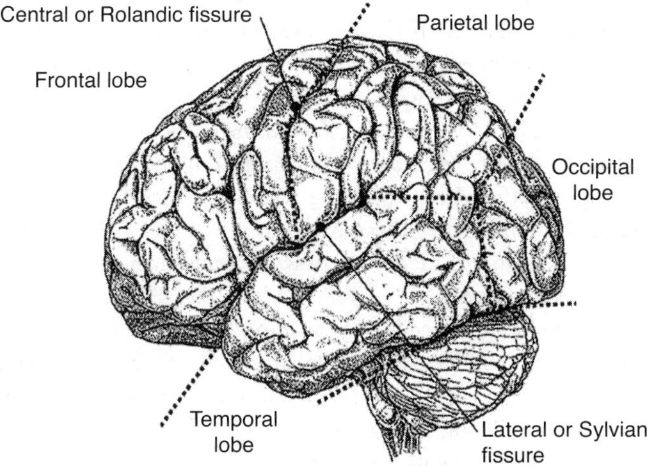

FIGURE 4.4 The major anatomical regions of the brain.

Source: Beaumont, 2008. Reprinted by permission of Guilford Press.

of the neuron travels down the axon where it synapses with the dendrite of an interconnected neuron. A postsynaptic potential then occurs in the dendrite and cell body of the interconnected neuron. This process occurs in all the millions of neurons interconnected into neuronal assemblies in the brain. Action potentials occurring in neuronal assemblies do not happen in a manner that allows the electrical activity of the network to sum up to a level that can be observed. Action potentials occurring in networks of neurons will actually often occur in a manner that cancels out their electrical potentials. Thus, EEG actually records the postsynaptic potentials that are longer lasting—in the range of milliseconds rather than microseconds as is the case for action potentials—and occur instantaneously, allowing the electrical potentials to be summed (Harmon-Jones & Peterson, 2009).

The ability to directly measure cortical activity in specific areas of the brain has led to extensive use of EEG in the psychological sciences to study social phenomena such as attitude formation, emotional disposition, motivational processes, stereotyping, and self-regulation (Bartholow & Amodio, 2009; Harmon-Jones & Peterson, 2009). Directly measuring brain activity when an individual is exposed to mediated messages also obviously has tremendous potential for generating exciting media psychology research. As mentioned in Chapter 1, the first application of *psycho*physiological measures to studying how the human brain processes media utilized EEG to study how different features of television advertisements impact attention and memory (Krugman, 1971; Reeves et al., 1985; Rothschild, Hyun, Reeves, Thorson, & Goldstein, 1988).

Subsequent media research utilizing EEG has been sparse, at least in the academic literature. Financial barriers as well as a lack of the required technical expertise may have limited the presence of EEG in most university media research labs. However, there have been some limited efforts recently to return to EEG measurement to gain insight into cognitive processing of mediated messages. It is also interesting to note that several corporate media research companies appear to have turned to EEG as a method for evaluating advertising executions for clients. For the most part, however, the potential for EEG measurement to contribute insight for rigorous communication theory building remains unfulfilled; however, the recent increase in published peer-reviewed research in which EEG has been used to study cognitive processing of mediated messages may suggest that these issues are beginning to be addressed.

In this section of the chapter the psychological meaning of different aspects of the EEG signal is discussed, as well as basic technical aspects of recording EEG. Experiments in which EEG is measured can range from very simple studies of brain hemispheric asymmetry utilizing only a few channels of data all the way to very extensive recordings from all of the major cortical areas involving high-density recordings of 256 channels. Thus, a highly detailed technical discussion of measuring EEG is beyond the scope of this book. The purpose is rather to give a general description of EEG measurement, one adequate for fundamental understanding of the measure and its potential. Readers who wish to pursue EEG recording in a media research laboratory are encouraged to consult more detailed sources on this measure (e.g., Andreassi, 2007; Bartholow & Amodio, 2009; Harmon-Jones & Peterson, 2009; Pizzagalli, 2007).

Psychological meaning of EEG

Embodied cognition theoretical perspectives, including LC4MP, propose that the phenomenon of attending to and remembering information is at its most basic level a concrete, physical process that can be observed in the workings of the human brain. Media psychology researchers, therefore, can record brain activity from all of the major cortical areas of the brain using EEG. The validity of EEG as a tool for studying how individuals cognitively process mediated messages, however, rests on the work done by psychophysiologists who operate under the theoretical assumption that specific patterns of electrical activity recorded from cortical areas reflect the physical activity of the brain that underlies unique cognitive processes evoked in processing environmental stimuli. Thus, deriving psychological meaning from EEG activity has involved psychophysiologists adamantly working to identify the unique patterns of electrical activity generated in the cortex that correlate with distinct cognitive processes.

The electrical potential recorded by EEG at the scalp appears as a sine wave with positive and negative deflections varying in frequency and amplitude. The temporal, spatial, and frequency domains of the EEG signal have been identified to have significant psychological meaning. Analysis of the temporal spatial characteristics of the EEG signal involves analysis of evoked response potentials

(ERP). This kind of research utilizes specific EEG waveforms occurring in the range of milliseconds after the onset of a stimulus that have been identified with meaningful psychological processes—e.g., fast-occurring attentional and evaluative processes (see Bartholow & Amodio, 2009 for a review of ERP methodology). For example, ERP analysis has often been conducted using basic and simple psychological stimuli such as the presence of an auditory tone appearing in the right side of a pair of headphones when the subject was told to listen for tones that would occur in the left. One hundred milliseconds after the "oddball" tone occurs in the unattended ear a significant increase in negative voltage (compared to a neutral site) is recorded at the top-center of the skull. This N1 (for "negativity at 100ms") is known as an auditory-ERP (Fabiani, Gratton, & Federmeier, 2007).

While the ERP is a very popular measure in basic psychophysiology, there are significant methodological challenges to applying ERP research protocols in experiments involving media use. Primarily, unlike most ERP experiments, media processing experiments involve exposure to complex stimuli that often change on a second-by-second basis over relatively longer periods of time. An additional challenge has to do with the fact that most of the evoked response potentials can only be reliably observed by averaging across hundreds of trials in an experiment. Sitting through the presentation of hundreds of single tones in headphones may take some time, but not nearly as long as sitting through hundreds of points of interest in real-time media messages. Nevertheless, a recent study integrated ERP methodology into the media psychology laboratory. Treleaven-Hassard et al. (2010) used an event-related potential known as the P300 to measure cognitive processing and working memory activation. The P300 is a reliably elicited increase in positive voltage occurring approximately 300ms following the stimulus onset. Quicker onsets of the P300 are indicative of "faster speed of information processing" (Treleaven-Hassard et al., 2010, p. 779).

In this experiment subjects were first presented with a block of 10 brand logos appearing on screen for one second each with one second of black between them. Of those 10 logos, four represented brands sponsoring interactive advertisements in a television program the subjects watched later in the experimental session. Four other logos represented brands sponsoring traditional ads in the program, and two were control logos. This block of 10 logos was presented 22 times while EEG data were collected.

After these pretest ERP measures were taken, subjects watched a television show that included 12 commercials. Eight were filler ads, and four were the target interactive ads. Of the four target ads, two were "impulse" ads which appeared at the top of the screen and could be interacted with while the television programming content continued to play on most of the screen beneath. The two other interactive ads were "Dedicated Advertiser Location (DAL)" ads which appeared originally as banners at the top of the screen but when interacted with (via a remote control device) would take viewers away from the television programming content to an entirely separate series of client-sponsored video screens.

After the television program, subjects once again completed the logo presentation task while EEG data were collected. Results show that the logos for brands sponsoring the DAL ads, which the authors argue provided a longer and more intrusive interactive experience than the impulse ads, elicited shorter post-interaction P300 latencies than pre-interaction while the impulse and control ad logos showed no significant difference between pre- and post-interaction measures.

Although Treleaven-Hassard et al. (2010) provide promise for how future researchers could include ERP in their work in the media laboratory, the difficulty in designing such studies is perhaps why most studies in which EEG has been used to study cognitive processing of mediated messages involve analysis of the brain biopotentials in the frequency domain. The EEG waveform has been separated into four distinct bands of frequency that have been associated with psychologically meaningful brain activity. As described by Stern et al. (2001) these frequency bandwidths are as follows:

- Alpha activity consists of relatively large amplitude, rhythmic waves in a frequency range of about 8–12 Hz and is generally associated with fairly deep relaxation;
- Beta activity consists of relatively lower amplitude waveforms that occur in a frequency bandwith of about 18–30 Hz and has been generally associated with alertness;
- Theta band activity, occurring in a frequency range of 5–7 Hz; and
- Delta, occurring in a range of 0.5–4 Hz. Delta activity is associated with sleep in healthy humans and therefore obviously has limited direct application to research on media message processing.

Alpha and Beta activity are the bands of the EEG waveform that have most commonly been observed in studies of how the mind processes media. Researchers conducting the earliest experiments in which EEG was used to study attention and memory focused on Alpha and Beta activity recorded in both hemispheres of the brain. An attenuation of Alpha activity, known as alpha blocking, and an increase in Beta activity came to be recognized as a response pattern in EEG activity that reflects an increase in effortful attention being paid to encoding information as part of a working memory representation of an environmental stimulus (Gevins et al., 1979). The goal of most of these experiments was to identify EEG activity in these bandwidths reflective of levels of attention that lead to successful learning and memory of presented stimuli.

Recording the EEG signal

The EEG signal is recorded through very careful and standardized placement of electrodes across the scalp in a pattern that reflects the region of the brain from which a researcher wishes to measure cortical activity. As previously mentioned, very simple EEG recordings can be made using just a couple of channels of data collection with electrodes placed over very broad regions of the brain (e.g., left and right frontal regions or left and right parietal regions) or very high density recordings can consist of up to 256 channels with electrodes placed within a few centimeters of each other across all cortical regions. The significant methodological strength of EEG recording over other brain imaging techniques has always been the ability to record brain activity in real time with a high degree of temporal precision while a weakness has been imprecise spatial resolution. High density recording of the EEG signal using significantly more channels of data collection compared to the earliest EEG research has significantly improved the ability to use EEG to identify more localized patterns of cortical activity (Pizzagalli, 2007). The tissue between the neo-cortex and the scalp acts as a high volume conductor—allowing for EEG biopotentials to be detected at the scalp. However, the skull distorts the electrical signal prior to its arrival at recording electrodes. Thus, even with high density recording it is best to assume that the EEG records activity from more general brain regions rather than highly specific cortical structures in the brain.

The most common form of EEG recording performed in contemporary research involves recording cortical activity from 32, 64, 128, or 256 Ag/AgCl electrodes mounted in a stretch Lycra electrode cap that is carefully positioned over the participant's head (Harmon-Jones & Peterson, 2009). The electrodes are positioned based on what has been termed the **international 10–20 system** (Jasper, 1958). A detailed description of this system of placing EEG electrodes is given in Andreassi (2007). Simply put, the system outlines standardized distances for electrodes to be placed from major anatomical landmarks—the nasion (an indent at the top of the bridge of the nose), the inion (a bump on the back of the head just above the neck), and indents located in front of the left and right ears, just above the cheekbone. The system allows for much more precise location of electrodes across individuals participating in an experiment as well as the standardization of electrode placement across laboratories where EEG is measured. The original 10–20 system has recently been modified to account for the development of high density EEG recording (Pizzagalli, 2007).

The EEG signal—in order to be detected from the surface of the scalp—must be amplified almost a million times because the original signal is only a few microvolts (Stern et al., 2001). This means that particular care must be taken to eliminate noise from the EEG signal. The EEG signal can only be reliably recorded when the electrical impedance between the skin and all attached electrodes is less than 5 kΩ (Pivik et al., 1993). Obtaining this low level of impedance requires fairly significant skin preparation prior to the placement of electrodes. The surface of the skin on the scalp where EEG electrodes are to be placed needs to be abraded and often, in practice, needs to be gently scraped with a blunt needle. Some psychophysiological supply vendors also sell skin prep gel specifically designed for EEG recording. The electrodes are also filled with highly conductive electrode gel. Harmon-Jones and Peterson (2009) provide a detailed description of the procedure for placing electrode caps on participants. In brief summary, this procedure involves using a metric tape to measure and mark with a wax pencil precise locations associated with the nasion and inion that can be used to align the placement of the electrode cap. It is also important to measure the size of the subject's head in order to determine the appropriate sized cap to use.

Appropriate skin preparation and careful placement of electrode caps improves the reliability of the EEG signal, however, there are several other sources of noise in the EEG signal that also must be dealt with. The frequency band of the EEG signal that is typically of most interest in studies of cognitive processing of mediated messages (0.5–40 Hz) overlaps with the frequency of signals associated with cardiac activity and eye movements. Controlling for these sources of physiological noise is recommended and is done by simultaneously recording ECG along with EEG and placing electrodes around the eye to record horizontal and vertical eye movements as well as eye blinks (Pizzagalli, 2007). Data analysis software that is customized for EEG applications is then often used to recognize and remove movement artifacts in the EEG signal that correlate with ECG and eye movements.

The biopotentials recorded by the electrodes placed on the scalp are passed to a bioamplifier that amplifies and filters the signal. EEG bioamplifiers should come with the ability to bandpass filter the signals so that only signals outside the frequency range associated with meaningful cortical activity are attenuated. Bioamplifiers might also come equipped with 50 or 60 Hz notch filters in order to reduce the likelihood of ambient electrical signal contaminating EEG measurement. The highest frequency of interest in most applications of EEG to study cognitive processing of media is 40 Hz; therefore the Nyquist function specifies that a sampling rate of 80 Hz should be adequate to reproduce the EEG waveform with a high degree of reliability. However, as mentioned in Chapter 2, published recommendations also suggest sampling as rapidly as 250 Hz to ensure accuracy (Pizzagalli, 2007). Keep in mind, however, that a higher sampling rate, multiplied by numerous channels if recording high-density EEG arrays, will result in a high demand for computer storage space. EEG recording with more than a handful of scalp locations in the media psychology lab will likely require specialized EEG systems.

Examples of research using EEG to study cognitive processing of media

The fact that EEG is a direct central nervous system psychophysiological indicator of cognitive processing makes this measure truly exciting to media psychology researchers wanting to study processing of mediated messages. We believe that EEG is currently an example of a psychophysiological measure that is on the brink of providing breakthrough scientific insight into the dynamic interaction between the human brain and media content. This measure, as mentioned earlier, is not frequently seen in a majority of media research labs housed at universities. There are, despite this fact, several recent examples of published research demonstrating the utility of EEG as a measure of cognitive processing of media.

Simons et al. (2003) conducted a spectral analysis of Alpha-wave power recorded in the EEG signal while participants viewed still and moving images in brief clips that varied in emotional content. They were specifically interested in the degree to which subjective reports of emotional arousal and image motion would impact Alpha activity—recall that a reduction in Alpha activity is believed to indicate higher levels of attentive encoding of a stimulus. Results of this experiment indicated that higher subjective ratings of emotional arousal were significantly related to reduced Alpha activity, particularly over the parietal lobe recording site. Further, viewing moving images resulted in lower Alpha activity in comparison to viewing still images. They concluded based on these results that image motion modulates attentive encoding of a mediated message by significantly boosting levels of arousal.

Another example was demonstrated by Smith and Gevins (2004), who specifically decomposed upper and lower frequency components of Alpha activity recorded from the frontal lobe and found that the lower frequency component was more attenuated when subjective interest in the television commercials was higher. Alpha activity in the upper frequency component was attenuated during the viewing of ads that had a greater probability of being recalled in subsequent memory tests. These findings point to the value of EEG in providing insight into perceptual and higher order cognitive processes related to encoding and subsequent recall of mediated messages.

Finally, Vecchiato et al. (2010) recently published a methodological study demonstrating the utility of analyzing EEG activity to observe variation in cognitive processes evoked by viewing commercials, political messages, and public service announcements. A particularly interesting finding from their study was that EEG activity was able to distinguish different patterns of cognitive processing in supporters of a political candidate compared to swing voters during exposure to a televised political speech.

We hope our brief review of recent research in which EEG was used to study cognitive processing of mediated messages has not only illustrated how this exciting psychophysiological measure has been applied to observing the dynamic interaction between the human mind and media but also sparks ideas for the future application of EEG in media psychology research. Overall, this section of this chapter should give you confidence that EEG can be a great tool for the media psychology researcher. We find it tremendously encouraging to see the recent resurgence of EEG in the study of cognitive processing of mediated messages after the early classic experiments conducted in the 1980s. This likely indicates that not only have EEG recording and analysis techniques become adaptable to be validly applied to studying mental processing of real world, complex stimuli, like mediated messages, but that EEG is becoming a measure that is more accessible to scientists interested in studying how the mind processes media.

Summary

Of all the measures discussed at any length in this book, the EEG is the only one which directly measures the activation of the central nervous system. EEG provides a direct measure of the electrical activity in the brain itself, and can do so with superior temporal precision if adequately time-locked to the presentation of a mediated stimulus. While EEG excels in terms of temporal dynamics, however, it suffers in localization of where the biopotentials are coming from in the brain itself. This is due to the minuscule amplitude of the signals, the distance they must travel to the scalp surface, and the blood, fluid, bone, skin, and hair they must travel through. Although the ability exists to more precisely localize the EEG signal using a statistical analysis technique known as Independent Component Analysis (ICA, Delorme & Makeig, 2004), this requires advanced statistical knowledge and recording from many (e.g., 256) scalp locations is preferable.

Perhaps for these reasons, most of the research employing psychophysiological methods to indicate cognitive activity uses the peripheral measure of cardiac activity. As we have mentioned, however, this important organ is innervated by both the "attention" mechanism of the ANS (the parasympathetic system) and the "emotion" mechanism (the sympathetic). For that reason, along with the complex interactions between attention and emotion that we acknowledged at the beginning of this chapter, heart rate is rarely collected as an isolated measure in the media laboratory. Instead, it is coupled with psychophysiological measures of emotional processing, to which we turn in the next chapter.

5

PSYCHOPHYSIOLOGICAL MEASURES OF EMOTIONAL PROCESSING OF MEDIA

The previous chapter covered psychophysiological measures used to index cognitive processes engaged during media exposure. We now turn to discussing the unique theoretical, conceptual, and operational issues associated with using psychophysiological measures to index emotional/motivational processes. The embodied motivated processing theoretical framework—discussed in the early pages of Chapter 4—provides a general conceptualization of emotion and cognition as highly integrated mental processes serving adaptive functions and accompanied by distinct patterns of measurable physiological activity. It is important for media psychology researchers who study how the human brain processes emotional media content to understand the distinct function and nature of emotion as well as the conceptual and operational details of specific psychophysiological measures of emotional processing. Thus, similar to Chapter 4, we begin with a theoretical consideration of human emotion and motivation in the context of media exposure and then proceed to discussing two specific psychophysiological measures of emotional processing—galvanic skin conductance and facial EMG—that are commonly applied in media psychology research.

Grounded in basic human/biological motivation, the emotional processes engaged during exposure to media content are not only fundamental to how the brain processes that content but also significantly determine the ultimate impact of it on individuals. The experience of consuming media content, after all, is fundamentally an emotional one. An extensive line of media research has demonstrated that individuals often turn to specific forms of media entertainment to manage and purposefully manipulate "real life" emotional experience (e.g., Carpentier et al., 2008; Chen, Zhou, & Bryant, 2007; Knobloch, 2003). Research on advertising and public health campaigns in the media indicates persuasion is significantly related to the emotionality of campaign messages (Dilliard & Nabi,

2006; Friestad & Thorson, 1993). Emotion also plays a huge role in news consumption with emotion-based explanations prevalent in studies of why individuals consistently attend to the violence and mayhem that occupies so much of the space and time in news reports (e.g., Shoemaker, 1996).

Scientific understanding of emotional processes engaged by media use is critical to understanding the impact of media on individuals; however, it was not until the latter half of the twentieth century that emotion attained its rightful place in media research. Dolf Zillmann was one of the earliest communication scholars to explicitly outline emotional processes that might underlie media effects when developing his Excitation Transfer Theory (Zillmann, 1983). More recently, Lang's LC4MP, which we introduced in Chapter 4, has been used as a theoretical foundation to directly study emotional processes engaged during media use (e.g., Lang, 2009; Lang, Park, Sanders-Jackson, Wilson, & Wang, 2007; Lee & Lang, 2009; Leshner & Bolls, 2005). It is interesting to note that the explicit inclusion of emotional processes in media theory occurred in the 1980s—a time that saw a resurgence of the use of psychophysiological measures in studying media audiences (Lang, Potter, & Bolls, 2009). Both Zillmann and Lang have made significant use of physiological measures of emotion in building their theories; however, as mentioned in Chapter 1 only the latter interpreted these measures using the *psycho*physiological paradigm.

The inclusion of emotion as a central theoretical concept has helped move media researchers beyond simply documenting static effects toward providing richer theoretical explanations of mental processes that dynamically build the impact media use has on individuals. Our colleagues in psychology have discovered that emotion and motivation—two very closely related concepts—are fundamental processes driving the mental activity that allows us to effectively process and adaptively respond to all forms of stimuli and information we encounter in our highly complex social world (Lang & Bradley, 2008). A significant portion of information and stimuli we encounter in our social world comes to us via media. It should not, therefore, be surprising that including emotion in the study of how individuals process and are impacted by media content has yielded insight that has advanced us beyond knowledge provided by the pioneers of media effects research.

These pioneers were not equipped with the knowledge or methods to scientifically study emotional processes engaged by media use and include insight gained from the study of emotion in their theorizing. Thankfully, the current scientific environment is vastly different for media psychology researchers and there is a growing body of research from which in-depth theoretical knowledge of the nature of human emotion can be gained. Researchers in neuropsychology have been engaged for several decades in intense study of the nature of human emotion—as evidenced by several psychological review articles which we highly recommend (Barrett, Mesquita, Ochsner, & Gross, 2007; Cacioppo & Gardner, 1999; Izard, 2009; Russell, 2003). Media psychology researchers must tune into the intriguing and powerful view of emotion emerging from this work if we are going to validly use psychophysiological measures of emotional/motivational processing in our efforts to advance knowledge of how the mind processes emotional media content.

The nature of human emotion

Emotion could be considered the lifeblood of human existence. Our ability to feel and then act on our emotional passions—when managed appropriately—enables us to live full and rich lives. Emotion flows through the most meaningful life experiences such as falling in and out of love, grieving the loss of a friend, or celebrating personal achievement. The impact of emotion on human behavior is of course not limited to the occurrence of major life events but extends into the minute details of our day-to-day existence. Many researchers now believe that there is likely a strong connection between the capacity to experience emotion and consciousness (Damasio, 1999). It has been proposed that as conscious human beings our daily life consists of a continuous stream of affect which we become more or less mindful of as we go about our business (Russell & Barrett, 1999).

It is useful to distinguish emotion from other forms of affective reactions we can engage in as we negotiate the complexities of our social world—including any media content we consume. **Emotions** are conceptualized as relatively fleeting, affectively valenced reactions evoked by encountering specific meaningful stimuli (Frijda, 1994; Larsen et al., 2008). This can be contrasted with **attitudes**—affective reactions that are more enduring (Eagly & Chaiken, 1993)—and **moods** which are also more enduring than emotional reactions but tend to be more diffuse rather than specifically directed at an affective stimulus (Frijda, 1994).

Researchers need to keep in mind the conceptual distinction between these three affective reactions—emotions, moods, and attitudes. All three could potentially influence physiological measures collected from experiment participants. Ongoing and enduring moods have physiological manifestations and have been shown to influence both the choice of and reactions to media content (Zillmann, 2003). There is also some interesting recent discussion of the use of psychophysiological measures as implicit measures of attitudes (Cunningham, Packer, Kesek, & Van Bavel, 2009). Media psychology researchers who use psychophysiological measures to study emotional processing are attempting to observe a unique, targeted, and temporally fleeting affective reaction evoked by specific psychologically meaningful stimuli occurring within the context of media exposure. This arguably makes it all the more important to study emotional reactions to media content as they unfold across time—as the use of psychophysiological measures enables. This also makes it important to conceptualize media content in a way that is consistent with these characteristics of emotional reactions by viewing media content as ongoing sensory streams of information that change from moment to moment in emotional tone and significance (Lang, 2009). Researchers have noted how any single instance of a media message—such as a specific ad, news story, or online game—can consist of a wide range of emotional stimuli (Dillard, Plotnick, Godbold, Freimuth, & Edgar, 1996) and have observed unique patterns of physiological responding to specific sections of emotional content within messages (Leshner, Bolls, & Thomas, 2009; Ravaja, Saari, Salminen, Laarni, & Kallinen, 2006a).

Our capacity to experience emotion through both media consumption and directly experienced events is so intertwined with our mental ability to perceive, think about, and make decisions based on information we receive that emotion probably impacts our day-to-day existence more than many of us consciously realize. Research into the neurophysiological basis of emotion has helped shatter the myth that emotion and cognition are completely separable processes by demonstrating that this distinction is not reflected in the workings of the brain (Duncan & Barrett, 2007). This line of research has revealed that emotional processes are implemented in an extensive, interconnected network that spans the sub-cortical areas of the brain—traditionally considered emotional areas— and cortical areas that have traditionally been considered cognitive areas of the brain (Tucker, Derryberry, & Luu, 2000). The brain areas that make up this emotion network are interconnected in both a top-down and bottom-up fashion—meaning that emotion helps construct cognition and cognition shapes emotion (Cacioppo, Gardner, & Berntson, 1999).

The media psychology researcher who wants to utilize psychophysiological measures to observe emotional/motivational processes engaged during media exposure must be aware of the interaction between emotion and cognition in how media content is processed. For example, a recent study of emotional processing engaged by televised anti-drug messages found young adults display less intense corrugator muscle activity during exposure to highly graphic messages than adolescents (Bolls, Miles, & Zhang, 2006). Corrugator muscle activity is a physiological indicator of negative emotional response (Larsen, Norris, & Cacioppo, 2003). One possible explanation for this finding is that young adults— compared to adolescents—have more information stored in memory concerning drug abuse messages, making them somewhat desensitized to such messages resulting in lower attention levels and less intense emotional responses. This illustrates how—as discussed in Chapter 4—researchers need to consider how the moment-by-moment mental processing of emotional media content engages complex interactions between emotion and cognition. Further, it also appears that the most rigorous and insightful models of how the human mind processes emotional media content will likely be built with data obtained from psycho- physiological measures of both cognitive processing—discussed in Chapter 4— and of emotional processing discussed in this one.

Another topic in our discussion of the nature of human emotion that has important implications for media psychology research concerns the role of consciousness in the expression of emotion. In theorizing about the human brain, neuropsychologists have highlighted just how much of cortical activity—including emotional processes—occurs with little to no conscious awareness (LeDoux, 1995). The obvious implication is that an in-depth understanding of the nature of human emotion cannot be achieved by simply asking individuals to self-report how they feel in certain contexts and situations. In the same vein, we should not expect to gain an in-depth understanding of the emotional impact of media content on individuals by only measuring emotion evoked by a message through self-report questionnaires—as much of the research on emotional media content has done (e.g., Dillard & Peck, 2001; Nabi, 1999). Researchers who have relied exclusively on self-report data to study emotional media content have provided valuable insight into highly conscious possible effects of various forms of emotional messages. Self-report data of emotional responses to media content, however, only reflects the surface output of what are likely highly complex, less conscious, emotional processes engaged over the time course of media exposure.

One is left to wonder how much more valuable theoretical as well as practical insight media researchers could contribute by more thoroughly studying emotional processes engaged by media content—obtaining multiple modes of data reflecting emotional activity. **Margaret Bradley** and **Peter Lang** (2007) noted three modes in which the "data" of emotion are expressed—physiologically, verbally, and behaviorally. A significant portion of emotional processing likely occurs in the physiological activity of central and peripheral nervous system structures whose output is hidden below explicit responses observed in verbal reports and behavioral actions (Larsen et al., 2008).

Theoretical understanding of the nature of human emotion ought to ultimately be grounded in an explicit acknowledgment that emotion is an extremely complex phenomenon experienced by living human beings. This is in essence a challenge to all who study human emotion—including media researchers—to approach our task from a conceptual foundation grounded in the fact that the essence of what we are studying is a complex interaction between the human body—made up of physiological systems—and an embodied human brain that produces all of our conscious experiences. At first glance this point seems obvious, but there is danger for media psychology researchers to conduct their work without fully appreciating this complex interaction. Researchers who study the emotional experience of consuming media by relying exclusively on self-report measures or, alternatively, believe that psychophysiological measures are more direct measures of emotional experience do not fully appreciate or reflect an understanding of the interaction of human mind and body in this complex phenomenon.

P. J. Lang and Bradley (2008) establish the importance of studying emotion in the context of media exposure by describing the complex interaction between body and mind during the consumption of media content. They claimed that during media exposure physiological responses that subserve real-world reactions to emotional stimuli are activated by emotional media content but are significantly modulated by mental activity reflecting our ability as humans to regulate our raw bodily responses to an emotional situation. If this is truly the case, media psychology researchers clearly need to approach this phenomenon for what it is—a continuous interaction between physiological systems activated by encountering emotional stimuli and the conscious, mental experience of experiencing and modulating an emotional response.

Conceptualizing emotion as involving an interaction between mind and body not only lays the theoretical foundation for applying psychophysiological measures in the study of how the mind processes emotional media content but should also make some intuitive sense. As humans we naturally associate bodily responses like sweaty palms and specific patterns of facial muscle movement with the experience of emotion. Some of the earliest theorizing about the nature of emotion delved into the connection between mind and body in emotional experience. We now turn to a more in-depth consideration of theorizing about the mind/body interaction that establishes a psychological and biological foundation for using physiological measures of peripheral nervous system activity to index emotional processing of media content.

Mind/body interaction in emotion

Barrett and Lindquist (2008) provide a historical review of how psychologists have approached understanding the nature of the brain/body connection in theories of emotion. Interested readers are encouraged to go to this source for a good review of how different perspectives on the mind/body interaction underlie theories of emotion. Here a general overview of this work is provided to give some theoretical context for the connection between emotion and peripheral nervous system activity—hereafter referred to as the psychophysiology of emotion.

William James launched one of the first formal theories of human emotion by proposing that specific bodily responses evoked by an encounter with an emotional stimulus produce distinct mental experiences of emotion (James, 1884). Alternatively, other emotion researchers proposed that conscious experiences of emotion evoke specific physiological activity (Cannon, 1927), or distinct experiences of emotional feelings are produced by a continuous interaction of both mind and body (Schachter & Singer, 1962). This last perspective is distinct from the others in that while proposing that the experience of emotion includes specific patterns of peripheral nervous system activity it discards the debate over whether bodily activity or mental experiences are dominant causes of emotion.

The tremendous amount of research conducted under these perspectives on the interaction of mind and body in the psychophysiology of emotion has laid down the base theoretical foundation on which media psychology researchers can depend in validly using indices of peripheral nervous system activity to measure emotional processing of media content. This theoretical foundation has been made even stronger by researchers studying the psychophysiology of emotion adopting an embodiment view of the body and mind in human emotion. The hallmark of an embodiment view of the body and brain in human emotion is that the concept of *the mind* is constituted in the form of brain activity influenced by afferent and efferent signals from the body. Under this perspective the problem of understanding mind/body interactions in the psychophysiology of emotion is reduced to the task of seeking insight into interactions between central and peripheral nervous system activity.

Before considering in detail how these two systems interact to produce emotional experience, let's briefly review the nervous system structures first discussed in Chapter 2. Remember that the broadest division of the human nervous system draws a distinction between the peripheral branch and central branch. The anatomical distinction drawn in the **central nervous system** is between the brain and spinal cord. Psychophysiological measures of emotion that focus on central nervous system activity are developed to directly index specific brain activity during emotional experiences. The **peripheral nervous system** is divided into the autonomic and somatic branches. The *autonomic branch* of the peripheral nervous system innervates the organs and glands through both the **sympathetic nervous system** and the **parasympathetic nervous system** pathways. Skin conductance—one of the specific psychophysiological measures of emotion we discuss later in the chapter—indexes sympathetic activation in the autonomic branch of the peripheral nervous system. The *somatic branch* of the peripheral nervous system innervates the skeletal muscles. Facial electromyography—the other specific psychophysiological measure of emotion we will discuss in this chapter— consists of somatic nervous system activity underlying facial muscle activity involved in emotional expression.

The entire nervous system is connected through both feed forward— **efferent**—and feed backward—**afferent**—pathways. An example of a behavior resulting from efferent nervous system activity during an emotional event would be a dog lover smiling while viewing a dog food commercial that features cute puppies playing. In this case the sensory perception of the advertisement creates a central representation of an emotionally pleasant stimulus—puppies—which feeds information forward through efferent nervous system pathways connecting the brain to the somatic nervous system resulting in the facial muscle activity that forms a smile. An example of emotional experience resulting from afferent nervous system activity would be if, while viewing an intense love scene in a movie starring a celebrity you find particularly attractive, you became *consciously aware* of your palms beginning to sweat, and this further heightened your arousal. In this case, afferent pathways connecting the autonomic branch of the peripheral nervous system to your brain feed information backward about the state of autonomic nervous system activity.

The earliest theorizing about this interplay between afferent and efferent signals, and therefore a psychophysiology of human emotion, dates back to the work of

Charles Darwin and William James. Darwin was one of the first researchers to formally document variations in facial expressions associated with specific discrete emotions (Darwin, 1897). **William James** articulated one of the first formal theories of human emotion, which came to be known as the James Lange theory of emotion (James, 1884). The work of both Darwin and James demonstrated a link between bodily response and emotional experience but James staked out the position that the conscious perception of highly specific and distinct bodily responses is in essence the emotion we experience. According to James experiencing an emotion begins when perceptual processes grounded in the central nervous system perceive an emotional stimulus and evoke a specific pattern of activity in the organs, glands, and muscles innervated by the peripheral nervous system. These "disturbances" in peripheral nervous system activity are then perceived by the central nervous system—creating the conscious experience of having an emotional response. The theoretical proposition that the body plays such a huge role in the conscious experience of emotion has had its opponents and adherents. One of the earliest opponents was Cannon, who collected evidence that changes in peripheral nervous system activity are definitely not a necessary condition for the conscious experience of emotion (Cannon, 1927).

Research since the time of James and Cannon has demonstrated that the strongest versions of either perspective are not tenable (Cacioppo, Berntson, & Klein, 1992). Peripheral nervous system activity does appear to play a significant role in the experience of human emotion but significant emotional experiences can occur centrally—only at the level of the brain. Furthermore, efforts to nail down the distinct peripheral nervous system patterns associated with discrete emotions—like happiness or sadness—have produced less than promising results (Bradley & Lang, 2007a). Rather than involving highly specific and consistent patterns of peripheral nervous system activity, the conscious experience of having a discrete emotional experience such as feeling angry more likely includes cognitive appraisal of physiological activity reflecting superordinate dimensions of emotional experience—arousal and valence—in relation to events and stimuli in one's environment (Barrett & Wager, 2006). Cognitive appraisal underlying discrete emotional experience could arguably result in a tremendously wide variety of interactions between the central and peripheral nervous system depending on numerous features of the environment, emotional stimulus, and characteristics of the individual. It seems possible, for instance, that depending upon variation in all three of the previously mentioned factors (environment, stimulus, and individual), the experience of viewing anger-inducing political content could evoke facial muscle activity indicative of either frowning or smiling. This may be why it has been difficult for psychophysiologists to identify distinct physiological responses that reliably distinguish between discrete emotional experiences. This also points out how important it is for media psychology researchers to collect both psychophysiological and self-report data in order to thoroughly observe the experience of consuming emotional media content.

Ultimately, theorizing about the nature of the mind/body interaction in the psychophysiology of emotion has led to a solid theoretical foundation concerning the embodiment of emotion that allows media researchers to confidently proceed in using psychophysiological measures to study emotion in the context of media consumption. This theoretical foundation clearly involves significant relationships between: mental representation of an emotional stimulus (e.g., a media message), our conceptual, centrally stored representation of emotion, and bodily states (Barrett & Lindquist, 2008). The activity measured by psychophysiological measures of emotional processes—including those engaged during media exposure—reflect the output of these dynamic relationships.

Arousal and valence as superordinate dimensions of emotion

Now that you have a theoretical foundation to draw upon in using psychophysiological measures to study emotional processes evoked by media, it is critical to understand the specific components of human emotion that psychophysiological measures such as skin conductance and facial EMG can validly index. In the psychological study of emotion, discrete feeling states refer to affective experiences such as anger, disgust, sadness, enjoyment, shame, fear, contentment, and surprise (e.g., Izard, 1972; Plutchik, 1980). From these discrete emotions, scholars have distinguished superordinate dimensions, the most widely recognized being arousal and valence (Bradley & Lang, 2007a; Lang, 1995).

Researchers interested in how the brain processes media have studied both dimensional and discrete aspects of the emotional experience of consuming media (see Bolls, 2010 and Nabi, 2010 for a recent discussion). As noted earlier, however, psychophysiological measures appear to most reliably and validly index superordinate dimensions of emotion rather than discrete affective feeling states (Larsen et al., 2008). Most media psychology researchers who utilize psychophysiological measures to study how the mind processes emotional content do so from what has become known as the dimensional theoretical perspective on human emotion—examining variation in the experience of arousal and emotional valence occurring during media exposure (see Lang et al., 2009 for a review).

The dimensional theoretical perspective conceptualizes emotion as affective experience that emerges from basic motivational processes (Lang & Bradley, 2008) organized according to two recognized dimensions of motivation—direction and intensity (Dickinson & Dearing, 1979). Direction refers to motivated behavior that ranges from approach to avoid; intensity refers to the strength of approach and avoidance responses. Under the dimensional approach to human emotion, direction of motivated behavior maps onto the dimensions of pleasant versus unpleasant emotional responding—the dimension of **valence**—while intensity maps onto the **arousal** dimension of emotion (Cacioppo & Gardner, 1999).

Recent theorizing about the nature of emotion—under a dimensional perspective—has led to the proposition that underlying the valence dimension are two separable motivational subsystems, the appetitive and the aversive systems (Cacioppo & Gardner, 1999). This is consistent with how emotion appears to be integrated at a neural level in the brain as there is substantial evidence of separable neural circuits involved in processing positive and negative stimuli (Cacioppo, Larsen, Smith, & Berntson, 2004). Arousal—under this perspective—is not conceptualized as a completely separate independent emotion concept but rather represents levels of activation within separable appetitive and aversive motivational subsystems underlying emotion (Cacioppo & Gardner, 1999). Moving away from simple bipolar conceptualizations of the valence dimension of emotion provides a more interesting and nuanced way to study emotional processes evoked by media content. Most relevant to media researchers is that this newer conceptualization expands emotion to allow the possibility that media content can simultaneously activate both positive and negative underlying dimensions of emotional experience to varying degrees. This has been reflected in interesting recent work incorporating psychophysiological measures of emotional processes engaged by media exposure in which media content coded as containing a mixture of positive and negative emotional tone has been shown to selectively activate psychophysiological indicators of appetitive and aversive activation (Lee & Lang, 2009; Potter, LaTour, Braun-LaTour, & Reichert, 2006).

Researchers who wish to utilize psychophysiological measures to provide in-depth, theoretically rigorous explanations of emotional processes engaged during media exposure—once equipped with a solid theoretical understanding of the nature of human emotion and aspects of emotion that can validly be observed in psychophysiological measures—are clearly positioned to make significant contributions to the growing body of media psychology research. The rest of this chapter will address the operational and technical knowledge required to employ these measures in a way that truly advances theoretical explanations of how individuals process emotional media content. We will present two psychophysiological measures extensively used in research on emotional processes evoked by media content—skin conductance and facial EMG. We will cover the physiological basis of these measures, their psychological interpretation, and technical knowledge necessary to implement them in a media research laboratory. We begin with skin conductance.

Skin conductance: an electrodermal measure of arousal

Skin conductance is a psychophysiological measure of emotional processing that is conceptually and operationally tied to what has been termed **electrodermal activity**—electrical activity that varies according to specific properties of the skin. Measures of variation in electrodermal activity have a long history in psychophysiology (Dawson, Schell, & Filion, 2007). This could very well be due to ease of measurement, quantification, and recognized sensitivity to variations in psychological states associated with electrodermal activity (Lykken & Venables, 1971). Noted French neurologist, **Charles Féré**, was one of the first to systematically observe changes in electrical activity of the skin (Andreassi, 2007). Féré passed a small constant current between two electrodes and measured conductance between the two recording sites on the skin, a procedure that became known as the exosomatic method for recording skin conductance, in contrast with an earlier technique used by psychophysiologists referred to as the endosomatic method which measures skin potential by recording electrical activity at the surface of the skin without introduction of an externally generated constant current. Not only did Féré recognize general skin conductivity, he also discovered differences in the amount of conductivity individuals had as a result of exposure to physical and emotional stimuli. This phenomenon captured the interest of psychologists working in the early twentieth century, including **Carl Jung**, and quickly became known as the galvanic skin response—due to the fact that a galvanometer was used to measure changes in skin conductance evoked by emotional stimuli (Andreassi, 2007).

In studying electrodermal activity in response to psychologically meaningful stimuli—such as emotional media content—it is important to distinguish between tonic and phasic activity. The difference between these two types of physiological activity—as discussed in Chapter 3—is that tonic electrodermal activity refers to baseline or continuously occurring activity, while phasic activity refers to a temporary response evoked by a specific known stimulus. A third type of electro-dermal activity—nonspecific—is also of interest. **Nonspecific electrodermal activity** refers to a temporary response that occurs without the presence of a known eliciting stimulus. The specific steps necessary to draw this distinction in measuring and quantifying skin conductance will be discussed later on, for now it is important to just note that the accepted practice is to use the term "level" in referring to tonic electrodermal activity and the term "response" when referring to phasic or nonspecific activity. Thus, four specific types of electrodermal activity are the focus of psychophysiological research—skin conductance level, skin conductance response, skin potential level, and skin potential response. Skin conductance—rather than skin potential—has become the most commonly used measure by psychophysiologists and most commercially available systems for measuring electrodermal activity are manufactured to directly measure skin conductance (Dawson et al., 2007). Skin conductance, as of the writing of this book, is the measure of electrodermal activity recorded in most media research labs so it is the specific measure we cover here.

Psychological meaning of skin conductance

Many of the psychological states demonstrated to reliably evoke detectable changes in skin conductance are tied to processing of the emotional characteristics of stimuli such as pictures (Lang, Greenwald, Bradley, & Hamm, 1993), music

(Grewe, Nagel, Kopiez, & Altenmuller, 2007), computer game avatars (Bailey, Wise, & Bolls, 2009), and emotional films (Codispoti, Surcinelli, & Baldaro, 2008). Galvanic skin conductance response has also been recognized as a possible physiological indicator of the orienting response (OR; Lynn, 1966), reflective of an automatic increase in attention paid to novel or signal stimuli in our environment. However, skin conductance responses associated with the OR could reflect the emotional-motivational component of orienting due to sympathetic nervous system activity evoked by motivationally meaningful stimuli. There is a strong, highly reliable association between activation of the sympathetic nervous system and skin conductance (Shields, MacDowell, Fairchild, & Campbell, 1987). This is why—despite the fact that skin conductance has been shown to vary with attention—we cover skin conductance as a psychophysiological measure of emotional processing.

The connection between skin conductance and emotional processing becomes clearer when you consider the biological and physiological basis of this measure. There are excellent descriptions of the anatomy and physiology underlying all forms of electrodermal activity (Andreassi, 2007; Boucsein, 1992; Dawson, Schell, & Filion, 2007; Stern, Ray, & Quigley, 2001) which you may wish to consult. Our purpose here is to describe these topics at a level that is adequate for giving the researcher interested in using this measure in the media research lab a basic foundation of conceptual knowledge necessary to validly measure skin conductance and confidently present the data.

The primary function of the human skin is to act as a protective barrier for our bodies. This barrier helps prevent entry of harmful materials into the bloodstream as well as passes substances from the bloodstream to the exterior of the body. Our skin also helps maintain proper hydration levels and regulate core body temperature. The processes that enable the skin to achieve these important bio-regulatory functions for us are **vasoconstriction/dilation** and the ability to produce sweat in varying amounts as needed. These processes are supported by extensive connections between the central and peripheral nervous system—more specifically connections between important brain areas involved in bio-regulatory processes and autonomic nerves in the skin. The arrival of brain signals at these nerve centers in the skin, for instance signals from the brain directing the production of sweat, are accompanied by measurable changes in the electrical properties of the outer layer of the skin. This is the biological basis of measurable electrodermal activity and, more specifically for our purposes, skin conductance. The specific bio-regulatory process underlying skin conductance is variation in the production of sweat in the eccrine sweat glands.

Underneath the outer surface of the human skin are two kinds of sweat glands— apocrine and eccrine glands. The **apocrine sweat glands** do not become fully mature until puberty and are primarily involved in thermal regulatory processes, giving these glands significantly less psychological significance. The **eccrine sweat glands** are believed to have the most psychological significance and as a result have been most extensively studied by psychophysiologists (Dawson et al., 2007). The eccrine sweat glands located on the palms of the hands and soles of the feet are believed to produce sweat that confers the adaptive advantage of supporting grasping behavior in support of fight or flight responses (Edelberg, 1972). These specific sweat glands, therefore, are of particular interest to psychophysiologists because of their involvement in what has been termed "psychological sweating," or the sweating that occurs in motivationally relevant contexts independent of sweat gland activity occurring purely for the purpose of regulating body temperature. The eccrine sweat glands on the palms and bottom of the feet are the object of measurement in utilizing skin conductance as a psychophysiological indicator of emotional processing. Thus, some understanding of the anatomy and innervation of these specific sweat glands is necessary for researchers who wish to use skin conductance as a psychophysiological measure of emotional processing of media content.

An eccrine sweat gland runs through the subdermis, dermis, and epidermis levels of the skin. The secretory portion of the gland—the part that actually produces sweat—is embedded in the **subdermis**. A duct, connected to the secretory portion of the sweat gland, provides a channel for sweat to flow through from the subdermis out to a sweat pore at the **epidermis** where sweat becomes noticeable on the outer layer of the skin. It is important to note that activity of the secretory portion of the eccrine sweat gland does not act like a pressurized fountain always producing sweat that gushes up through the duct all the way to the outer surface of the skin. Instead, the levels of sweat may only partially rise through the sweat gland duct. Nevertheless, any level of sweat production, or increase in the level of sweat within the sweat gland duct, will change the electrical properties of the skin underlying observable patterns of electrodermal activity like skin conductance.

Eccrine sweat gland activity is ultimately driven by the interconnection of peripheral and central nervous system activity; therefore it is important to outline what is known about the specific involvement of both of them in generating activity within these glands. In the case of the peripheral nervous system, eccrine sweat glands are entirely innervated by the sympathetic branch of the autonomic nervous system (Boucsein, 1992); however, the neurophysiology underlying sympathetic activation of these glands is a bit unusual. The neurotransmitter involved in activation of the eccrine sweat glands is **acetylcholine**—a neurotransmitter that is most typically involved in parasympathetic activation (Shields, MacDowell, Fairchild, & Campbell, 1987). This biological fact further highlights the potentially important role eccrine sweat gland activity plays in processing and responding to psychologically meaningful stimuli rather than just simply responding to variation in core body temperature. Central nervous system involvement in psychologically meaningful activity of the eccrine sweat glands is not entirely known. There are, however, some specific brain areas whose activity appears to show a consistent relationship with eccrine sweat gland activity and specifically skin conductance (Tranel, 2000). Parts of the brain that have been associated with eccrine sweat gland activity range from sub-cortical to cortical structures. Tranel and Damasio (1994) specifically studied brain areas involved in generating skin conductance responses and found the most important areas to be the right inferior parietal and dorsolateral frontal regions, the anterior cingulate, and the ventromedial frontal region. Other research has identified the amygdala and hippocampus as brain areas that underlie skin conductance (Dawson et al., 2007).

The specific way in which the central and peripheral nervous systems are involved in generating eccrine sweat gland activity underlying skin conductance supports using this specific psychophysiological measure as an indicator of emotional processing. An examination of a recent meta-analysis of research focused on discovering the neuroanatomy of emotion (Barrett & Wager, 2006) reveals that many of the brain areas believed to play an important role in observed changes in skin conductance are also involved in generating emotional experience. Further, sympathetic nervous system activation—under the dimensional theory of emotion—is believed to reflect emotional arousal (Bradley & Lang, 2007a). Thus, we believe that the specific innervation of eccrine sweat gland activity that underlies skin conductance makes this a reliable psychophysiological measure of emotional processing—more specifically emotional arousal. Emotional arousal—under our embodied motivated processing theoretical framework—reflects the level of activation within the appetitive and aversive emotional/motivational systems.

Measuring skin conductance in the media research lab

We now proceed to a discussion of the skin conductance signal and specific procedures in measurement and analysis of the data. The Society for Psychophysiological Research has published a committee report detailing technical recommendations for the measurement of skin conductance (Fowles et al., 1981). The recommendations offered in this report have been incorporated into more recent books on psychophysiological methods and are followed by most researchers who use skin conductance as a measure of emotional arousal. Thus, the technical details we offer here concerning skin conductance coupler settings, skin prep, and application of electrodes are primarily based on this published committee report.

Skin conductance varies according to changes in electrical resistance across the surface of the skin due to eccrine sweat gland activity. Conductance is the reciprocal of electrical resistance and is how the signal is most commonly quantified in psychophysiological research. The electrical principle involved in measuring skin conductance is **Ohm's Law**. According to Ohm's Law resistance equals the voltage applied between two electrodes placed on the skin surface divided by the current being passed through the skin. Electrical conductance is expressed in Siemens with skin conductance being reported in units of microSiemens.

The biological basis of this change in electrical resistance detected at the surface of the skin has to do with the manner in which the eccrine sweat glands act like a series of electrical resistors wired in parallel. As activation within the sympathetic branch of the autonomic nervous system increases, the secretory portion of the sweat gland produces sweat, causing the level to rise in the duct of the gland. This, in turn, lowers the electrical resistance of the outer layer of the skin. Conductance is the reciprocal of resistance. Therefore, as the sweat increases in the ducts the resistance at the skin level goes down, resulting in higher levels of recorded skin conductance.

Researchers studying emotional media content should be very thankful the physical presence of sweat on the outer layer of the skin is not required for skin conductance to be a psychologically meaningful measure of emotional arousal. Even the most arousing media content is extremely unlikely to lead to such high levels of sympathetic nervous system activation that participants in an experiment will visibly sweat. The obvious possible exception could occur when a participant is engaged in a highly interactive, emotionally intense gaming experience. The fact that even low levels of sweat—completely contained in the sweat gland duct—can lead to observable changes in skin conductance indicative of significant changes in emotional arousal makes it all the more necessary for researchers studying emotional processing of media to pay extra attention to technical and procedural aspects of measuring skin conductance. Significant changes in emotional arousal evoked by the features of media being investigated can be due to very subtle changes in sympathetic nervous system activation. These changes can be ever so subtle because often our research environment involves participants sitting comfortably while they consume the media we are studying, further relaxing them. This makes any changes in skin conductance occur within a background of relatively low levels of sympathetic activation. Further, the day-to-day media use of some participants may make them somewhat desensitized to all but the most extreme emotional media content. Thus, detecting small, yet meaningful changes in skin conductance evoked by emotional media content requires detailed attention to equipment and procedures that are necessary in order to obtain the best signal-to-noise ratio during data collection.

Skin conductance recording equipment and supplies

The primary instrument for recording skin conductance is a **skin conductance coupler** that consists of an electrical circuit that generates the necessary electrical signal for recording changes in the electrical properties of the outer layer of the human skin. It is important to note that recording systems have been manufactured in two different ways to measure change in electrical activity across the skin surface. Some recording systems pass a small electrical current between two electrodes—

recording and storing electrical resistance. Other systems pass a small voltage between the electrodes—directly recording skin conductance. In an influential article, Lykken and Venables (1971) provided a strong argument in favor of directly measuring skin conductance rather than skin resistance and this is what researchers have measured in studying emotional processing of media content (Lang et al., 2009). Most equipment vendors sell recording systems that directly measure skin conductance rather than electrical resistance and this kind of recording is currently recommended for psychophysiological research investigating electrodermal activity (Dawson et al., 2007). One specific advantage of directly measuring skin conductance rather than electrical resistance is that skin conductance has been shown to be less susceptible to the law of initial values that has been shown to affect responding in other physiological channels (Stern et al., 2001). The law of initial values refers to the fact that the degree to which physiological activity recorded by a psychophysiological measure can be expected to vary at any point in time is constrained by the level of preceding activity (Stern et al., 2001). The fact that skin conductance may not be as susceptible to the law of initial values means that the magnitude of skin conductance responses evoked by media content being studied in an experiment might not be significantly influenced by baseline levels of skin conductance occurring prior to the onset of stimulus messages. It is important for media researchers to know this important difference between electrodermal activity recording systems to make sure that when setting up a lab they order the appropriate equipment—a skin conductance coupler that directly measures skin conductance by generating a small voltage rather than electrical current between recording electrodes.

The voltage generated by a skin conductance coupler in order to directly measure skin conductance level is referred to as the **excitation voltage**. The recommended excitation voltage for a skin conductance coupler is 0.5 volts. Skin conductance couplers offer the option of generating an AC or DC excitation voltage. We recommend measuring skin conductance using an AC excitation voltage in order to minimize polarization of the recording electrodes which can introduce noise into the skin conductance signal. Skin conductance couplers will also offer the option of recording skin conductance in either a DC coupled or AC coupled manner. AC coupling will measure skin conductance response over a set time constant. DC coupling will constantly measure skin conductance level over an entire recording session. In our own research we have used DC coupling to record skin conductance level during exposure to any media content we are interested in studying and then have performed any analysis of skin conductance responses offline, after data collection. The final technical detail of the skin conductance coupler concerns sensitivity or amplification of the skin conductance signal. The amplification needs to be adequate in order to observe phasic skin conductance responses but not so high that the skin conductance signal goes off scale—exceeding the measurement capabilities of the range of the coupler. Stern et al. (2001) offer the following recommendation for how to set an appropriate level of amplification. At the beginning of a recording session the researcher can have a participant take a deep breath. This action on the part of the participant should result in an observable skin conductance response. If no response is seen, obviously amplification needs to be increased. On the other hand if the signal goes off scale then the researcher should decrease the amplification.

In our own research on emotional processing of media content we have measured skin conductance utilizing 8mm, Ag/AgCl, shielded, floating electrodes attached to skin surfaces with double-sided adhesive electrode collars. It is critical to use Ag/AgCl electrodes in order to minimize polarization—where one of the electrodes can become positively charged relative to the other recording electrode. Avoiding polarization in measuring skin conductance is critical because any difference in the electrical charge of the recording surface of electrodes will significantly change conductance levels recorded from a participant's skin surface. The size of electrodes used to measure skin conductance can also potentially affect conductance values recorded from a participant. It is not a good idea to use electrodes smaller than 8mm—such as those recommended for the measurement of facial EMG—because extremely small electrodes can cause current density to become high enough to inflate skin conductance levels and can potentially stimulate the skin tissue under the surface of the electrodes (Stern et al., 2001). **Current density** refers to the amount of current being passed per unit of area under the recording surface of the electrode. Measuring skin conductance involves passing a constant voltage between electrodes—regardless of the size of the electrodes being used—therefore, current density is inversely related to the size of electrodes being used. Floating electrodes are particularly good for measuring skin conductance because the double-sided adhesive collar used to attach the electrode to the surface of the skin not only holds the electrode in place but also helps control the size of the area of the skin that comes into contact with the electrode gel—yielding more reliable recorded levels of skin conductance. It is important to keep in mind that it is actually the size of the area of skin coming into contact with electrode gel that impacts recorded skin conductance rather than the size of the electrodes being used. The bottom line is that the contact area of the gel needs to be strictly controlled across participants and ideally across research labs in order to promote comparison of results across experiments conducted in different laboratories. This is accomplished by the appropriate selection of electrodes and careful application of an electrode gel.

Electrode gel is the medium that makes contact between the recording surface of the electrode and the surface of the participant's skin. In all other psychophysiological measures electrolyte gel is used. However, the signal recorded by skin conductance electrodes is made up of changes in the electrical properties of the outer layer of the human skin rather than a direct electrical signal generated by nervous system activity. Therefore, it is critical that electrode gel used to measure skin conductance not substantially change the electrical properties of the human skin. This is why under no circumstances should the electrolyte gel used to obtain other psychophysiological measures like heart rate and facial EMG be used in measuring skin conductance. The best electrode medium for that purpose will be a non-conductive gel that is as close as possible in its chemical makeup to human sweat. In our own work we have obtained satisfactory results using the water soluble K-Y Jelly® brand personal lubricant. However, it has also been widely recommended that researchers make their own skin conductance gel. Fowles et al. (1981) gave instructions for making skin conductance electrode gel using a skin care cream called Unibase combined with a mixture of sodium chloride and distilled water, which they referred to as physiological saline. Unibase is no longer commercially available, however, a brand of skin cream named Velvachol has been recently identified as a suitable substitute (Dormire & Carpenter, 2002). It may also be possible to find vendors of psychophysiological supplies that offer skin conductance gel, sometimes referred to as paste, in addition to their standard line of electrolyte gels.

Skin conductance electrode gel must be carefully placed in the cups of recording electrodes such that the cup is entirely filled, without air bubbles or excess gel seeping over the rim of the electrode and under electrode collars. This is especially critical for the measurement of skin conductance because, as noted earlier, any seepage of the gel outside the cup of the electrode changes the contact area affecting the recorded measurement. One tip that has been offered to tightly control the contact area by eliminating gel seepage is to place adhesive electrode collars on the recording surfaces of participants' skin before attaching them to electrodes and then place filled electrodes on the adhesive collars (Boucsein, 1992). It is also worth noting that some vendors sell disposable, pre-gelled electrodes for recording skin conductance.

Skin conductance electrode placement

Skin conductance can be reliably measured by placing electrodes on the palm of the hand or near the sole of the foot. As noted earlier, there is a particularly high concentration of eccrine sweat glands on these skin surfaces, making it particularly easy to detect changes in skin conductance due to any "psychological sweating" evoked by emotional media content. Skin conductance is most commonly measured from the palm; however, the choice of measurement location should be driven by the tasks a participant will be required to perform during the course of an experiment. If they require extensive grasping or other significant activity requiring the use of both hands it is probably best to measure skin conductance from the foot. Both measurement locations involve a bipolar placement of recording electrodes—meaning that two, active recording electrodes are placed on the skin surface. The specific recording sites that electrodes are placed on when recording skin conductance from the palm are the Thenar eminence—located near the base of the thumb—and the Hypothenar eminence—located on the pinky side of the palm or, alternatively, on the middle phalanges of the ring finger and pinky. Electrodes are typically placed on the palm of the non-dominant hand because this hand usually has the least amount of scarring or callusing, which can interfere with recording. If it is necessary to measure skin conductance from the foot, the recommended recording sites involve placing electrodes on the medial side of the foot down from the big toe near the arch of the foot. Electrode placements for these recording locations are displayed in Figure 5.1.

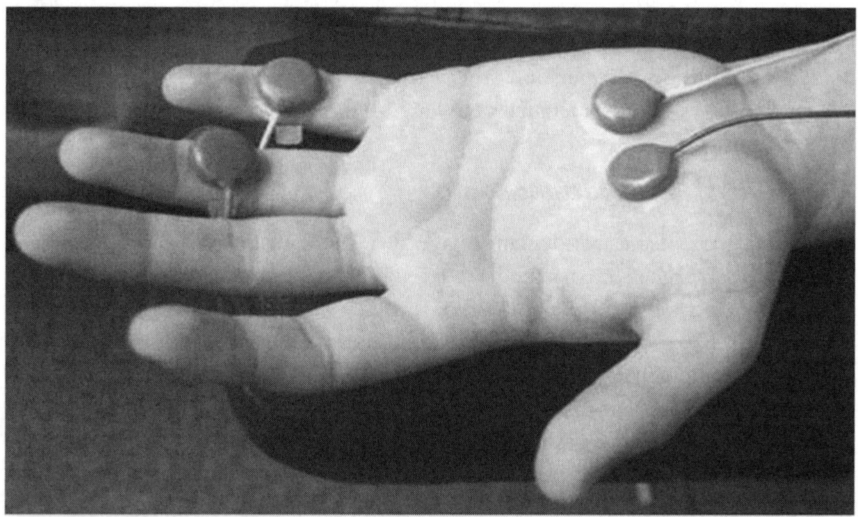
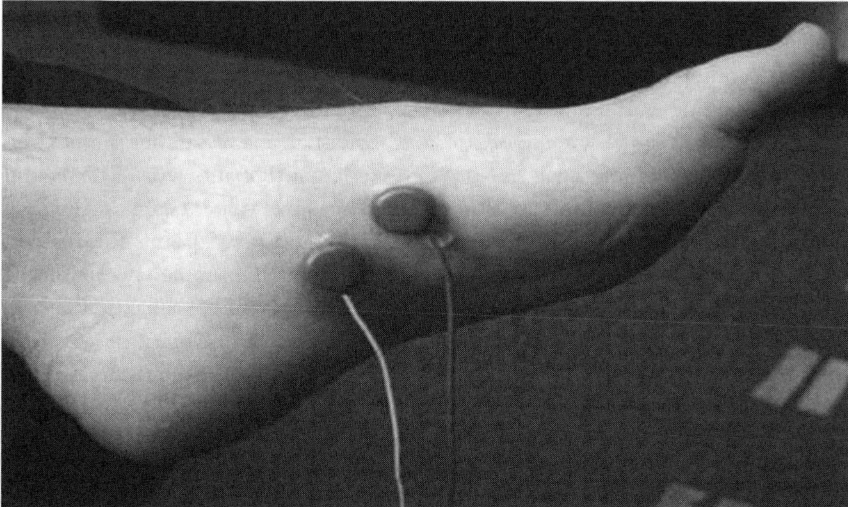

FIGURE 5.1 Alternative skin conductance electrode placements; middle phalanges of ring and pinky finger, Thenar eminence and the Hypothenar eminence, and medial side of foot.

Prior to placing electrodes on the recording surface of a participant's skin some preparation of the recording site is necessary. It is important that skin preparation for recording skin conductance not substantially change the physical makeup, and as a result the electrical properties, of the outer layer of the human skin prior to electrode placement. Researchers should absolutely not abrade skin conductance recording sites with abrasive skin prep pads as is done in preparation for the recording of other psychophysiological measures. The only required skin preparation for the measurement of skin conductance is to have participants simply wash their hands with a non-abrasive soap and warm water. Once the skin surface is prepped, skin conductance electrodes can be placed on the recording site in a bipolar fashion and plugged into the active receptacles on the electrode cable attached to the skin conductance coupler.

Analysis of skin conductance data

Two parameters of skin conductance have been the focus of a majority of research on emotional processing of media content—skin conductance level and skin conductance response. In the context of studying emotional processing of media, analyzing skin conductance level (SCL) involves analysis of skin conductance averaged over a determined period of time during which participants were exposed to the media content under study. A skin conductance response (SCR) analysis typically involves assessing the amplitude and frequency of nonspecific skin conductance responses occurring during media exposure. Data obtained from both SCL and SCR analyses are most commonly analyzed using a general linear model procedure such as repeated measures ANOVA.

The first step in conducting an analysis of skin conductance level across exposure to media content is to perform data reduction by obtaining an average SCL for the time increment of interest. In our own work, we have typically sampled the skin conductance signal at a rate of 20 Hz. If for instance, a researcher is interested in a second-by-second analysis of SCL while participants view 30-second advertisements, the 20 samples of skin conductance level values taken during each second of recording time will be averaged, yielding 30 data points for analysis. The time period over which SCL data is averaged is completely up to the researcher. Data collected during a hypothetical experiment in which participants view 30-second advertisements could just as well be averaged over the entire 30 seconds of viewing time yielding a single measure of skin conductance level for each stimulus advertisement. This form of data reduction should broadly be governed by consideration of the time period over which one might expect to see meaningful change in SCL given the nature of emotional content in experimental stimuli as well as the presence of different emotional events within the media content being examined. For example, most media content approved for broadcast in the United States is unlikely to evoke extremely quick meaningful change in skin conductance level across message exposure. Thus, in conducting a skin conductance level analysis it may not be necessary to average skin conductance over one-second epochs, rather a researcher might want to further reduce the data by averaging across larger time epochs of say two or five seconds.

The second step in conducting an SCL analysis is to compute a change score for each time epoch the skin conductance data has been averaged over. Despite the fact that skin conductance level has been found to not be substantially influenced by the law of initial values it is still important to collect baseline data prior to any stimulus messages in an experiment because the change scores in the skin conductance level analysis are based on change from baseline activity. The measurement of baseline activity for psychophysiological measures was discussed in Chapter 3. Skin conductance level change from baseline is a simple calculation. The researcher just subtracts baseline skin conductance level—typically averaged over some time epoch prior to stimulus onset—from the skin conductance level data recorded during media exposure at each aggregated time epoch determined to be most theoretically relevant. The skin conductance level change scores from baseline are then submitted for statistical analysis.

A second way of analyzing skin conductance is to perform analysis of skin conductance response by examining the amplitude and frequency of nonspecific SCRs occurring during media exposure. Recall that a nonspecific skin conductance response is a phasic response reflecting sympathetic nervous system activity occurring in the absence of a discrete, known stimulus. To help clarify this distinction it is useful to note that skin conductance level analysis is considered an examination of tonic skin conductance evoked during an entire episode of exposure to a media stimulus. Skin conductance response analysis is an examination of phasic responses of very brief length that occur during exposure to the same stimulus. More frequently occurring and larger nonspecific SCRs observed during exposure to media content are taken as evidence of a higher level of emotional arousal. These responses are considered nonspecific because they occur against the background of media exposure rather than to other specific, known stimuli in the environment.

The first issue to be dealt with in an SCR analysis concerns the identification of the responses themselves. Recall that skin conductance response occurs against the background of tonic skin conductance level, therefore, the identification of skin conductance response requires a criterion for defining the phasic increase in skin conductance level that will be considered to be meaningful. A widely accepted criterion for the identification of a meaningful skin conductance response is an observed change in skin conductance of at least 0.1 microSiemens over a maximum time course of three seconds (Dawson et al., 2007). This issue is also entangled with data collection procedures in that amplification, or sensitivity, set on the skin conductance coupler must be high enough to observe meaningful skin conductance responses occurring within tonic activity. Some skin conductance couplers will offer the option of balancing—in essence zeroing out—participants' tonic skin conductance level prior to the onset of each media stimulus in an experiment.

In theory the advantage to this is that it allows higher amplification of the skin conductance signal yielding better identification of skin conductance responses. The problem with this is that in zeroing out participants' baseline tonic skin conductance prior to the onset of a stimulus the researcher loses the data required to do a skin conductance level analysis as previously described and, therefore, can only conduct a skin conductance response analysis on the recorded data.

The valid identification of nonspecific SCRs enables researchers to measure the amplitude of each response and count the frequency of responses occurring during exposure to each stimulus message used in an experiment. Obtaining the frequency of nonspecific skin conductance responses during a media stimulus is as "simple" as counting the number of times the predetermined meaningful increase in amplitude occurs during the stimulus. This is indeed what researchers do, however, counting the frequency of skin conductance responses is complicated in the media research lab by the fact that the dynamic nature of the stimuli means a new nonspecific SCR can be evoked before the previous response has completely unfolded to the point that skin conductance returns to the level at which it was prior to the onset of the response. This is illustrated by the hypothetical skin conductance waveform in Figure 5.2.

One way that we have dealt with this issue in our own work is by marking separate nonspecific skin conductance responses according to the presence of a decrease in skin conductance of some standard minimum. For example, you could claim that a decrease of at least 0.1 microSiemens—the same degree of increase considered to be a meaningful response—is the necessary criterion for differentiating separate SCRs. The application of this criterion is illustrated in Figure 5.3. It should be noted, however, that the definition of the increase in amplitude necessary to constitute an SCR is somewhat arbitrary (Dawson et al., 2007), and the diminishing criterion should be as well.

Stern et al. (2001) describe an additional criterion for the identification of separate skin conductance responses occurring over tonic activity. Recording the

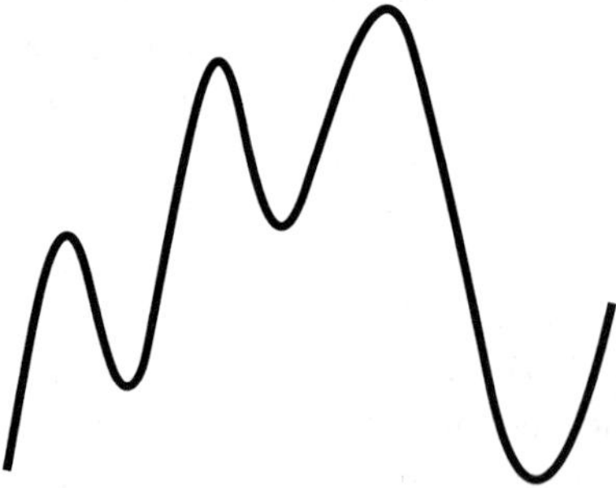

FIGURE 5.2 Hypothetical skin conductance waveform illustrating multiple nonspecific skin conductance responses evoked prior to completion of the previous response.

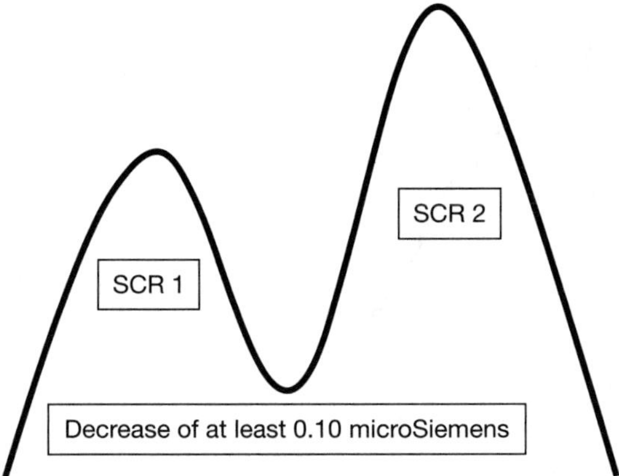

FIGURE 5.3 Hypothetical skin conductance waveform illustrating application of common criteria for scoring frequency of non-specific skin conductance responses.

amplitude of nonspecific skin conductance responses is a much simpler matter. To do so, a researcher simply measures amplitude as the increase in microSiemens from the onset of a response to the peak of the response. Measurement of the amplitude of an SCR is illustrated in Figure 5.4.

Examples of the use of skin conductance in media research

Skin conductance is indeed an extremely exciting psychophysiological measure of emotional processing of media content. The ability to dynamically record emotional arousal—activation within the appetitive and aversive motivational systems—on a dynamic basis during media exposure using skin conductance has provided tremendous insight into mental processing of emotional media content. We do not have the space here to review all of the intriguing lines of research being done in labs across the world so we merely offer a couple of examples of scholars using skin conductance data to study emotional processing of various forms of media.

Skin conductance data have been used to gain useful insight into the impact of specific features of the ever-changing new media environment on emotional arousal. Ravaja (2009) used SCL analyses to examine the arousal effect of different kinds of opponents on players of an online digital game. He recorded skin conductance level while participants played a digital game against a computer or a human that was either co-located or not co-located with the participant. Furthermore, the human opponent was also either a friend or stranger. Skin conductance data was reduced by averaging SCL across an entire game session. Results indicate that playing a digital game against a human is more emotionally arousing than playing

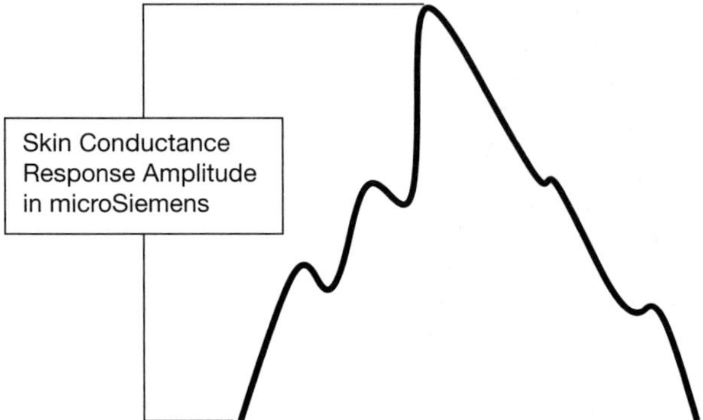

FIGURE 5.4 Hypothetical skin conductance waveform illustrating scoring non-specific skin conductance response amplitude.

against a computer—as evidenced by higher skin conductance level—but whether or not the opponent is a friend or stranger or is co-located in the same physical space does not have a significant impact on emotional arousal.

An additional significant area in which skin conductance data has contributed useful insight is in the study of persuasive media messages. One such study involved an examination of how sensation seeking and age impacts emotional processing of televised substance abuse public service announcements that vary in terms of arousing content and production pacing (Lang, Chung, Lee, Schwartz, & Shin, 2005). In this experiment the researchers used SCR analysis to determine emotional arousal evoked by the messages. Results show that low sensation seekers exhibit more frequent SCRs and therefore higher levels of emotional arousal during exposure to substance abuse public service announcements compared to high sensation seekers. Further, adolescents may require higher levels of production pacing in messages to exhibit strong skin conductance response indicative of emotional arousal when compared to college students.

These are merely two examples of how electrodermal activity, in the form of skin conductance, has recently been employed to better understand emotional response to media. As mentioned earlier, however, arousal is only one of the two primary dimensions underlying experienced emotion. The second is valence, or how positive and/or negative the emotional experience is. For that reason, SCR and SCL data are often reported in parallel with a physiological measure of valence: facial electromyography.

Facial EMG: a measure of emotional valence

Facial electromyography (EMG)—the recording of the electrical signal associated with facial muscle activity—has been extensively used as a psychophysiological indicator of the valence of emotional processing evoked by motivationally meaningful stimuli. Although the relevance of facial activity to emotion traces back to Darwin, Duchenne, and even earlier, the development of this physiological measure gained wide acceptance in the mid-1970s when psychophysiologists began extensive investigations mapping relationships between the experience of pleasant and unpleasant emotional states and the activation of specific facial muscles. Some of the earliest research in this area was conducted by Schwartz and colleagues who recorded facial EMG while individuals engaged in pleasant and unpleasant mental imagery (Brown & Schwartz, 1980; Schwartz, Fair, Salt, Mandel, & Klerman, 1976). Since that pioneering work, an impressive body of psychophysiological research has mapped variation in electrical activity recorded from specific facial muscles to emotional processing of a wide variety of pleasant and unpleasant emotional stimuli, including pictures of emotional scenes, faces, as well as pro- and counter-attitudinal messages (for a review see Larsen, Berntson, Poehlmann, Ito, & Cacioppo, 2008).

For the media psychology researcher, the extremely valuable scientific outcome of the work of psychophysiologists studying facial EMG has been the identification of specific facial muscles that are consistently activated according to variance in the valence of emotional processing during media use. The specific muscles are the **corrugator supercilii, orbicularis oculi**, and **zygomaticus major**. Facial EMG recording sites that overlie the anatomical location of these facial muscles are displayed in Figure 5.5.

Researchers studying emotional processing of media have almost exclusively focused on measurement of activity within these specific facial muscles (Lang et al., 2009). Therefore we will focus our discussion on these muscles—the psychological meaning of their activity as well as how to collect and analyze data from them in the media research lab.

Psychological meaning of facial EMG

A solid understanding of the psychological meaning of facial EMG—as is the case with any psychophysiological measure—begins with an understanding of the biological basis of the signal being measured. Several excellent sources exist that discuss the biology and physiology underlying the EMG signal in greater detail than we will cover in this chapter (e.g., Hess, 2009; Stern et al., 2001; Tassinary, Cacioppo, & Vanman, 2007). Our purpose here is to draw on these sources to discuss this topic at a level of detail that gives researchers studying emotional processing of media basic knowledge of the biological process that leads to variation in muscle activity observed during the recording of facial EMG. After all, it is these biological processes—according to an embodied theoretical perspective of human emotion—that are the foundation of emotional processing.

The biological process underlying muscle activity is the generation of action potentials that travel down the axons of the neurons that make up the somatic

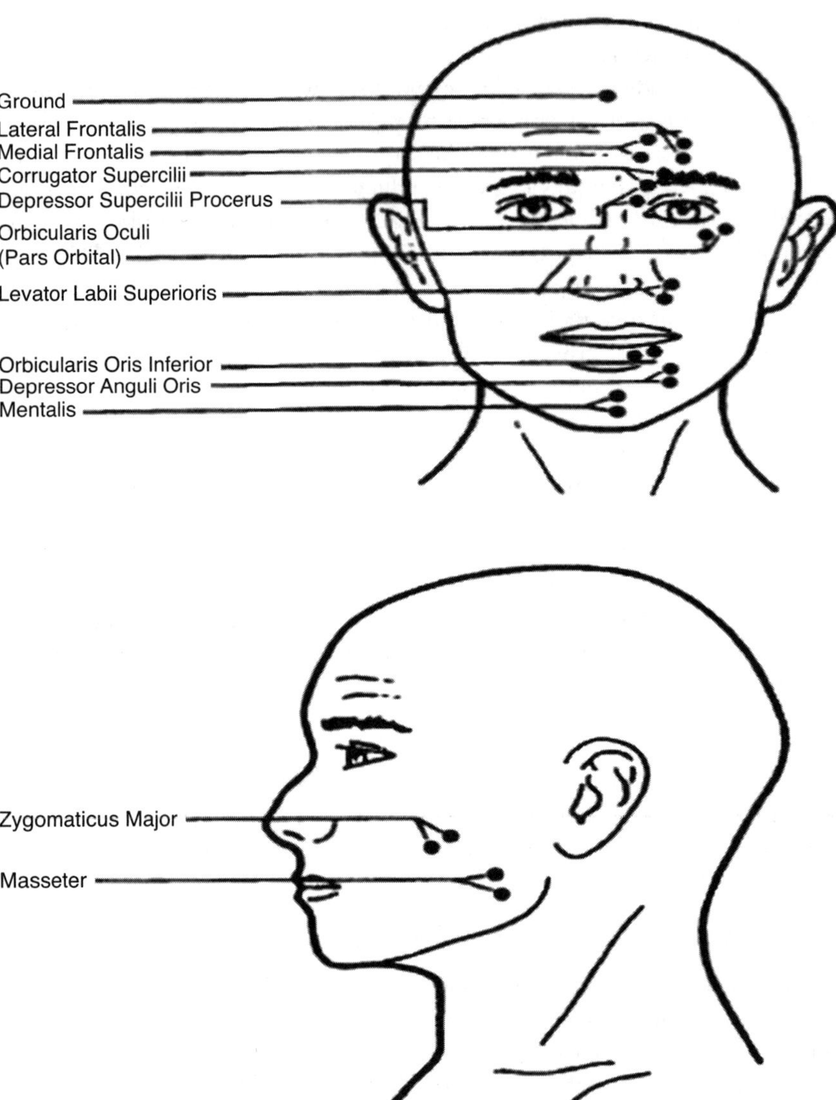

FIGURE 5.5 Facial EMG recording sites that overlie the anatomical location of specific facial muscles. Corrugator supercilii, orbicularis oculi, and zygomaticus major are muscles most commonly recorded in the media psychophysiology lab.

Source: reprinted from Fridlund & Cacioppo, 1986, courtesy of Blackwell Publishing.

branch of the peripheral nervous system. The somatic nervous system innervates all of the skeletal muscles, which are voluntary striated muscles, meaning that they consist of longitudinal fibers. Each muscle has numerous striated fibers that are bundled into **motor units**. Every motor unit is innervated by a single motor neuron axon. All of the muscle fibers within a motor unit are activated together when an action potential travels down the motor neuron axon causing a muscle contraction. This specific form of action potential is termed a **motor unit action potential** (MUAP). Contraction of an entire specific muscle is accomplished by the summative effect of numerous MUAPs. Action potentials are bioelectrical signals; therefore, the occurrence of numerous MUAPs within a specific muscle not only results in muscle contraction but also an electrical signal strong enough to be detected by electrodes placed on the surface of the skin over the site where the muscle is located. The difference in electrical potential across the two electrodes is transduced into voltage amplitude.

The voltage amplitude recorded from the skin surface over a muscle site has been found to reliably represent the force with which a muscle is contracted (Tassinary et al., 2007). However, it is important to emphasize here that the facial EMG signal that is recorded is electrical activity representative of muscle contraction, not actual muscle movement. This makes facial EMG a very sensitive measure of emotional processing because electrical activity in a facial muscle that is reflective of meaningful emotional experience can be recorded without visibly observable movement of facial muscles used to express emotion. The nature of much media content may not lead research participants to contract their facial muscles to a degree resulting in visible facial expressions yet processing of that content may still evoke meaningful variation in emotional processing that can be detected by recording the electrical signal generated by MUAPs. This fact confers some advantage to facial EMG over other methods of indexing emotional processing such as videotaping participants in an experiment and coding their visible facial expressions to measure the emotional experience associated with mentally processing various forms of media content.

The psychological connection between activation of facial muscles and emotion dates back to the work of Darwin, who systematically observed visible patterns of facial muscle action associated with different emotional states (Darwin, 1897). Psychologists building on the work of Darwin have concluded that variation in facial muscle activity is not only a means through which we externally express emotions to others but fundamentally shapes our own emotional experience (Neumann, Hess, Schulz, & Alpers, 2005). As proponents of a dimensional theory of emotion, which emphasizes patterns of motivational activation reflecting variance in the valence of emotional experience, we understandably believe that the fundamental psychological meaning of variance in facial muscle activity is variability in the valence of the current situation being processed. This means that from our perspective the most important theoretical and operational application of facial EMG is to index variance in the valence, the extent to which a media exposure activates appetitive and aversive motivational systems.

The muscles of the face that have been most extensively studied by psycho-physiologists in the context of emotional processing—corrugator supercilii, orbicularis oculi, and zygomaticus major—have proven to be most consistently activated according to the valence of emotional stimuli. The corrugator supercilii and zygomaticus major muscles have been found to automatically activate according to whether a stimulus is unpleasant or pleasant (Neumann et al., 2005). It appears that, at least for now, the media psychology researcher who wants to use facial EMG as a psychophysiological measure of emotional processing is on the strongest theoretical and operational ground in using this measure to index variance in the valence of emotional processing. Although some work has been conducted using facial EMG as physiological indicators of discrete emotions, it is recommended that this bioelectrical measure be paired with the existing reliable and valid self-report scales to index discrete affective feelings states that may have been evoked by media content (Bolls, 2010).

Now that we have established the psychological meaning of facial muscle activity recorded by facial EMG we can proceed to a more detailed discussion of specific muscles and how to record facial EMG in the media research lab.

Specific facial muscle activation as an index of emotional valence

The use of facial EMG to validly index the valence of emotional processing of media content is built on foundational work by psychophysiologists mapping out specific facial muscles that are selectively activated according to the experience of pleasant and unpleasant emotional/motivational activation. This work informs media researchers wondering which specific muscles they should record in order to study the emotional impact of media content. It also can assist in determining the inferences that can validly be drawn from variance in the activity of these muscles. The majority of work in this area indicates that activation of the zygomaticus major and orbicularis oculi muscles increases according to the pleasant dimension of emotional valence and activation of the corrugator supercilii muscle increases according to the unpleasant dimension of valence (Cacioppo, Petty, Losh, & Kim, 1986).

Previous research on emotional processing of media content in which facial EMG was measured indexed pleasantness by recording activity over the zygomaticus major muscle and unpleasantness by recording activity over the corrugator supercilii muscle (e.g., Bolls, Lang, & Potter, 2001; Hazlett & Hazlett, 1999). Research in which zygomaticus major muscle activity is recorded as the only facial EMG signal used to index pleasantness, however, does not reflect a full appreciation of the nature of facial muscle activity in the experience of emotion. Activation of the zygomaticus major muscle does indeed pull the corners of the lips up in order to form a smile; however, not all smiling reflects pleasant emotional experience. Ekman and Friesen (1982) distinguished smiles that reflect the genuine experience of pleasant emotion from smiling that can actually occur during the experience of unpleasant emotion. The distinguishing feature of facial muscle activity that reflects genuinely pleasant emotional experience is the simultaneous activation of the zygomaticus major muscle along the cheek and the orbicularis oculi muscle at the base of the eye socket (Ekman, Davidson, & Friesen, 1990). Smiling formed by this pattern of muscle activity across both the zygomaticus major and orbicularis oculi muscles has been termed the **Duchenne smile** (Ekman, 1989). It would appear that media researchers are well advised to record activity over both the zygomaticus major and orbicularis oculi muscles in order to index emotional activation that truly reflects pleasantness, as has been done in some more recent research (Ravaja, Saari, Kallinen, & Laarni, 2006b). Interestingly, there is some indication that the corrugator supercilii muscle is reciprocally activated by unpleasant and pleasant emotional experience, theoretically making it possible for variation in the activity of this specific muscle to index both dimensions of emotional valence (Larsen et al., 2003). The most common theoretical interpretation of corrugator supercilii muscle activity, however, remains that it indexes increases and decreases in unpleasant emotional experience.

The clear impression from the previous paragraph is that for most experiments in the media research lab it is important to record facial EMG by measuring activity from more than one muscle location. Recall that according to more recent conceptualizations of emotional valence, variation in this dimension of human emotion consists of activity within separable motivational subsystems—the appetitive and aversive systems—and activity within these systems can be reciprocal, coactive, or uncoupled (Cacioppo & Gardner, 1999). This means that to truly understand the valence of emotional activation a researcher must simultaneously observe both positive and negative activation in the human affect system (Cacioppo et al., 2004). The implication for the measurement of facial EMG is that in using this psychophysiological measure of emotional processing of media content it is wise for researchers to simultaneously measure activity over a facial muscle that has validly and reliably been tied to the experience of positive emotional activation and a facial muscle that has been associated in the same way with negative emotional activation. Simultaneously measuring both positive and negative emotional activation also makes sense in light of the emotional complexity and variation that can exist in various forms of media content. Recent research on emotional processing of media messages has noted how persuasive health campaign messages often consist of both positive and negative emotional content (Leshner et al., 2009). Practically speaking this means setting up the media research lab to measure at least two, and more ideally three, channels of facial EMG—enabling the simultaneous measure of orbicularis oculi, zygomaticus major, and corrugator supercilii activity. We now turn to a discussion of the technical details of recording the facial EMG signal.

Recording the facial EMG signal

The facial EMG signal is a very small bioelectrical signal generated prior to muscle contraction that can be detected at the surface of the skin over the site of the muscle group. The nature of the facial EMG signal requires researchers to be extremely diligent concerning technical procedures required to get the best signal-to-noise ratio in the recorded data. The frequency range of the facial EMG signal is comparatively wide, ranging from just a few Hertz to approximately 500 Hz. This range overlaps with the range of frequency generated in powering other AC electrical equipment—50–60 Hz—that might be present in the lab. Unfortunately this means ambient electrical noise generated by other AC electrical equipment can contaminate the recorded facial EMG signal if researchers are not careful to take steps to eliminate it. Further exacerbating the problem of electrical noise in the facial EMG signal is the fact that this signal is very small in amplitude, ranging up to only several hundred milliVolts by the time it reaches the surface of the skin. Thus, detecting the facial EMG signal requires high gain amplification of at least 50K and often as much as 100K. Amplifying the signal increases the entire signal—electrical noise and all—so without careful attention to procedures designed to eliminate noise in the signal the old adage "garbage in, garbage out" will be true of any data collected with this measure. The Society for Psychophysiological Research has published recommended guidelines for the measurement of facial EMG (Fridlund & Cacioppo, 1986), most focusing on reducing signal noise, further illustrating the heightened degree to which electrical noise can be a problem for this specific psychophysiological measure. Our discussion of the technical procedures for measuring facial EMG in the media research lab is grounded in the guidelines offered by Fridlund and Cacioppo (1986) and we pay particular attention to steps media researchers can take to eliminate electrical noise in the facial EMG signal.

Clearly the best way to deal with ambient electrical noise in the laboratory environment is to minimize it as much as possible before ever even attempting to record facial EMG from participants in an experiment. Minimizing electrical noise in the media research laboratory is discussed in Chapter 8; however it is worth also discussing briefly here due to the fact that this is particularly a problem in measuring facial EMG. One of the most likely sources of electrical noise in the media research laboratory comes from computer monitors and older televisions. The best way to eliminate this source of noise is to completely avoid the use of cathode ray monitors in favor of newer flatscreen monitors and televisions which will not leak 60 Hz noise that can potentially show up in the facial EMG signal. Electrical noise can also result from lighting used in the lab. Fluorescent and halogen bulbs are notorious sources of electrical noise and should be avoided in favor of regular lightbulbs when lighting the lab. Ultimately, all electrical equipment, outlets, and cables—except for electrode leads—should be well shielded. Fortunately, this is the case for most commercially available psychophysiological measurement systems so it is mostly other electrical equipment in the lab that the researcher needs to be attentive to. It is also a good idea to seat participants as far as possible away from electrical equipment so the leads are less likely to pick up any stray signal from equipment.

Electrode placement for recording facial EMG

The recommended electrodes for recording facial EMG are 4mm, Ag/AgCl floating electrodes. The advantage of using smaller electrodes rather than the standard 8mm ones recommended for heart rate and skin conductance is that they allow for a much more precise placement over the site of the facial muscle from which activity is being measured. There are over 30 bilaterally symmetrical pairs of muscles in the human head and face (Hess, 2009). This means that the facial EMG signal recorded from one muscle can contain cross-talk in the form of electrical activity generated by the contraction of other muscles that are anatomically close to the recording site. This cross-talk is obviously unwanted noise and can be minimized by using smaller electrodes, placing them very carefully over the desired recording site. The advantage of using floating electrodes is that the electrode gel placed in the electrode cup acts as a flexible cushion helping to maintain a more stable contact area between the recording surface of the electrode and skin. The double-sided adhesive colors used with floating electrodes also help in this regard. Facial EMG electrodes should be filled with a commercially available electrolyte gel. The electrode cup should be entirely filled, air bubbles removed, in order to make solid contact between the recording surface of the electrode and skin surface. Researchers also need to be careful not to overfill electrodes— causing the gel to seep across the electrode collar. Not only can this possibly cause electrodes to come off during recording but the gel can make an electrode bridge across the two sensors. This essentially turns the two electrodes into one, preventing the comparison necessary for bipolar measurement. The close proximity of facial EMG electrodes makes this an even more important concern.

Electrode site preparation and placement is critical to obtaining a high quality facial EMG signal, one that can be expected to reliably vary according to the valence of emotional processing during exposure to media content. It is nearly impossible to place surface electrodes such that they are practically guaranteed to pick up activity from one and only one specific facial muscle. For this reason, it has been recommended that in referring to electrode site location researchers refer to the region from which facial muscle activity was recorded rather than claiming to have recorded activity of one specific muscle (Tassinary et al., 2007). That being said, thorough electrode site preparation that minimizes electrical impedance and standardized placement of electrodes to record corrugator supercilii, zygomaticus major, and orbicularis oculi muscle activity will enable the media researcher to have confidence that significant differences in the activity of these muscles reflect variance in the valence of emotional processing evoked by media content being studied.

Electrode site preparation for the measurement of facial EMG involves the researcher abrading the skin surfaces where electrodes are going to be placed. We recommend using pumice alcohol skin prep pads that should be widely available from psychophysiological supply vendors for corrugator supercilii and zygomaticus major electrode site preparation. It is important, however, to explicitly inform participants that you are going wipe down their skin with an alcohol-soaked pad as some participants may have sensitive skin that is easily irritated. For orbicularis oculi some subjects find the alcohol vapor to be too irritating due to the close proximity to the eye. Using a paper towel dampened with distilled water is therefore a good option. Some vendors also sell dry abrasive pads, specifically made for abrading the skin for electrode site preparation. What is most critical for sufficient EMG electrode site preparation—regardless of the specific material used—is that the skin surface be abraded to a degree that removes dead skin cells, oil, dirt, and makeup to the extent necessary to obtain very low electrical impedance between the skin and recording surface of electrodes. One additional tip for reducing impedance is to rub a small amount of the electrolyte gel used in facial EMG electrodes into the skin surface where electrodes are being placed. The potential problem in doing this is less precise control over the size of the contact area from which electrodes record the facial EMG signal. In our own work, we have found that adequately abrading the skin surface achieves sufficiently low impedance levels.

The impedance level of electrodes at each facial EMG recording site must be directly measured prior to data collection using an impedance meter—not indirectly measured by recording resistance using an ohmmeter. Close attention to impedance levels helps minimize noise in the facial EMG signal, significantly improving the likelihood that the potential difference recorded by the electrodes from the surface of the skin more accurately represents muscle activity that the researcher wishes to measure. Originally it was recommended that impedances of facial EMG electrodes not exceed 10 k ohms (Fridlund & Cacioppo, 1986). The higher quality of more modern psychophysiological recording systems has made slightly higher impedance levels more tolerable so a more recent recommendation is that electrode impedances should be less than 30 k ohms (Hess, 2009). This low level of electrical impedance must be achieved prior to any data collection. If electrodes placed on a participant exceed this level of impedance it is highly recommended that the electrodes be removed and the researcher completely begin again the process of electrode site preparation and placement— re-measuring impedance of the newly placed electrodes.

The facial EMG signal is most commonly measured using a three-lead, bipolar electrode placement on the skin surface over the muscle whose activity is being recorded. Two recording electrodes are placed on the skin surface over the muscle and are referenced to a third, ground electrode. It is important for both safety and signal quality issues that all recording electrodes placed on a participant are referenced to only one ground electrode. Generally speaking, electrodes should be placed near the middle of the muscle on a line that runs parallel to muscle fibers. Fortunately, standardized electrode placements for the measurement of facial EMG from the zygomaticus major, orbicularis oculi, and corrugator supercilii muscle regions are well-established (Fridlund & Cacioppo, 1986). Figure 5.6 contains photographs displaying electrode placement for recording facial EMG from these facial muscle regions along with description of these electrode placements taken from the facial EMG guidelines paper by Fridlund and Cacioppo (1986).

The primary piece of recording equipment for facial EMG is a differential bioamplifier. A bioamplifier is needed for every channel of facial EMG a researcher wishes to record during an experiment. This obviously means that in ordering equipment to measure facial EMG, researchers need to order at least two and ideally three bioamplifiers in accordance with our earlier recommendation that activity from at least two different muscles needs to be simultaneously recorded in order for facial EMG to be a useful measure of the valence of emotional processing engaged by media content. The bioamplifier not only amplifies the signal recorded by the electrodes at the skin surface but also has filtering capacity that allows the attenuation of electrical signals falling outside the frequency range of the desired facial muscle activity. An amplifier gain setting of at least 50 k and possibly as much as 100 k is necessary in order to reliably record facial EMG. The primary frequency range of the facial EMG signal is approximately 10–500 Hz and low-pass and high-pass filters should be set accordingly (Fridlund & Cacioppo, 1986). In fact, Hess (2009) suggests a band pass filter range of 30–500 Hz allows researchers to remove extraneous electrical noise that might not reflect true EMG signal. Practically speaking, this would be accomplished by setting the high-pass filter to 30 Hz and low-pass filter to 500 Hz.

The facial EMG signal directly recorded by the bioamplifier is a pseudorandom waveform with both positive and negative deflections around an electrical mean of zero. This raw EMG signal is fed into some form of an integrator/contour follower—depending upon the specific psychophysiological recording system being used—that rectifies and smoothes the signal. **Rectification** involves mirroring the amplitude of the negative portion of the electrical signal to the positive scale. **Smoothing** the signal rounds off the momentary peaks in the raw EMG signal and is typically accomplished by selecting a time constant on the integrator/contour follower. Selecting too long of a time constant for smoothing may lead to the loss of peaks in the rapidly changing facial EMG signal but too short a time constant loses efficiency gained in data collection and can lead to an analog waveform that is difficult to interpret. In our own work we have found that a time constant of 500ms yields an easily interpretable analog waveform that captures variation in the facial EMG signal evoked by emotional media content.

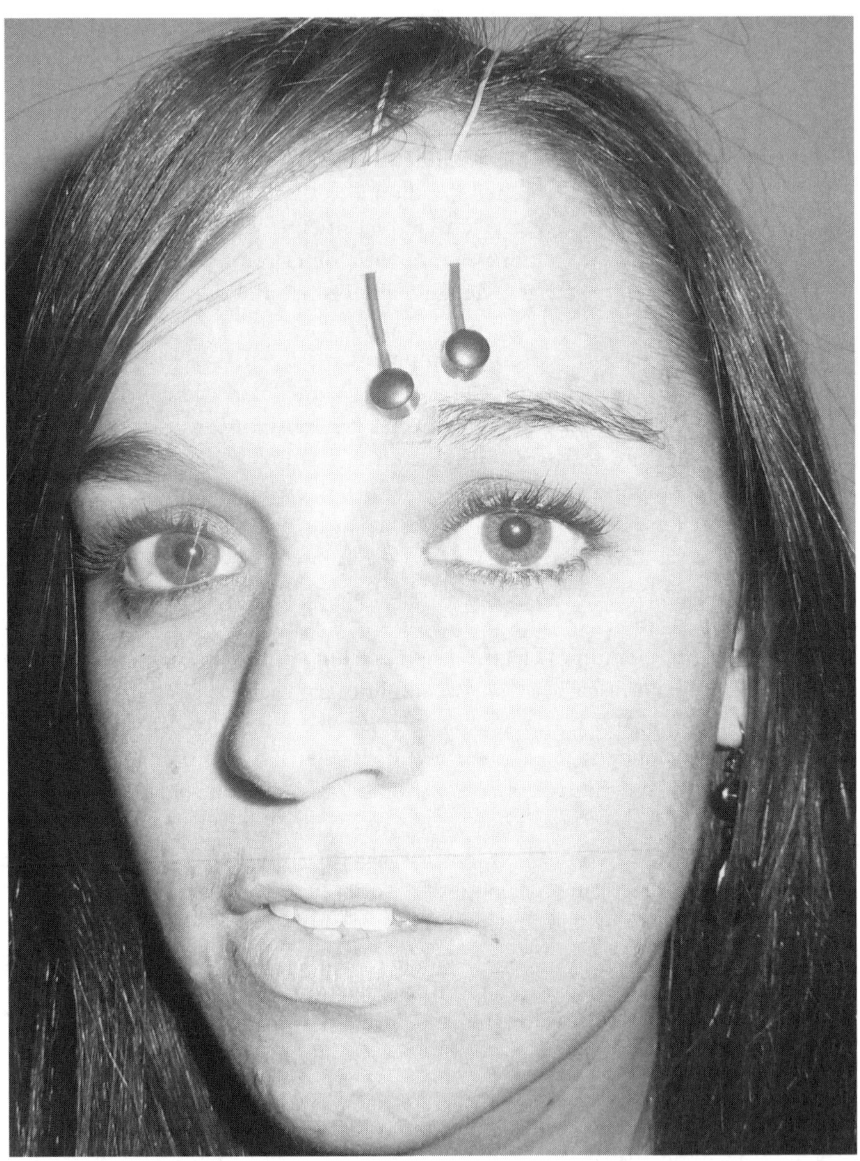

FIGURE 5.6a Electrode placement for recording activity from the corrugator supercilii region. "One electrode is affixed directly above the brow on an imaginary vertical line that traverses the endocanthian (the inner commissure of the eye fissure. The second electrode is positioned 1cm lateral to, and slightly superior to, the first on the border of the eyebrow." Fridlund & Cacioppo, 1986, p. 572.

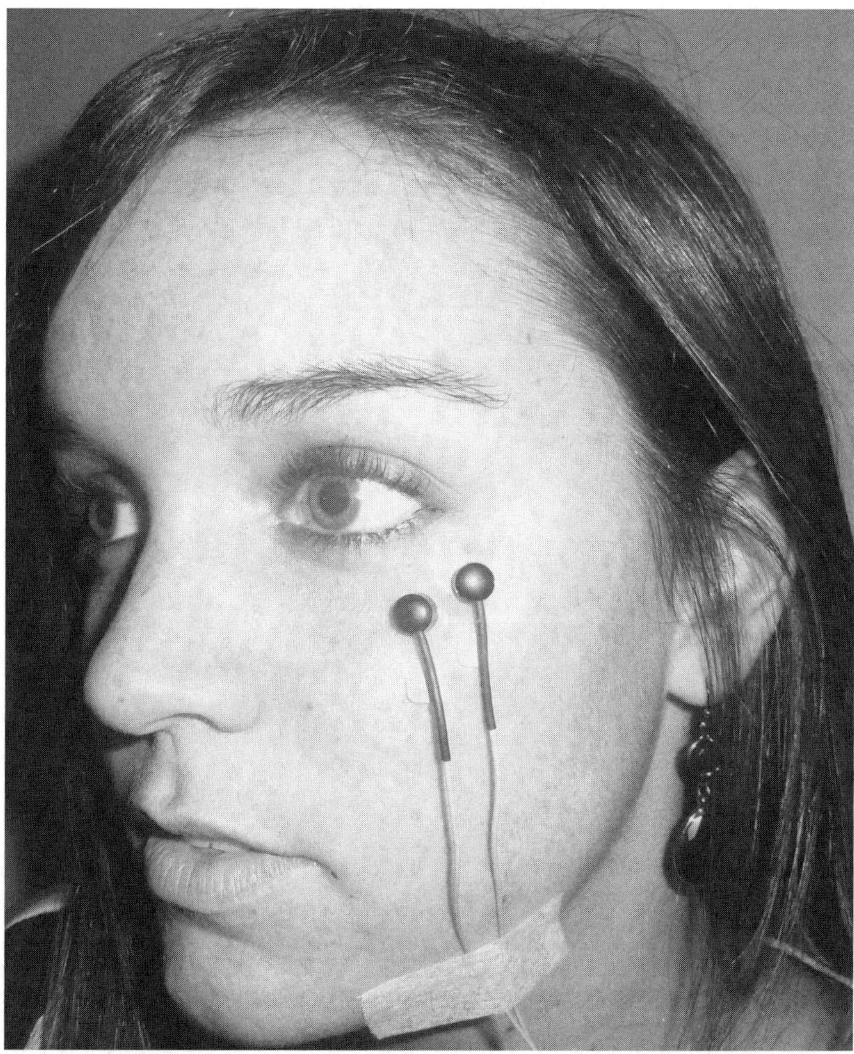

FIGURE 5.6b Electrode placement for recording activity from the orbicularis oculi region. "The first electrode is affixed 1cm inferior to the exocanthion (outer commissure of the eye fissure). The second electrode is placed 1cm medial to, and slightly inferior to, the first, so that the electrode pair runs parallel to the lower edge of the eyelid." Fridlund & Cacioppo, 1986, p. 572.

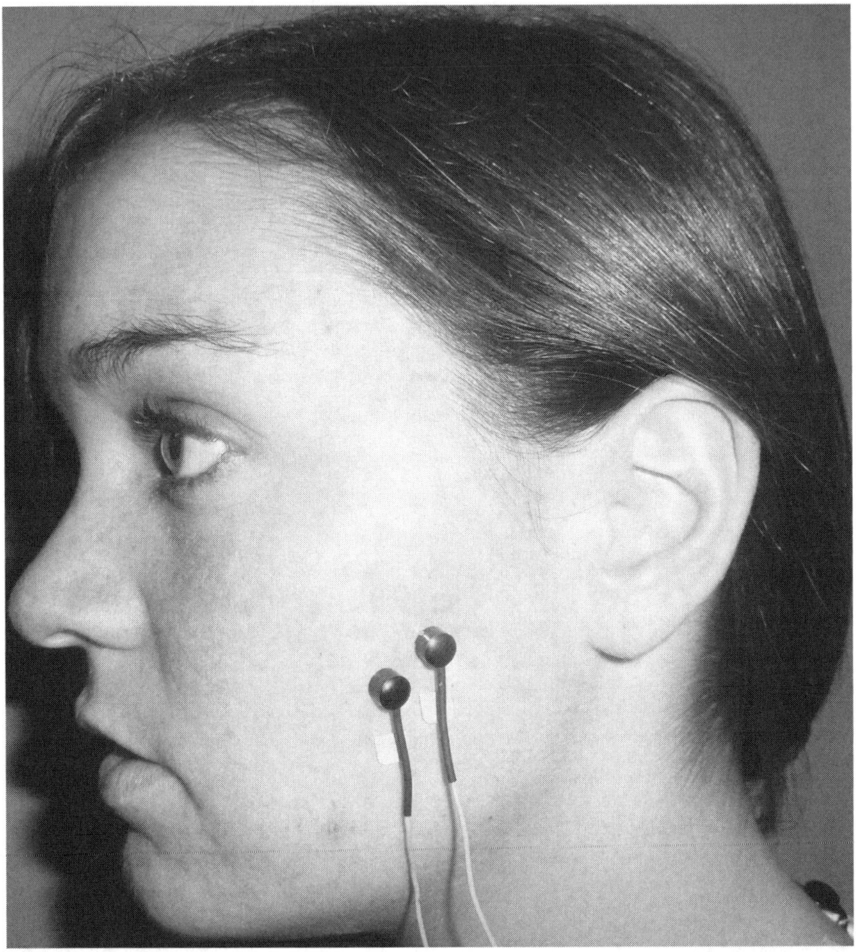

FIGURE 5.6c Electrode placement for recording activity from the zygomaticus major region. "One electrode is placed midway along an imaginary line joining the cheilion and the preauricular depression (the bony dimple above the posterior edge of the zygomatic arch), and the second electrode is placed 1cm inferior and medial to the first (i.e., toward the mouth) along the same imaginary line." Fridlund & Cacioppo, 1986, p. 572.

Analysis of facial EMG data

Media psychology researchers who use facial EMG to index the valence of emotional processing evoked by media content are typically interested in analyzing changes in the experience of pleasant and unpleasant emotion across time during exposure to some form of media content. The rectified and smoothed facial EMG signal is typically sampled and digitized by the AD/DA board and the choice of sampling rate should be driven by the need to capture meaningful variation in muscle activity. In our own work we have used a sampling rate of 20 Hz. Researchers then typically average the digitized signal over a selected period of time. Signal averaging was previously discussed in the section on skin conductance data analysis. Here the same principle applies: researchers choose a time period over which to average data that captures meaningful variation in the facial EMG signal, given the media content being studied.

The analysis of facial EMG data, regardless of the time period over which data is to be analyzed, should be conducted using change scores. Facial EMG change scores should be calculated as change from some initial baseline level of electrical activity in the muscle region from which activity was recorded. It will never be the case that a participant's facial muscles are completely inactive so some thought must be given to how to obtain a useful indicator of baseline activity that can be used to calculate change scores. One possibly useful way to obtain a measure of baseline activity could be to record facial EMG during a resting session prior to participants being exposed to any experimental stimulus messages. The length of this resting time should be long enough to obtain a good indicator of resting levels of activation when participants are not processing any media messages but not so long that participants become bored and begin to get restless and even experience unpleasant emotional states. The other potential problem with this is that early on in an experiment participants may still be somewhat uncomfortable with having electrodes on their face such that this resting period does not represent a true baseline level of muscle activity. In our own work we have attained measures of baseline activity prior to the onset of each stimulus message in an experiment. This has the advantage of providing a comparison point for each individual stimulus in the study. A third alternative to obtaining baseline activity would be to measure facial EMG during exposure to some neutral media stimulus to which you might not expect significant levels of pleasant and/or unpleasant emotional experience. The overall point of this discussion is that the valid analysis of facial EMG data does require significant thought ahead of time to obtain the best indicator of baseline activity from which to calculate change scores.

Facial EMG data collected as a psychophysiological indicator of the valence of emotional processing engaged by media content is typically analyzed by submitting it to a repeated measures ANOVA. Analyses can be performed on data averaged over a meaningful time period for each message or averaged across entire messages in an experiment. The emotional complexity of most media content presents an argument in favor of analyzing facial EMG across multiple discrete units of time for every stimulus message; however analysis of facial EMG data collapsed across entire messages has also proven insightful in previous research. Theoretically it could also be interesting to perform a peak analysis on facial EMG data—analyzing the highest level of corrugator supercilii, zygomaticus major, and orbicularis oculi muscle activity evoked by messages in the different independent variable conditions in an experiment.

Review of recent facial EMG research on emotional processing of media

The use of facial EMG as a psychophysiological indicator of the valence of emotional processing evoked by media content has substantially taken off since the initial work by Hazlett and Hazlett (1999) and Bolls et al. (2001) which sought to demonstrate the value of facial EMG as a psychophysiological measure of emotional valence evoked by television and radio advertisements. This initial media research on facial EMG did indeed demonstrate the validity and reliability of facial EMG by showing that zygomaticus major muscle activity increased during exposure to messages with pleasant emotional tone and corrugator supercilii muscle activity increased during exposure to messages with unpleasant emotional tone.

Since this initial work, scholars have used facial EMG to investigate the emotional impact of numerous content and structural features of media. For example, Ravaja et al. (2006b) examined the influence of mood on processing of media messages presented on small screens that are typical of modern mobile devices used to access the Internet. They found participants in a depressed mood displayed higher orbicularis oculi muscle activity while reading text messages on smaller screens compared to viewing video and that the reverse was true for participants in a joyful mood. Zygomaticus major, orbicularis oculi, and corrugator supercilii muscle activity has also been used to study the emotional experience of participants playing a first-person shooter video game. This line of research has found significant differences in the phasic activity of these muscles for different segments of the game. Wounding and killing an opponent was found to result in a decrease of zygomaticus major and orbicularis oculi muscle activity while the wounding and death of one's own character was found to result in a decrease of corrugator supercilii activity and simultaneous increase in both zygomaticus major and orbicularis oculi activity (Ravaja et al., 2008). Lee and Lang (2009), in an interesting experiment that merged both the dimensional and discrete theoretical perspectives of emotion, investigated how facial EMG as an indicator of emotional valence varied during exposure to video messages with content reflecting discrete affective feelings—joy, fear, sadness, and anger. They found significantly higher levels of corrugator supercilii activity compared to a neutral message during exposure to video content reflecting fear and anger. This is only a small sample of experiments where facial EMG has been used to gain deep insight into the valence of emotional processing as it unfolds across time according to very specific components of media content and structural features. Other researchers have also used facial EMG to identify the presence of discrete affective feelings like happiness, anger, and disgust (Ekman, Friesen, & Ancoli, 1980; Ekman, Levenson, & Friesen, 1983). Of all the psychophysiological measures, facial EMG does indeed show the greatest promise in terms of being able to distinctly identify the occurrence of discrete affective feelings. One particularly interesting stream of psychophysiological research targeted at identifying specific patterns of facial

EMG associated with discrete affective feelings has been focused on discovering specific facial muscles activated according to the experience and expression of disgust (Stark, Walter, Schienle, & Vaitl, 2005; Vrana, 1993). Media psychology researchers can be excited about the promise of facial EMG to possibly identify the presence of discrete affective feeling states because ultimately a significant part of our emotional experience evoked by media includes the presence of affective feeling states—things that make us angry, sad, disgusted, or happy.

Summary

In this chapter we have outlined a detailed theoretical perspective on human emotion and the value of studying emotion as motivational activation in media psychology research. We have covered two important psychophysiological measures of emotional processing—skin conductance and facial EMG—that have been proven to be extremely valuable in understanding the emotional impact of media. Skin conductance reflects variation in sweat gland activity due to activation of the sympathetic nervous system and is a valid and reliable measure of emotional arousal. Facial EMG involves recording summed motor unit action potentials underlying facial muscle activity and is a highly sensitive measure of emotional valence due to variation in appetitive and aversive motivation activation.

We see numerous opportunities for future research to use these measures to gain in-depth insight into mental processing of media content in an increasingly emotional and constantly changing media environment. The best research will not only validly apply the measures that we have discussed in this chapter to studying processing of emotional media content but will also draw on the exciting work being done by our colleagues in neuropsychology who are constantly learning more about the physiological and experiential basis of human emotion. This approach will position researchers at the forefront of understanding emerging issues and trends in psychophysiological measurement so that their work can tap psychophysiological measures in theoretically exciting ways that have yet to be extensively applied in media psychology research—a topic we turn to in the next chapter.

6

EMERGING PSYCHOPHYSIOLOGICAL MEASURES FOR MEDIA RESEARCH

The most common psychophysiological measures utilized in the media psychology laboratory were discussed in the previous two chapters. When researchers want to obtain a dynamic indicator of cognitive processing of mediated messages they turn to heart rate and, occasionally, the EEG. When emotion is the construct of interest skin conductance and facial EMG are often used. As the field grows, however, media researchers are discovering new measures by reading publications arising from psychophysiological experiments conducted in cognitive psychology and neuroscience labs. While many of these measures have been validated within a more basic research experimental paradigm, their applicability to longer-form stimuli such as media messages is only beginning to be explored.

This chapter is designed to introduce you to several of these emerging measures or techniques. It will follow the same general format of Chapters 4 and 5: first briefly discussing the conceptual understanding and biological basis of the measure, then providing some basic operational information about how data are collected using the measure, and finally presenting a summary of several recent media psychology studies that utilize the measure to help open the black box of mediated message processing.

The eye-blink startle response

Picture this: it is late October and a fraternity house on your campus has decided to host a Halloween haunted house. They have taken an all-purpose ballroom in your student union and created a makeshift maze through which you must weave your way, as an array of zombies, ghosts, and ghouls jump out at you. At the front entrance you and your friends pay the charity donation and enter into the darkened first corridor. Inching along the dark passageway you *know* that something is soon to happen . . . will it jump out at you . . . or drop from the ceiling . . . or scream . . . or *what?!?* And then, from the depths of a formerly hidden corner, a strobe light starts spasmodically flashing, revealing a blood-stained skeleton! At exactly the same time a loud cackling scream blurts at full volume from a set of speakers behind the artificial wall. What do you and your friends do? That's right, even though you *knew* it was coming you likely jerked in a full-body startle. *That's* the Startle Response (SR). Just like the Orienting Response (OR), discussed at some length in previous chapters, the SR is an automatic response—meaning that you can't keep it from happening. (Which is why, at the haunted house, you shouldn't believe your friend who says, "It didn't scare me!" It did . . . even if only for a few milliseconds.)

Conceptual understanding of startle

The SR is similar to another automatic response we extensively covered in earlier chapters—the Orienting Response (OR)—which you'll remember was a momentary automatic allocation of cognitive resources to encoding something new in the environment. The SR is like the Orienting Response in that it is automatic and pre-conscious. However, startle is marked by important differences —both conceptually and physiologically—from orienting responses (Graham, 1979). Conceptually, while the OR is all about information intake to the cognitive system, the SR is designed as a system interrupt, bringing a halt to all processing in order to martial resources required to protect the organism from something dire and threatening in the environment. Physiologically, the SR is different, too. While the OR was identified by heart rate deceleration following the eliciting stimulus, the SR is primarily a sympathetically driven response and as a result heart rate levels significantly increase when the organism is startled (Graham, 1979; Bradley & Lang, 2007a). Other bodily indications of a startle response were well documented by Landis and Hunt (1939) who took high-speed photographs—anywhere from 200 to 3,000 frames per second—of research subjects startled by the firing of a pistol into the air just behind their heads! Their responses were marked by a "blinking of the eyes, head movement forward, a characteristic facial expression, raising and drawing forward of the shoulders, abductions of the upper arms, bending of the elbows, pronation of the lower arms, flexion of the fingers, forward movement of the trunk, contraction of the abdomen, and bending of the knees" (Landis & Hunt, 1939, p. 21). The most consistent indicator of an SR is the rapid and defensive closing of the eyelid— the blink. In fact, the eye-blink is such a strong indicator of the startle response that it is measurable even when an aversive stimulus is not strong enough to evoke other noticeable bodily responses (Lang, Bradley, & Cuthbert, 1990).

While almost universally recognized as an interrupt system, there has been some debate about what generally causes changes in the amplitude of the startle eye-blink. The discussion centers on whether the startle indexes attention being paid to the environment or the emotional valence associated with it. In accord with the underlying assumptions of the psychophysiological approach covered in Chapters 1 and 2, the answer depends upon where in the dynamic cognitive processing task you place the startle probe itself. A brief but chronological presentation of some early startle research will show how this is the case.

In the 1970s and 1980s, **Frances Graham** conceptualized the SR as an indicator of the amount of attention a subject paid to an external stimulus (Anthony & Graham, 1985; Graham, 1975, 1979). Thankfully, the methodology had advanced considerably since the time of Landis and Hunt, and the pistol had been replaced—most often by a brief pulse of white noise or flash from a strobe light. Many of Graham's experiments utilized an experimental design known as the *pre-pulse paradigm*. In it, something occurred—such as the onset of a quiet tone— just before the startle pulse. This occurrence was the pre-pulse and it provided just enough environmental novelty to produce a cardiac orienting response (Bohlin & Graham, 1977). The associated automatic allocation of cognitive resources to encoding, in fact, was found to impact the magnitude of a subsequent startle response. However, the direction of that impact—whether it made the startle response get larger or smaller compared to control conditions without pre-pulse—depended upon how much time elapsed between the pre-pulse and the startle probe (Graham, 1975). On the one hand, if the lead time was extremely short (< 250ms) the startle response was smaller than controls. Graham interpreted this finding by suggesting the initial automatic allocation of cognitive resources to encoding elicited by the OR was "protected" from interruption. In other words, the brain had evolved in such a way that the first 250ms following an OR was devoted exclusively to the processing of the novelty the eliciting stimulus had evoked and not even a noxious burst of white noise could penetrate.

In other studies, however, Graham and colleagues found intriguing and somewhat opposite results when the time interval between the pre-pulse and the startle probe was longer (1,200 or 2,000ms). If the long durations were allowed to vary, the startle response to the white-noise probe was substantially larger than controls and did not habituate. However, if the startle probe always occurred after a standard long duration the eye-blink was initially larger but eventually habituated to such an extent that the overall mean showed no differences compared to controls without pre-pulses (Graham, Putnam, & Leavitt, 1975). Here the interpretation was that when the intervals were allowed to vary the pre-pulse informed subjects that a startle probe was coming but not when it would occur. As a result, they devoted sustained controlled attention to anticipating its arrival, which led to a potentiated eye-blink. In experiments where the interval was constant, however, the subjects eventually learned that the pre-pulse signaled exactly when a startle probe was coming. This resulted in less anticipatory attention being paid by subjects and a lack of potentiation in the startle response.

In the early 1990s, **Peter J. Lang** and colleagues at the University of Florida (Lang et al., 1990) began to explore if other variables could impact eye-blink amplitudes at long intervals following onset of a startle probe. Hopefully you remember Lang from Chapter 5 as a key figure in the dimensional view of emotion. Also remember that in this approach the central components of any emotional experience are best viewed using a biological framework of organism motivation. In other words, we are motivated to approach things that are good and avoid things that are bad. "*Valence* refers to the organism's disposition to assume either an appetitive or defensive behavioral set. *Arousal* refers to the organism's disposition to react with varying degrees of energy or force" (Lang et al., 1990, p. 380, italics in original). Suggesting "that attentional effects [of startle] cannot be clearly assessed if the emotional valence of foreground and probe are ignored" (Lang et al., 1990, p. 380) they conducted an experiment to explore the impact of valence on eye-blink. In it subjects sat in front of a computer screen and viewed pictures for six seconds that were either pleasant (smiling baby, chocolate sundae, nude), unpleasant (starving child, slashed face, snake), or neutral (rolling pin, neutral face, city building). The eye-blink startle responses were measured using both auditory and visual probes. The results showed that compared to neutral images, eye-blink magnitude was suppressed during positive image viewing and enhanced during negative image viewing. This was even the case when there was a modality mismatch; that is, when the startle probes were an auditory burst during the visual stimulus.

It may be of interest to media psychology researchers that these valence-based hypotheses were subsequently tested using longer duration motion picture clips instead of still images. Jansen and Fridja (1994) explored startle responses to white noise bursts during neutral travel films, climactic scenes from horror films, or pornographic films designed to appeal to women. The startle probes occurred either 10, 30, or 50 seconds after the beginning of the film segments. Results showed that, similar to Lang et al. (1990), the startle response was enhanced for the probes occurring in the horror films but smaller during the erotic and neutral films. Interestingly, the startle responses during erotica were not significantly different than those during travel films—contrary to the prediction that would be suggested by Lang et al. (1990). Jansen and Fridja suggest that this may be due to negative affective response that some subjects associated with watching the pornography in an experimental setting. Kaviani, Gray, Checkley, Kumari, and Wilson (1999) added support for this by showing smaller startle responses during clips of ice dancing or the slapstick comedy *Mr. Bean* compared to neutral clips of household items and street scenes. Interestingly, they also found a different response to negatively valenced film clips, with startle responses during them actually reduced in a manner similar to the positive film clips. An analysis of responses to the two individual scenes used as negative content showed that a *fictional* scene taken from a commercially-available gangster film elicited the predicted increase in startle response but a clip from an educational film showing actual toe surgery resulted in smaller startle responses. Media researchers may find this an interesting launching point for future studies looking at startle responses elicited during the affective processing of media events believed to be fictional compared to those believed factual or that examine nuances in mediated portrayals of threat such as severity and vulnerability.

So, does the eye-blink startle response assess attention or emotion? More recent research (Bradley, Cuthbert, & Lang, 1993; Vanman, Boehmelt, Dawnson, & Schell, 1996) confirms Graham's notion of inhibited startle as a result of increased attentional resources applied to processing a complex stimulus—such as the onset of a still image—as long as the probe occurs quite quickly after the onset (Graham, 1980). Bradley et al. (1993), for example, administered startle probes to subjects at 300ms, 800ms, 1,300ms, and 3,800ms while they looked at pleasant, neutral, and unpleasant still images for six seconds. Results show that early in the dynamic processing of the content—at the 300 and 800ms point—the attentional task of making sense of the image onset suppressed the eye-blink for the complex emotional images compared to the simple neutral ones. However, late in the process—at 1,300 and 3,800ms—the valence manipulation predominated with eye-blinks increasing linearly from pleasant to neutral to unpleasant images. So, this brief "zone of protection" concept following an OR is widely accepted. There is about 250ms after a pre-pulse when the encoding subprocess cannot be disturbed by the interrupt function of the startle response (Graham, 1980). Similarly recognized is that outside this time window the amplitude of an eye-blink provides an index of the emotional valence of the foreground situation the subject finds themselves in (Bradley, Maxian, Wise, & Freeman, 2008).

Measuring eye-blink startle

There are researchers who have spent a career investigating the startle response and perfecting measurement techniques. It is, therefore, impossible for the entire list of considerations to be covered in this section. You should be sure to consult other excellent discussions of the measure prior to beginning your own startle data collection research program. Suggestions for further reference include the chapter on EMG from *The handbook of psychophysiology* (Tassinary, Cacioppo, & Vanman, 2007) and the published official guidelines from the Society for Psychophysiological Research (Blumenthal, Cuthbert, Filion, Hackley, Lipp, & Van Boxtel, 2005). Still, what follows are basic measurement considerations implemented in our own labs which have been influenced by these larger instructional sources.

Electrode preparation—much of what could be said about the selection of electrodes for the eye-blink startle measure is a reiteration of the section on EMG recording in Chapter 5. The electrodes used to measure eye-blink are collecting the motor unit action potentials of the orbicularis oculi muscle located just below the eye. Because of its placement in proximity to the eye (and the importance of *seeing* mediated messages when cognitively processing them), the small 4mm diameter Ag/AgCL electrodes are recommended for this measure. Remember that the skin conductance measure is the only one where you do not want to artificially inflate the electrical signal in the electrode; in all the others—including the eye-blink measure—your goal is to boost the very tiny bioelectrical signal that comes from deep within the body as much as you can. So, just like other EMG recordings you fill the cup electrode with high-conductivity electrolyte gel or use disposables that are pre-gelled.

The electrodes are attached with double-sided adhesive collars. It is recommended that you trim the edges of these collars as closely as possible while still allowing for good adhesion to the subject's skin. This is because, as noted in Chapter 5, electrodes are placed between one to two centimeters from each other in order to minimize cross-talk from other muscle activity in the very crowded area surrounding the eye. Be careful that when adhering the collars to the skin surface you do not allow them to touch as this may result in unnecessary movement artifact in the data as the collars scrape against each other during the recording session. A similar caution concerns the combination of close proximity of the startle electrodes, their small size, and the very tiny amount of electrode gel needed to fill them. Because the electrode cup used around the eye is so small, when filling it with gel it is easy to have the feeling "that can't possibly be enough." It is. Do not overfill the cups and be sure to have a toothpick handy to scrape off excess. If you have too much gel spilling out of the cups and onto the collars, and you place those collars very close to each other, the possibility exists of making a bridge of gel between the two. This, in a sense, turns them into a single electrode taking one reading. Remember, in almost every media psycho-physiology lab you will be taking bipolar measurements, where the bioamplifier is comparing the readings across two electrodes. This is very hard to do if the presence of too much gel makes the bioamplifier think there is only a single one there.

Skin preparation—the general skin preparation procedures for EMG discussed in Chapter 5 should be followed when measuring startle, with a few addendums. When preparing the skin *above* the eyebrow for measurement of the corrugator muscle as an index of valence, Chapter 5 suggests using a skin preparation pad soaked in isopropyl alcohol and pumice specifically designed to remove dead skin prior to physiological recording. The SPR recommendations for preparing the skin *below* the eye for measuring the orbicularis, on the other hand, stress that while isopropyl alcohol may be a fine preparatory agent—provided you tell the subjects before applying it and have them close their eyes to avoid fume irritation—the abrasive pumice is too harsh for the area. This is particularly of importance given the influence of negative affective states on the startle amplitude mentioned above. For this reason, some researchers also forego the use of isopropyl alcohol as an agent for orbicularis skin preparation as well.

The goal of thorough skin preparation is to reduce the impedance in the signal coming from the electrode to as low a level as possible. Getting low impedance is sometimes difficult and one must weigh the amount of time spent on skin preparation against a number of other factors such as the total number of electrodes you must apply, the duration of your experimental protocol, and the demeanor of the research participant. Here is a suggested skin preparation procedure for the eye-blink startle:

1. gently rub the lower lid with a paper towel dampened with distilled water, removing makeup and dead skin;
2. dry the area with a few more passes of a dry paper towel;
3. rub a *very small amount* (e.g., the size of an unpopped corn kernel) of electrolyte gel into the area using your finger, allowing it to begin penetrating the skin to the level of the motor neurons;
4. once again take a dry paper towel and use it to dry the excess gel from the surface of the skin to avoid making a bridge between the two electrodes.

Again, this is certainly a fair number of steps and it is not guaranteed to result in acceptably low impedance levels. However, taking the time to prepare the skin for the best possible signal strength—when measuring *any* EMG signal but particularly eye-blink startle—will result in much cleaner and easier to interpret data in the end.

Electrode placement—when putting the electrodes on a subject in a startle experiment it is probably best to first make a mental note of what their eye does while it blinks. Make this observation casually, perhaps while explaining the nature of the study to the subject. This is because everyone's anatomy around the area of the eye is different and individual adjustments to the general placement guidelines may be necessary (Blumenthal et al., 2005). But, generally speaking, begin the application of the electrodes by asking the subject to look straight ahead. Place the first electrode on the lower portion of the eyelid on the muscle just below the pupil. Be sure the electrode is on the OO muscle itself and above the bone of the eye socket. The second electrode will be placed in the direction of the subject's ear, along the half-moon shape of the muscle. The recommended distance between the center of the two electrode cups is 1–2cm (Blumenthal et al., 2005).

The electrodes may be placed under the left or the right eye as long as the audio startle probe is delivered to both ears. However, it is also suggested that for the sake of unified experimental protocol that the same eye is used across subjects. It is interesting to note that most published studies seem to use the subject's left eye, likely because the researchers are right-handed and have easier access.

Probe elicitation—although the startle response can be elicited by a variety of stimuli such as visual strobe or tactile stimulation, the majority of startle studies rely on auditory bursts delivered through headphones or speakers (Blumenthal et al., 2005). The duration of the burst is extremely short, usually 50ms, and contrary to what you may think the important attribute of the burst is not only its volume (technically referred to as the *intensity* of the sound) but also how long it takes the probe to reach its full level of intensity—a concept known as *rise time*. Auditory probes with as close to instantaneous rise times as possible, and an intensity level of 100 decibels (db) are often used to evoke the startle. Most psychophysiological equipment vendors (see Chapter 8) can provide noise generators that produce both pure tones and white noise bursts fitting these criteria. However, work by Blumenthal has shown that the white noise is more reliable at generating the startle response (Blumenthal & Berg, 1986; Blumenthal & Goode, 1991). He has also shown that bursts need not be as loud as 100 db to reliably elicit startle, suggesting that intensities in the area of 50–85 db should be sufficient (Blumenthal et al., 2005). Individual researchers should pretest their equipment to determine how the acoustic properties of the lab space, the headphones being used, and the media stimuli interact in order to find the intensity level that reliably results in eye-blink.

The use of headphones to deliver startle response seems to be most common in the media psychology literature. Although headphones may physically interfere with electrode leads and result in problematic movement artifact, this allows for assurance that the audio portion of the media content, along with the probe itself, is heard by the subject in what may be a busy lab environment. Furthermore, the task of pointing speakers to ensure a startle probe of the proper intensity and frequency range for each individual subject can be a trickier proposition than just having them wear headphones.

Signal acquisition—much of what was discussed about EMG signal acquisition in Chapter 5—amplification, rectification, and integration—also applies to the collection of startle response data. However, the initial amplitude of the eye-blink can be much greater than the signal generated by the corrugator or zygomatic muscles. Therefore, special attention must be paid to the amount of amplification you give to the signal. This has to do with the conversion of the analog bioelectrical signal to a digital signal by the AD/DA converter. Essentially, AD/DA converters have ceiling thresholds, and if you amplify the startle response too much the upper end of the response will be "maxed out" if it is amplified to a level above what the converter can handle. Blumenthal et al. (2005) offer two suggestions to avoid this. The easiest is to make sure, if you plan to measure startle response in your lab, that you purchase a high-resolution AD/DA converter—one that is 16 or 24 bits will be sufficient. The second suggestion is to present sample startle trials to the subject. This not only familiarizes them with the phenomenon prior to the actual experiment, but allows you to decrease the amplification if the startle responses obtained in the sample trials are too great to be properly converted to digital data.

Another issue concerning the AD/DA converter when measuring startle is the sampling rate. As mentioned in Chapter 5, a common sampling rate for typical EMG recording is 20 Hz. However, the startle response occurs so rapidly after the probe onset that sampling this slowly may result in missing the response altogether. Sampling rates of at least 1,000 Hz are recommended to capture the eye-blink startle response. If storage capacity is an issue . . . and it likely would be if, for example, you sampled all your EMG data at 1,000 Hz for the duration of an episode of a sitcom . . . you can sample at a lower rate for most of the stimuli and shift to a greater sampling rate for the 1,000ms before and after the startle probe.

Quantifying the startle response—most researchers quantify startle with the assistance of a computer algorithm written to detect significant increases in the slope of the EMG signal within a specific time window. Remember in Chapter 1 we mentioned how easy it is to forget that a person's physiological activity has a lot more to do with keeping them alive than with responding to your media stimuli. That's important to mention at the beginning of this discussion because human beings blink for a wide variety of reasons other than to respond to a burst of white noise. That is why the first thing to do when looking at a presumed startle response identified by any computer algorithm is to explore its temporal relationship to the probe onset. If the eye-blink is in response to the burst of white noise, you will see the EMG signal starting to increase between 21 and 80ms in adults (Blumenthal, Elden, & Flatten, 2004). Other research suggests a slightly longer window, up to 120ms, for wider age ranges (Balaban, Losito, Simons, & Graham, 1986). If you have a blink that happens earlier or later than that in relation to the probe onset, you just happened to record a blink that was more likely due to moistening eyeballs than a measure of emotion or attention.

Not every startle probe results in an identifiable or quantifiable eye-blink. Sometimes there is no response at all; other times there is too much noise or movement artifact to be able to determine the peak amplitude of the response from baseline. Either of these cases is referred to as **non–response trials** or flat responses. However, when there is a consistent baseline and a peak that satisfies some substantial increase in slope then the response is scored by quantifying that increase. Definitions for "substantial increase" vary from multiples of a baseline level to a set increase in microVolts within specific time windows (Blumenthal et al., 2005). Sometimes there will be multiple increases in slope following a single trial and Blumenthal et al. (2005) suggest that the maximum amplitude be counted as a peak "unless the EMG response line has returned to baseline for a long enough time that the later peaks are not considered components of the stimulus–elicited response" (p. 10). Because of the subjective nature of this determination, rules should be established as to what constitutes significant amplitude to justify response and how to deal with multiple peaks. Ideally, also, scoring of startle responses should be done blind to treatment condition.

Mean startle response is calculated for subjects across levels of independent variables. These means can either include a value of 0 for non-responses (in which case the mean is called the average **magnitude**) or can exclude non-responses from the calculations altogether (called the average **amplitude**). For reasons that are not yet understood, there is a substantial difference between individuals on the size of the startle response and some do not respond at all. For that reason, many researchers reduce the risk of having results unduly influenced by a few individuals by transforming startle data into standardized values—most typically z or T scores.

Recent startle research in media psychology

Several studies have recently applied the eye-blink startle measure to the understanding of media message processing. For example, in a series of studies S. D. Bradley and colleagues (Bradley, 2007a; Bradley, Maxian, Wise, & Freeman, 2008) showed subjects one of two episodes from the primetime medical drama *ER*. These episodes had been previously coded for emotional valence by pretest subjects using a Continuous Response Measurement tool (CRM is discussed in further detail in Chapter 7). This identified the most positive, the most negative, and the most neutral scenes in the episodes. They then located 12 points in scenes from each of these valence levels and placed auditory bursts to elicit the startle response. The results overall confirmed the ability of startle to be used as an indication of valence, or more specifically motivational system activation, during television viewing (Bradley, 2007a). Overall, the largest eye-blinks were during negative emotional scenes, the smallest during positive, and neutral scenes resulted in responses somewhere in the middle.

Bradley (2007a) also tests another interesting hypothesis, namely whether the presence of a camera change in a television program can be considered a pre-pulse stimulus with the resulting startle responses indexing attention more than emotional valence. This is a theory-based question, of course, because previous work has shown that people orient to camera changes (Lang, 1990; Lang, Geiger, Strickwerda, & Sumner, 1993), and that startle probes immediately following orienting to a pre-pulse are attenuated due to the so-called "zone of protection." So, Bradley varied the location of the auditory startle probes to occur either more quickly (133 and 267ms) or slowly (1,000 and 1,300ms) after a camera change. Results show that there was a significant interaction between where the probe was placed in regards to a camera change and the emotional valence of the programming in which it was placed. Essentially, the ability to differentiate motivation system activation got less precise the closer the probe was placed to the preceding camera change. In a subsequent study (Bradley et al., 2008) the camera change was replaced by a more traditional auditory pre-pulse with similar results. The takeaway point from this pair of early studies using the measure to assess television processing is that it seems to be a robust index of motivational/emotional state rather than attention—with increases in startle response associated with aversive activation and decreases (compared to neutral) associated with appetitive activation. A methodological matter worth remembering from Bradley's work, however, is that researchers should be diligent and methodical in the placement of their auditory startle probes, ensuring onset occurs between 800–1,000ms after a camera change or other structural feature thought to result in an orienting response.

The auditory startle probe has also been recently shown to adequately index emotional response to auditory stimuli (Roy, Mailhot, Gosselin, Paquette, & Peretz, 2009). In this study, six 100s excerpts of music that had been pre-rated for arousal and valence were selected so that three were arousing/pleasant and three were arousing/unpleasant. Results show larger startle responses occurred during the unpleasant music compared to the pleasant. Furthermore, negative music resulted in startle responses with faster **latency**—in other words, the increase in EMG slope occurred sooner following the probe bursts—than the positive music.

The post-auricular startle response

Another measure elicited by a startle probe has recently appeared in the media psychophysiological literature. The **post-auricular muscle** is located behind the ear, attaching the **pinna** to the skin of the head. When activated, the muscle pulls the ear up and to the back. It has been shown that the muscle activates in a reflexive manner to an auditory startle probe (Benning, Patrick, & Lang, 2004), a phenomenon known as the Post-Auricular Response (PAR). In comparison to a neutral emotional setting, the PAR has been shown to be larger when elicited during positive emotional foreground and smaller during negative (Benning et al., 2004; Hess, Sabourin, & Kleck, 2007).

Although they can be collected concurrently, measuring the PAR is slightly different than measuring the eyeblink startle at the orbicularis oculi. First, there are practical considerations such as special disposable ear-bud style headphones must be used due to the placement of the electrodes on the post-auricular muscle. The electrodes themselves must be smaller than the typical EMG recording electrodes and are designed specifically for PAR measurement. There are differences in data cleaning and analysis, too. The PAR is considered a "micro-reflex," in that it cannot be seen in a single trial (Sparks & Lang, 2010). This means that the aggregation of many more trials is necessary to separate the PAR from the noise in the EMG signal. In that way it is similar to the Event-Related Potential in the EEG signal discussed in Chapter 4. The latency is also much shorter for PAR than for the eye-blink, with responses occurring 9–11ms after the startle probe.

In a recent study, Sparks and Lang (2010) applied the findings from still-image studies to the question of what the PAR could be measuring when elicited during television viewing. One possibility was that the PAR could be simultaneously measuring the appetitive and aversive systems just like the eye–blink startle measure: when a subject was in a positive state the PAR would go up, when in a negative state it would go down. The other possibility was the PAR assesses activation of only the appetitive system. If that were the case Sparks and Lang expected the data to show that PARs during arousing positive messages should be greater than those during calm positive messages, and both arousing and calm negative messages. In the experiment they showed subjects 30 television commercials. Twelve of them had been selected by pretest to be in one of the four valence/arousal categories. The data support the interpretation that PAR indexes appetitive motivation activation only, uninhibited by the presence of aversive activation. Obviously, with only a single published study in media psychology, substantial potential remains for investigating how this measure can help peer into the "black box."

Another facial EMG measure: Levator labii

Recall from the discussion in Chapter 5, psychophysiological measures of emotional processing appear to be more reliable and valid indicators of dimensions of emotion rather than specific affective feelings. The psychophysiological measure of emotional processing that does appear to have much promise in the ability to discriminate the presence of discrete affective feelings is facial EMG. Some of the most extensive theorizing about the connection between facial expressions and emotion has been done by **Paul Ekman**, who proposed that there are groups of distinct facial muscle movements which are representative of the expression of specific affective feelings such as anger, sadness, and disgust (Ekman, 1993). In theory, this means that a media psychology researcher wishing to study the experience of specific affective feelings evoked by mediated messages could use facial EMG to index activity in specific facial muscles reliably associated with discrete affective feelings. It should be noted, however, that there is still significant debate over the theoretical and practical possibilities of this approach (Hess, 2009). That being said, there have been some notable examples of impressive efforts by psychophysiologists attempting to identify specific patterns of facial EMG response that reliably reflect specific feelings (Scherer & Ellgring, 2007). Unfortunately for media researchers who wish to use facial EMG to index specific feelings, most of this work has ended up primarily offering further support to the notion that psychophysiological measures primarily respond to the arousal and valence dimensions of emotion. On the other hand, there is one facial muscle that seems to reliably index the presence of a specific emotion. The Levator labii muscle group connects your lower nostril to the upper lip and has been found to be activated in response to disgust eliciting stimuli (Chapman, Kim, Susskind, & Anderson, 2009; Vrana, 1993; Yartz & Hawk, 2002).

Disgust is a theoretically interesting specific emotion emerging from aversive motivational activation. It represents a unique form of defensive response to stimuli perceived as revolting or impure (Woody & Teachman, 2000). Nabi (2002) further described disgust as an important theoretical concept for media psychology researchers by distinguishing it from a form of disgust that is more akin to anger than actual disgust—that is, more related to the colloquial notion of being "grossed out" or "nauseated." Psychologists who study disgust have identified specific categories of elicitors related to food contamination, certain animals, body products, violations of the body envelope (e.g., wounds), certain sexual acts, and hygiene (Haidt, McCauley, & Rozin, 1994). The levator labii muscle, along with the corrugator supercilii discussed in Chapter 5, appears to selectively respond to disgust. Given that images of stimuli that fall into established categories of disgust-elicitors appear with a fair amount of frequency in media content, media researchers may be very interested in a specific psychophysiological measure of this discrete emotion. One specific area of media research where this measure might be particularly useful is in studying cognitive and emotional processing of health campaign messages that seem to be including graphic negative visual images of disgusting nature (e.g., blood, wounds, diseased organs, etc.) with more frequency.

All the issues raised in Chapter 5 concerning the measurement of other facial EMG signals apply to the valid and reliable recording of activity from the levator labii. Bipolar recording of this muscle also involves the use of miniature electrodes placed as closely as possible without the housings touching. High conduction electrolyte gel is used. The general anatomical area where electrodes are placed for recording levator labii activity is just to the side of the nostril and above the corner of the lips. Fridlund and Cacioppo (1986) recommend placing the first electrode about 1cm lateral from the base of the nostril and the other approximately 1cm above the first (see Figure 5.5).

To date, no published studies exist that have purposefully measured levator labii muscle activity from a media psychology perspective. The most related work has measured activity in this muscle in response to disgust-related pictures with the objective of specifically drawing conclusions about the nature of human emotion rather than drawing conclusions about mediated message processing (Chapman et al., 2009; Yartz & Hawk, 2002). For example, Yartz and Hawk (2002) should give media psychology researchers some hope that this specific muscle might be useful in purposefully studying disgust-related content in mediated messages. However, researchers should also be prudent in applying the measure as disgust is a specific emotion for which the potential for significant individual variability has been noted (Haidt et al., 1994). Not to mention the fact that the very proposition of using the measurement of activity in any facial muscle to reliably index discrete emotion can be somewhat unpredictable. These limitations aside, the potential promise for a specific facial muscle like the levator labii to index discrete emotions represents a truly emerging application of psychophysiological measures that media psychology researchers ought to be aware of.

Heart rate variability (HRV)

An important characteristic of psychophysiological measures you may recall from earlier chapters of this book is that—with the exception of skin conductance which is solely innervated by the sympathetic nervous system—all the measures collected by a media psychophysiologist are simultaneously influenced by both the sympathetic and the parasympathetic nervous systems. One place where this is particularly problematic is when measuring cardiac activity in the form of beats-per-minute (Ravaja, 2004a). The parasympathetic influence on heart rate is one of deceleration due to attention increases, while the influence of the sympathetic nervous system is acceleration due to arousal increases. When considering mediated messages like television dramas, rock music, and computer games, understanding of any particular beats-per-minute value would certainly be improved by knowing the relative contribution of the two systems. This is, in fact, what measures collectively known as *heart rate variability* (HRV) provide.

As mentioned in Chapter 4, the collection of cardiac data often centers on the duration between the QRS-complex spikes in the bioelectrical signal generated by electrical activity of the beating heart. This duration is known as the Inter-beat Interval (IBI). Now, consider a string of these IBIs collected over a period of time while a person is exposed to a media message. Such a string might look something like this: 713, 777, 779, 812, 801, 756, 766, etc. Unlike an analog recording procedure, where the amount of time between signals is identical (e.g. at 20 Hz) there is a lot of variability in the duration between QRS peaks. HRV analyses explore the meaning behind that variability with a number of different metrics used to determine the different sympathetic and para-sympathetic influences. A good way of differentiating these metrics is by placing them into one of two categories described by Allen, Chambers, and Towers (2007) as "time-domain measures" or "frequency-domain measures."

Time-domain indices of HRV essentially calculate some measure of variation in the IBI values as a dataset. There has been a wide range of different time-domain quantifications employed. Some have been as simple as the standard deviation in the mean IBI value (Murray, Ewing, Campbell, Neilson, & Clarke, 1975), others slightly more involved such as that by Ewing, Borsey, Bellavere, and Clarke (1981) designed to calculate the percentage of occurrences when the absolute difference between successive IBIs in the series is greater than 50ms. Still others are complex and inaccessible like "the patented Porges–Bohrer algorithm with a moving polynomial that filters out nonrespiratory frequencies and removes non-stationarities" (Allen et al., 2007, p. 245). Allen et al. (2007) provides a web address to download the CMetX shareware program written especially to input IBI data and calculate a wide array of different time-domain HRV measures discussed in the literature as indicators of parasympathetic or sympathetic nervous system contributions.

In an early secondary analysis utilizing these HRV measures Koruth, Potter, Bolls, & Lang (2007) submitted the IBI data for subjects who listened to radio advertisements that were either positively or negatively valenced. Their results suggested that what had been previously interpreted as greater attention to the negative ads than the positive due to slower heart rates in beats-per-minute (Bolls, Lang, & Potter, 2001) actually resulted from significantly greater sympathetic activation for the positive ads compared to the negative. Koruth et al. (2007) suggest that this indicates a re-interpretation of the original data. However, their findings should be viewed cautiously as the design of the original experiment did not comply with established guidelines suggesting that the IBI data series for HRV analyses be at least two minutes in duration (Task Force, 1996).

Koruth (2010) addressed that design issue in an original study exploring the impact of increases in the number of camera changes in two-minute movie clips that were either positive or negative in emotional valence on time-domain HRV measures. Findings were less than promising for the HRV analysis, however, as "the results were incongruent with both the traditional [BPM] analysis and theory" (p. vii). Koruth suggests that this may be due to time-based HRV indices being summative and therefore not allowing for analysis of moment-to-moment change in emotional nuance indicative of television programming.

Frequency-domain indices of HRV take the series of IBI values and submits them to what is known as a **Fast-Fourier Transform** or FFT. Describing the intricacies of the FFT is beyond the scope of this chapter. But briefly, any complex waveform can be represented as the combination of simple periodic waveforms at different amplitudes. An FFT decomposes a complex waveform into the amplitudes—or strengths—of the specific frequency bands that make it up. When conducting an FFT analysis for heart rate variability the strengths of two frequency bands are of primary interest. The first is referred to as the Low Frequency (LF) which ranges from 0.04 to 0.15 Hz. There is debate over what LF actually measures (Task Force, 1996). Some believe it reflects sympathetic activation (Kamath & Fallen, 1993) while others feel that it continues to be the same intertwined contribution of sympathetic and parasympathetic influences (Akselrod et al., 1985).

The second band of interest, and one which is less controversially interpreted, is High Frequency (HF)—also referred to as Respiratory Sinus Arrhythmia (RSA). RSA, which ranges from above 0.15 to below 0.40 HZ, is considered an indication of parasympathetic control of the heart by the vagus nerve (Porges, 2007). A decrease in RSA compared to baseline suggests a period of sustained attention (Porges, 1991; Weber, Van der Molen, & Molenaar, 1994). From the field of psychophysiology several studies have attempted to use media messages as emotional stimuli to impact the strength of RSA with unclear results (Baldaro, Mazzetti, Codispoti, Tuozzi, Bolzani,

& Trombini, 2001; Kreibig, Wilhelm, Roth, & Gross, 2007). For example, Codispoti, Surcinelli, and Baldaro (2008) collected a variety of psycho-physiological responses, include RSA, while subjects watched three film clips: a nature film scene, a scene from a medical training film showing a thoracic surgery, and a sexual scene. Their results show significant decelerations in beats-per-minute for both the positive and negative arousing scene compared to neutral. As you might expect after reading Chapter 4, the decelerations were even deeper for the negative scene. However, there were no significant differences in RSA changes between the three types of film clips. Instead, the only significant RSA finding was a decrease from baseline to film viewing for all films. They suggest that "[f]urther studies are needed to clarify the role of parasympathetic and sympathetic branches of the autonomic nervous system on the development of the heart rate response to highly arousing pleasant films" (Codispoti et al., 2008, p. 94).

One media psychology researcher who has been able to obtain results with frequency-based measures of HRV is Nikolas Ravaja who first called for the use of RSA as a way to disentangle sympathetic and parasympathetic influences on cardiac response to media messages (Ravaja, 2004a). In one experiment (Ravaja, 2004b) subjects watched 32 news stories on a small screen video player. The stories were narrated by a newscaster shown on screen. One of the independent variables, though, was whether the image of the newscaster was moving or a still frame. Among the results was significantly lower RSA while watching the moving news anchor compared to the still frame for subjects who had scored high on a self-reported scale of Fun Seeking. There were also significant LF results across several independent variables in the study, which are open to interpretation due to the exact nature of that frequency-domain measure as mentioned above.

Within both the time- and frequency-domains a lot of possibilities exist in the media lab. Another aspect of HRV which has yet to be applied by media psychology researchers in any form is the impact of known differences on *resting* cardiac variability on subsequent cognitive processing tasks such as sustained attention and working memory (Hansen, Johnsen, & Thayer, 2003). Hansen and colleagues, for example, took cardiac recordings for five minutes from male adults and then divided them into high- and low-variability groups based on median split values of the time-domain index root-mean-square standard deviation (rMSSD). Subjects then completed a series of mental tests. Results showed that those with higher resting HRV levels answered the test questions faster and scored better than those with low resting HRV. This raises a theoretical interest: the possibility of investigating whether differences exist in the attentional processing of, and memory for, media messages based upon baseline HRV levels. However, the theoretical question becomes even more practical considering resting HRV has also been linked to a variety of health concerns in later life. If HRV can be used to identify those who are both prone to certain types of heart disease *and* process mediated warning and prevention messages differently, suggestions can be made about how best to design messages to maximize knowledge acquisition and behavior change.

Functional magnetic resonance imaging (fMRI)

Recently a number of publications have appeared in the academic literature—and even the popular press—showing "blobs on brains," where translucent human heads have been cut away to show an image of the brain with brightly colored areas upon it. These images are created through a data collection and analysis technique known as functional magnetic resonance imaging (fMRI), and fMRI methodology is becoming more frequently used to report brain activity while people process media messages. We expect that the number of studies utilizing fMRI to investigate media message processing will increase in the future, particularly as the world of "neuromarketing" takes off (Penn, 2010). And, while it is important to be aware of the basics of the measure, this section of the chapter will be kept purposefully short for two reasons. First, the intricacies and complexities surrounding fMRI measurement are enough to fill volumes and space will not allow too much focus on the topic here. The second reason for brevity is that unlike all the other measures in this book, an MRI machine is not something that you'll likely be acquiring for your media psychology lab anytime soon. With price tags in the millions of dollars, most researchers who conduct fMRI research—be it related to media psychology or otherwise—must access their MRI machine by booking time in one when it is not in use in a medical school or hospital. If you are lucky enough to have access to an MRI, as well as neuroscientists and physicists as colleagues who are willing to collaborate with you, it is suggested that you also read many of the excellent chapters and books on the topic of fMRI recording to provide you with the depth you need (Heuttel, Song, & McCarthy, 2008; Johnstone, Kim, & Whalen, 2009; Wager, Hernandez, Jonides, & Lundquist, 2007).

But, for the rest of us, just what is an fMRI? As you might expect from the name, it is a very large magnet—generating a magnetic field that is at *least* 30,000 times stronger than that of the earth! How does a huge magnet translate into cognitive and emotional processing research? If you remember back to your early days of chemistry, each atom contains a certain number of protons that hover in a type of orbit around a nucleus. Each proton has a positive magnetic charge. When conducting fMRI experiments the subject lies on their back and is slid inside a large tube that houses the magnet. By placing their brain in the middle of the strong magnetic field, many of the protons become aligned along the magnetic pole. But remember, they aren't just aligned they are also orbiting around the nucleus of their respective atoms. The recording of data begins when the fMRI operator turns on a second magnetic signal in a direction perpendicular to the original one.

This second signal is often in the radio frequency range and therefore called an **RF pulse**. The RF pulse knocks the protons out of their initial magnetic alignment. So, although they are still in a spinning orbit around the nucleus, they are spinning out of alignment to the original magnetic field. When the operator turns off the RF pulse, these protons don't automatically snap back into their original magnetized positions. Instead, they wobble and slowly *precess* back to the original direction. The rate at which they return depends on several things, two of which are important for the measure. The first is the level of water density of the microscopic environment they are rotating in. Certain RF pulse sequences are designed to determine the presence of bone, white and grey matter that forms the structure of the brain. Recording the rate of precess in response to these RF pulses is what creates the anatomical scan of an fMRI study. This is what provides the picture of the brain geography itself—the *brain* part of the "blobs on brains" images. Other RF pulse sequences are designed to measure proton precession based upon the ratio of oxygenated to deoxygenated blood in the brain. (You're right, that's what creates the *blobs*.) So, the more oxygenated blood that is in a region of the brain, the stronger the fMRI signal will be. That is why most researchers utilizing fMRI methodology will talk about recording the **BOLD signal**. BOLD stands for Blood Oxygen-Level Dependent. Most fMRI results are actually presenting comparisons of the amount of BOLD signal in certain areas of the brain during one type of stimulus compared to another. If there are significantly more oxygenated blood cells in an area of the brain, say in the prefrontal cortex, in one stimulus condition than in the other, the extent of the increase is represented by different colors on the anatomical map of the brain surface.

As you may surmise, the benefit of the BOLD technique to the media psychology researcher is that it is quite precise at identifying particular structures of the brain activated by cognitive and emotional processing of media. What it isn't very good at—or at least not as good at as the other measure that directly indexes activation in the human brain, the EEG—is identifying precise moments in a message that cause the brain activation. So, for example, a recent fMRI study (Langleben et al., 2009) explored how different areas of the brain were activated by watching Public Service Announcements that were high in Message Sensation Value (MSV). MSV is a composite variable comprised of the number of visual changes (camera changes, special effects, vivid colors), audio changes (sound level, music and voice onsets), and sensational content (surprise endings, etc.). In this study eight anti-smoking PSAs were selected, four that were hiMSA and four that were lowMSA. Also selected were eight segments from a documentary about arctic wildlife. Eighteen people who smoked regularly were shown the video messages inside an fMRI. Afterwards they completed a visual recognition task where they had to answer whether they had seen single frames of video that were either taken from the video stimuli or not. Below is an excerpt from the discussion of Langleben et al. (2009), presented as a typical example of the spatial-based type of data one reads in fMRI studies:

As predicted by our primary hypothesis, the hiMSV PSAs produced less recognition than the lowMSV PSAs. This behavioral indication of reduced cognitive processing of the content of the hiMSV PSAs is further supported by the corresponding imaging data; the hiMSV PSAs were associated with extensive activation in the occipital (including the fusiform gyrus) cortex and the parahippocampus, while the loMSV PSAs were accompanied by the higher prefrontal, temporal, and posterior parietal activation.

(p. 224)

As you can tell, one has to become quite fluent at brain anatomy to make sense of fMRI results. But, that's what the measure does best, locate blood flow in the brain and assume a correlation between it and cognitive processing. FMRI would not have been the best measure in the anti-smoking PSA study if Langleben and colleagues had been interested in determining the response to a single attribute of a hiMSV message—such as a specific camera change. That's because although it is recognized that the dynamic flow of blood into the brain in response to an external stimulus is likely something which is variable and highly dependent upon interactions between the internal and external environment of the embodied cognition system, most fMRI analysis programs estimate this variable and dynamic response using a single curve called the *canonical hemodynamic response function*. The typical shape of such a function predicts that the maximum blood flow into a brain region increases slowly to a peak level six seconds after an eliciting stimulus (Heuttel et al., 2008).

To many, the fMRI is so exciting because it provides the ability to literally measure the central cortical processing—accessing the insides of the "black box" itself. However, this measure is prohibitively expensive to most and burdened with concerns that must be seriously considered. For the media researcher a pressing issue associated with fMRI is that of ecological validity. Recording sessions are tremendously noisy due to the processes associated with generating the magnetic field and keeping it of a uniform intensity across the surface of the brain. This noise means that any audio associated with a media message must be boosted to intensities above that of the magnet itself. This is certainly achievable, but can be fatiguing to the subject and should not be forgotten. Also of consideration is the claustrophobic and clinical environment associated with most fMRI recording sessions as well as certain populations that are ill-advised to participate in fMRI research.

Finally, mention should be made that simply because fMRI (and EEG for that matter) is a more direct measurement of brain activity—as opposed to heart rate or skin conductance which are peripheral nervous system measures—does not mean that it is not still subject to the basic assumption of psychophysiological measurement mentioned in Chapter 1. The activity of blood flow to the brain is associated with so much more than merely media message processing. Careful interpretation of results, scrutiny of experimental design and research protocols are necessary to prevent a return to the days of the more linear S-R approach to the use of psychophysiology. Nowhere does this seem to be more of a threat than in the application of psychophysiological research measures to advertising effectiveness. Consider, as an example of puffery surrounding the fMRI approach, this quote from the president of a major global advertising agency in the recent trade publication *Admap*:

> a cursory study of the literature shows that it's possible to predict behavior from brain scans. Within a couple of decades, brain scan research will have evolved to answer questions about brand empathy and brand learning from a communication just by studying mirror neurons in the brain—and without having to rely on the inaccuracy of consumer self-reporting.
>
> (Wight, 2010, p. 16)

Because we are sensitive to coming across as academic elitists, let us be clear that our implication is *not* that university professors are the only ones who can be trusted to properly interpret fMRI data. However, research shows that "blobs on brains" can be used as a heuristic cue positively impacting both the perceived validity and appropriateness of a study design compared to other forms of data presentation (McCabe & Castel, 2008). Proprietary business ventures that are not subjected to the scrutiny of peer review may present the method as capable of providing the "magic bullet" to their clients . . . something which is counter to the very assumptive underpinnings of how the body's signals contain psychological meaning.

Summary

The use of psychophysiological measures to index the processing of media messages has never been so widespread. And, as this chapter has tried to illustrate, the methodological toolbox available to the media psychology researcher continues to expand with new ways of correlating bodily signals to psychological states experienced during media message exposure and processing. You may have noticed that these new measures frequently migrate from work done in cognitive and biological psychology as well as basic psychophysiology. This trajectory should become even clearer during the next chapter's discussion of self-reported measures of human cognition and emotion that are frequently used in conjunction with psychophysiology to explore media processing. Beyond the useful overview information about the methods mentioned in these two chapters, the overarching theme which cannot be stressed enough is that those interested in keeping their eye to the horizon and recognizing measures that could be applied to the cognitive and emotional processing of media would be well-served to read widely across this array of disciplines. Furthermore, attend colloquia in these fields on your campus as ways of making both intellectual and methodological connections between them and your own media research lab.

7

CONNECTING PSYCHOPHYSIOLOGY TO OTHER MEASURES OF MEDIATED MESSAGE PROCESSING

The previous six chapters of this book have provided knowledge of how psychophysiological measures can be an exciting addition to the media psychology researcher's toolbox for investigating mental processes engaged during media use. We have discussed well established psychophysiological indicators of cognitive and emotional processing as well as measures that have yet to be extensively applied in media psychology research but have tremendous potential to significantly increase our understanding of how the mind processes mediated messages. The goal of this chapter is to place psychophysiological measures of cognitive and emotional processing of mediated messages in the proper perspective by discussing the connection between physiological indicators of mental processes engaged during media use and other measures that provide valuable self-report and behavioral data. We begin by discussing how media psychology researchers can gain a proper perspective of the need for data obtained from multiple measures of mediated message processing. Relationships between psychophysiological and other measures of mediated message processing will then be discussed. This chapter concludes with a review of specific self-report and behavioral measures of mediated message processing, many of which were first covered in Annie Lang's (1994b) foundational book, *Measuring psychological responses to media*. This chapter expands upon and updates that resource by explicitly discussing important methodological issues that must be considered when studying mediated message processing through a combination of psychophysiological and self-report measures. The seminal volume edited by Lang, however, should be considered an important resource in the library of any media psychology researcher.

Such a researcher is dedicated to systematically investigating some of the most complex and dynamic social phenomena that exist—the human mind as it consumes and is influenced by media. The complexity of this phenomenon appears on both the independent and dependent variable side of experiments on mediated message processing. The complexity of the stimulus being studied—mediated messages—has exponentially increased since the days of the first experiments on media effects. In addition to studying more traditional media content, media psychology researchers currently investigate independent variables that researchers involved in the birth of media effects research likely could not even imagine would exist, such as features of online avatars, social media, and multimedia platforms. Further, the dependent variables of interest in media psychology research—attention, emotion, memory, attitudes, decision-making, etc.—emerge from the operation of multiple dynamic, embodied mental processes that ultimately yield numerous forms of meaningful experiences reaching varying levels of consciousness. The entire set of conscious and unconscious mental processes and experiences engaged by media use contains data that reveals the impact of mediated messages on individuals. Thus, advancing knowledge in this area requires media psychology researchers to ground their research programs in conceptual and operational thinking that results in a coherent analysis of multiple forms of data obtained from a range of interconnected measures that are capable of indexing mental processes and experiences varying in the level to which they rise to consciousness. This will require clear understanding of the role of data obtained from multiple measures in providing insight into the mind "on" media.

Gaining a proper perspective on data obtained from multiple forms of measurement

The extent to which psychophysiological measures have already been used to gain insight into mediated message processing has helped create an extremely exciting research environment in which today's media psychology researchers can build upon the growing body of existing knowledge through data collected in their own experiments. The challenge is that in a research environment where some scholars emphasize understanding mental processes engaged across time during media use over documenting more static outcomes of media use, it can be easy for a media psychology researcher to become overly enthralled with psychophysiological measurement. After all, a primary strength of psychophysiological measures is the ability to index cognitive and emotional processes in real time during media exposure. However, failing to understand the unique insights that can be gained from specific forms of data—psychophysiological, self-report, and behavioral—and over-emphasizing one form of measurement over another is unlikely to lead to research capable of producing in-depth and thorough insights into mediated message processing.

Media psychology researchers who understand the unique insights that can be gained from specific forms of data have a proper perspective on the value of studying complex phenomena—like mediated message processing—through the combination of multiple forms of measurement. This perspective is grounded in the realization that each specific measure provides data that yields a partial glimpse of dynamic mental processes and experiences. The ability to gain this proper perspective and understand the unique insights that can be gained from multiple measures of mediated message processing requires careful consideration of the nature of the phenomenon being studied—the mental experience of consuming and being influenced by media—as well as solid concept explication that includes a high degree of attention to operational strengths and weaknesses of specific measures.

Let's start by considering the phenomenon being studied—an embodied human mind consuming media—with an eye toward the challenge of measuring the functioning of representative constructs. The LC4MP—a model of mediated message processing presented in Chapter 4—describes all communication as a continuous, dynamic interaction between a message and a message recipient (Lang, 2009). In the context of mediated message processing it is the continuous interaction between a mediated message and a message recipient—an individual that dynamically acts, reacts, and interacts in a social environment across time— that is the catalyst for the mental experience of media consumption. It is important to note that labeling this phenomenon a "mental experience" is not meant to diminish or deny behavioral components of media consumption. Rather, behavioral components of media consumption can be viewed as reflecting motor responses enacted by the embodied human mind that produces mental experience.

A significant component of a motivated cognition theoretical perspective on mediated message processing is the assumption that physiological activity of the central and peripheral nervous system creates an embodied mind, from which the mental experience of consuming media emerges. A belief that central and peripheral nervous system activity underlies and produces mental experience is the core belief that allows a researcher to apply psychophysiological measures to the study of mediated message processing (Lang, Potter, & Bolls, 2009). It would be a mistake, however, to believe that embodied mental processes—as revealed by psychophysiological measures—fully describe or actually are the entirety of media-evoked mental experiences generated by the embodied mind. Our hearts slow down as we allocate more cognitive resources to encoding important news stories and our palms sweat when playing a particularly arousing online game; however, observing this physiological variance indicative of cognitive and emotional processing of media structure and content only allows researchers to scratch the surface of the complete dynamic experience of consuming and being influenced by media.

Media consumption clearly evokes engaging and gratifying conscious mental experiences that, while produced by specific patterns of nervous system activity constituting an embodied mind, are completely outside description provided by psychophysiological measures. For instance, playing a violent online game may be an extremely arousing experience as indicated by skin conductance data, however, psychophysiological data cannot describe conscious gratifications that might be obtained from playing violent games such as those that might deal with escaping into a fantasy world. The embodied human mind as it interacts with mediated messages produces much more than just biological, physical activity reflective of the cognitive and emotional processes discussed earlier in this book. Our mental experience evoked by consuming media includes a host of discrete emotional feelings as well as sensations such as being entertained, informed, and fascinated. Therefore, the study of the embodied human mind interacting with mediated messages requires researchers to conceptually and operationally define a wide range of relevant constructs in practically every experiment.

In Chapter 1 we were critical of media effects research for not including mental processes as relevant constructs and taking a "black box" approach to studying how individuals consume and are influenced by media, an approach that was consistent with the dominant paradigm grounded in behaviorism. The shift away from behaviorism to considering mental processes as valid objects of study burst open the "black box" and was absolutely a catalyst for advancing knowledge of the experience of consuming and being influenced by media. This shift, however, in no way decreases the importance of measuring variables that appear to be outcomes of media exposure. Rather, the ability to study mental processes evoked by media exposure enables media psychology researchers to study the dynamic interaction between psychological processes and states representative of the entire mental milieu accompanying mediated message processing occurring across time. Under this approach, "outcome" measures—representative of beliefs, attitudes, feelings, and behaviors—should not be viewed as indexing stable and predictable "effects" of media exposure. The media psychology researcher should rather view self-report and behavioral measures of so-called "media effects" as indexing psychological states that dynamically interact with mental processes as well as other psychological states across time in a broad complex social environment that includes media use.

Figure 7.1 contrasts the early "black box" approach to studying media effects with a dynamic processes approach that is theoretically grounded in the LC4MP (Lang, 2009). A dynamic processes approach to understanding the media–mind interaction encapsulates multiple concepts representative of interacting psychological processes and states that operate and emerge into consciousness to varying degrees over time. A core epistemological assumption of a dynamic processes approach to understanding the media and mind interaction is that mediated message processing at any point in time is impacted by prior events and interactions as well as anticipated events and interactions (Lang, 2009). Thus, embodied mental processes and emerging psychological states are continuously fluid throughout time rather than static. Advancing knowledge of dynamic mental processes and emerging psychological states in the context of mediated message processing requires researchers to address the complexity of this phenomenon at both the conceptual and operational level in conducting research. This seems more likely to occur through a dynamic processes approach that provides a description of this phenomenon that is more analogous to looking through a kaleidoscope than the traditional input/output model applied to early media effects research.

Taking a dynamic processes approach to investigating mediated message processing, grounded in a consideration of a wide range of relevant constructs

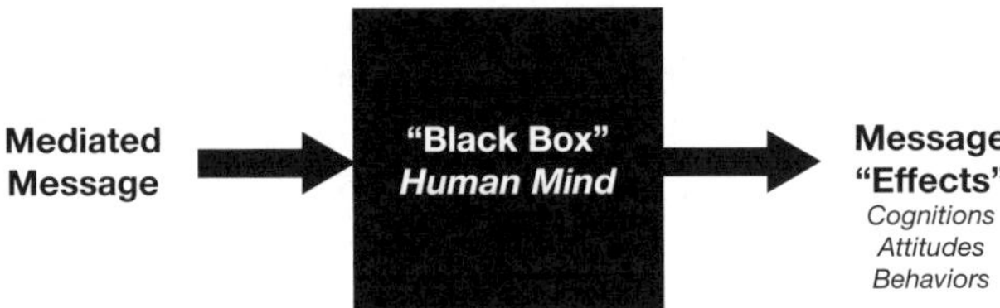

FIGURE 7.1a This diagram depicts the traditional media effects research paradigm in which mental processes are considered a form of "black box" phenomenon that researchers cannot validly observe.

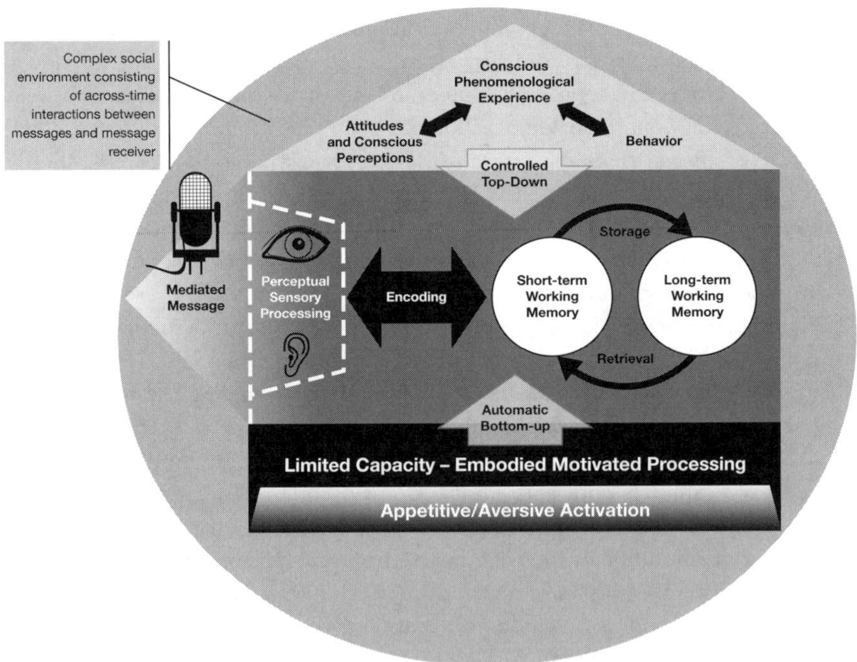

FIGURE 7.1b This diagram depicts a dynamic processes perspective for studying mental processes and states that operate and emerge into consciousness to varying degrees across time during interactions between mediated messages and message recipients.

in any given experiment, requires solid concept explication. Solid concept explication in this context requires going beyond conceptualizations rooted in the lowest, biological process level of the embodied human mind and returning to a higher level view of the phenomenon. The ultimate research objective of media psychology researchers is to draw conclusions about the interaction between mediated messages and message recipients—not merely the functioning of their embodied mind. Thus, the explication of multiple concepts relevant to the mental experience of a message recipient consuming and being influenced by media is needed. This fundamentally means connecting conceptual definitions of the relevant concepts to multiple measures of mediated message processing—in other words just good, plain, solid concept explication as described by Chaffee (1991). We will do that here in a general way, beginning with a discussion of conceptualizing "message recipient," ultimately teasing out concepts—relevant to mental experiences evoked by media use—to be explicated in a way that provides insight into the roles and interconnections of psychophysiological and other measures of mediated message processing.

The ability to connect multiple measures of mediated message processing in a way that provides a complete description of the mental experience of consuming and being influenced by media can only emerge through a strong connection between the conceptual definition of message recipient and specific measures indexing psychological processes and states engaged and experienced through media consumption. Message recipient has been conceptualized as an individual consisting of an embodied mind that dynamically acts, reacts, and interacts in a complex social environment across time (Lang, 2009). Measures of mediated message processing that are strongly connected to this conceptualization of message recipient must be capable of describing psychologically meaningful patterns of nervous system activity as well as phenomenological experiences occurring as a result of action, reaction, and interaction engaged by media use across time. These measures must be sensitive to change across time as well as a host of changing features of a complex social environment—including more than just specific content and structural features of mediated messages.

The psychophysiological measures of mediated message processing discussed in this book are sensitive measures of psychologically-meaningful patterns of nervous system activity that can be used as valid indicators of this dimension of cognitive and emotional processes engaged by media use. Self-report and behavioral measures—many of which have an extensive history of being applied to studying the mental experience of media consumption—have tremendous potential to be sensitive indicators of phenomenological experience constructing psychological states emerging from the interaction between message recipients and mediated messages. Thus, the unique role of psychophysiological measures in understanding the mental experience of consuming and being influenced by media is to describe the embodied processes of human cognition and emotion while the role of self-report and behavioral measures is to describe conscious psychological states reflective of phenomenological experience and potential behavioral action that might emerge from media use.

It should be clear now that under the previously mentioned conceptual definition of "message recipient" any concept the media psychology researcher wishes to study represents a more specific explication of the broader concepts *embodied cognitive and emotional processes, phenomenological experience,* and *behavior.* Figure 7.2 illustrates this idea, listing specific examples of concepts media psychology researchers might need to explicate in their research that fall under each broader concept. This form of explication is consistent with a view of the phenomenon to be studied by media psychology researchers as a dynamic interaction between mediated messages and an individual with an embodied mind that produces emerging mental experiences that reflect and support action, reaction, and interaction across time. Thus, as required by solid concept explication, there is a tight relationship between concepts and their measurement.

The media psychology researcher who studies mediated message processing by connecting psychophysiological measures with self-report and behavioral measures—as we advocate here—needs to understand the relative strengths and weaknesses of each of these measures. Psychophysiological measures of mediated message processing are true process measures in that they can be used to observe embodied mental activity as it unfolds across time. Self-report measures reflect the output of a conscious state of a message recipient at a given moment in time. Thus, psychophysiological measures possess the relative strength of describing

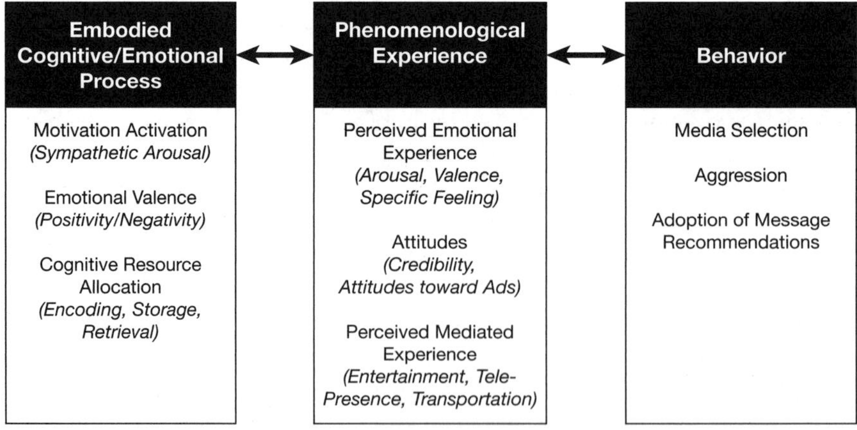

FIGURE 7.2 This diagram depicts examples of specific concepts that represent explication of the broader concepts, embodied processes, phenomenological experience, and behavior.

instant-by-instant fluctuations in the temporal dynamics of relevant concepts. Self-report and behavioral measures possess the relative strength of describing relevant concepts in a way that captures the experientially meaningful summation of mental activity over time that can be difficult to discern in psychophysiological data.

A significant amount of the mental activity and experience of individuals is unconscious, incapable of being reported by the individual (Cacioppo & Decety, 2009). Psychophysiological measures of mediated message processing are capable of capturing the less conscious dimensions of processes underlying the mental experience of consuming and being influenced by media. Alternatively, it is important to note that there are significant psychological states for which no meaningful, reliable, observable physiological footprint, as would be required for psychophysiological measurement, has been identified (Strube & Newman, 2007). The implication of this fact for the media psychology researcher is that psychologically-meaningful features of mediated messages may evoke patterns of mental processing that may be difficult or impossible to observe through psychophysiological measures. Researchers need to evaluate whether a construct under investigation can be validly distinguished according to a specific pattern of embodied mental activity reliably observable with a specific psychophysiological measure or response pattern. For instance, facial EMG may reliably distinguish between generally positive and negative attitudes evoked by an advertisement; however, there is not a psychophysiological measure that can distinguish whether those attitudes vary due to perceived attractiveness or perceived trustworthiness of a spokesperson.

A final consideration here concerns challenges to validly drawing conclusions based on data obtained with different measures of mediated message processing. Weaknesses of self-report and behavioral measures that can impact the validity of conclusions drawn from data include **social response bias** and the fact that responses on these measures are influenced by ease of memory retrieval. Psychophysiological measures are not as susceptible to these weaknesses but, as discussed in Chapter 1, are monstrosities—meaning that removing what should be considered physiological noise and isolating variance in physiological activity due to mental processing is difficult and poses a very real threat to the validity of conclusions drawn from data. Once equipped with an understanding of the role of data obtained from multiple measures of mediated message processing, researchers are ready to consider how psychophysiological measures are related to other measures of processing.

Understanding relationships between psychophysiological and other measures of processing

A discussion of relationships between psychophysiological and other measures of mediated message processing begins by considering the degree to which one ought to expect measures of embodied cognitive and emotional processes, conscious phenomenological experience, and behavioral actions to be correlated with each other. This involves moving beyond a consideration of simple correlation to thinking more broadly about theoretical coherence between measures of mediated message processing in obtaining data that describes multiple processes and states emerging from media use. Researchers who do not fully understand the embodied motivated cognition theoretical framework and psychophysiological measurement—as described earlier in this book—can be tempted to limit their understanding of the relationship between psychophysiological and self-report measures to an analysis of the degree to which they are correlated. We would strongly caution against such a mindset because when these two types of measures are found to not be significantly correlated, an easy default is to assume that one of the measures must be invalid. Unfortunately, our experience suggests the physiological response measure is usually thought to be at fault. This kind of thinking reflects a rather shallow view of the relationships between measures of mediated message processing,

Limiting your consideration of relationships between measures of mediated message processing to the degree to which they are correlated is misguided for several reasons. First, simple correlation between these measures glosses over the temporal dynamics of the concepts being measured. Psychophysiological measures of mediated message processing are often employed to observe cognitive and emotional processes that unfold instant-by-instant during media use. Self-report measures, on the other hand, are obtained post hoc and often used to assess participants' conscious perception of cognitive and emotional processes that were engaged by a mediated message. Averaging across the dynamic activity indexed by psychophysiological measures yields data for which the degree of correlation with a conceptually related self-report scale of message processing will depend on specific patterns of temporal fluctuation in physiological activity. For instance, if the emotional intensity of a mediated message varies widely within the message skin conductance level recorded during exposure to the message will likely also show a high degree of variation across the message. This variation in the instant-by-instant recorded data will impact averaged skin conductance collapsed across the entire message but may or may not impact the average level of self-reported arousal for the same message. The fact that averaged psychophysiological data will be impacted by instant-by-instant variation in mental processes that are engaged during message exposure, but averaged ratings obtained on a related self-report measure may not, has implications for any observed correlation between these measures. Researchers should keep these temporal dynamics in mind particularly in cases where either no or very modest correlations between psychophysiological measures and self-report measures are found.

Second, the complexity of the phenomenon under study, the media–mind interaction, makes obtaining strong intuitive correlations between psychophysiological, self-report, and behavioral measures a chancy proposition. Mediated messages have a tremendously wide and complex range of both structural and content features executed across multiple modalities that are capable of evoking widely varying patterns of embodied cognitive and emotional processing observed in psychophysiological measures. These defy expectations associated with simple correlational relationships between measures of mediated message processing. Finally, examining the relationship between these measures only through the lens of correlation at best severely limits theoretical development, and at worst can lead to rejection of psychophysiological measures as valid indicators of embodied cognitive and emotional processes evoked by media use.

There are theoretically interesting reasons why distinct measures of mediated message processing—that are believed to be conceptually related—may or may not be significantly correlated. Let's imagine you wanted to study arousal evoked by a specific feature of mediated message content—for the purpose of this example let's say it's the degree to which participants are able to customize an avatar that they use to play an online videogame. Two measures of arousal that you might obtain in such an experiment could be skin conductance (see Chapter 5) and a self-report measure which asks participants to rate how calm or exciting they perceived playing the game to be. There are interesting theoretical reasons why you may or may not expect these measures of arousal to be correlated. For one, previous research has indicated that arousal is not a unitary concept—there are distinct types of arousal that have been identified including autonomic, cortical, and behavioral (Stern, Ray, & Quigley, 2001). Skin conductance and a self-report measure of arousal could be indexing different forms of arousal while individuals play online video games and these distinct forms of arousal may or may not be correlated with each other. Further, specific features of mediated messages can easily have differential impact on these distinct forms of arousal, making the relationship between skin conductance and self-reported arousal much more dynamic and complicated than can be described by consideration of the simple correlation between these two measures. If you found only a very weak correlation between these measures or, more clearly, if the ability to customize an avatar was found to only significantly affect one of the measures of arousal, it would be misguided to conclude that one of the measures must be a poor measure of arousal. When considering the relationship between measures of mediated message processing obtained in specific experiments, media psychology researchers should find it quite fascinating to consider the theoretically exciting reasons why measures may or may not be correlated and reveal a consistent pattern of results. This requires thinking of measures of embodied cognitive and emotional processes, phenomenological conscious experience, and behavioral action associated with mediated message processing as measures of distinct concepts representative of, and emerging from, related but unique underlying mental processes.

The importance of viewing psychophysiological, self-report, and behavioral measures as indexing related yet distinct concepts can be illustrated by considering previous research that offers evidence that embodied motivated processing of a mediated message—as reflected by cardiac activity—is a distinct phenomenon from the conscious experience of attending to a message—as measured on a self-report scale. According to previous research on radio advertising, individuals self-report paying more attention to high versus low imagery ads but high imagery ads evoke a pattern of cardiac acceleration rather than deceleration (Bolls, 2002, 2007; Bolls & Lang, 2003; Bolls & Potter, 1998). At face value this pattern of results suggests a lack of correlation between the self-report and psychophysiological data as—consistent with our discussion of heart rate in Chapter 4—one might expect an increase in self-reported attention paid to a message to be associated with cardiac deceleration. However, if one considers that the conscious perception of paying attention to an ad is a distinct concept from embodied motivated processing of the ad, then a very interesting theoretical explanation emerges. Bolls and colleagues interpreted cardiac acceleration during exposure to high imagery radio ads as reflecting an increase in cognitive resources allocated to retrieving information already stored in memory that is needed to support visual mental imagery. *This* mental process results in cardiac acceleration and is arguably evoked during exposure to high imagery ads. The fact that individuals report paying more attention to high imagery ads may indicate that the conscious perception of attending to a message is not sensitive to changes in the relative allocation of cognitive resources to encoding, retrieval, and storage. This kind of in–depth theorizing about how the mind processes media is more likely to come from researchers viewing psychophysiological and self-report measures as indexing distinct, independent concepts that are related in ways that go beyond simple correlation.

It is important to note that correlation between physiological activity and self-report measures of psychological states has played a critical role in the development of the psychophysiological measures media psychology researchers use to study mediated message processing. Psychophysiologists in validating the psychophysiological measures directly assess the correlation between physiological responses and psychological states within individuals. Cacioppo and colleagues provide a very good description of the process of validating psycho-physiological measures by considering the correlation between physiological activity and other measures of psychological states (Cacioppo, Tassinary, & Berntson, 2007b).

The task of validating psychophysiological measures, however, is a completely different task than what media psychology researchers do in studying the media–mind interaction. Media psychology researchers are engaged in a unique activity that requires a more nuanced and in-depth theoretical analysis of possible relationships in experimental data obtained through various measures of mediated message processing than considering simple correlations among these measures. Media psychology researchers use psychophysiological and self-report measures to study an interaction between distinct concrete entities—mediated messages and individual human beings. This is a fundamentally different task than the task of validating psychophysiological measures—which is properly based on a significant degree of correlation between specific patterns of physiological activity and self-report measures of psychological states.

Media psychology researchers use psychophysiological measures that have already been validated by psychophysiologists to conduct research on mediated message processing. The results of this research consist of data—ideally obtained by multiple measures of mediated message processing—reflecting processes and states that can exist in a wide, dynamic constellation of relationships depending on features of media messages and message recipients. When the relationship between measures of mediated message processing does not appear to make intuitive sense researchers simply need to roll up their sleeves and do the difficult theoretical work of figuring out what interactions between features of individuals and of the mediated messages under study may be responsible. This has certainly been the case in work on understanding cognitive processing of emotional radio content where research has found that cognitive resources allocated to encoding, as measured by cardiac deceleration, does not necessarily translate into better message recognition (Bolls, Lang, & Potter, 2001; Potter, Koruth, Bea, Weaver, Lee, Rubenking, & Kim, 2008).

Now that we have considered the nature of general roles of psychophysiological and other measures of mediated message processing, as well as the relationships between them, we turn to a more specific methodological discussion of combining psychophysiological and self-report measures in studying mediated message processing. An overview of several forms of measures commonly used to study mediated message processing will be provided: self-report, continuous response measurement, thought listing, secondary task reaction time, and measures of memory. While many reading this chapter will be already familiar with these measures, perhaps even having used them in their own research, we will point out some specific methodological considerations necessary when combining them with psychophysiological measures that may not have been thought about. Several studies will also be presented to highlight the usefulness of combining data from these measures with psychophysiological data in order to gain a better understanding of mediated message processing.

Combining self-report and psychophysiological measures of mediated message processing

Truly understanding the phenomenological experience of individuals when they consume mediated messages requires an assessment of how features of mediated messages impact well-established psychological states. Put more directly, there is no other way to capture psychologically meaningful aspects of the phenomenological experience evoked by mediated messages then having participants, themselves, describe—or self-report—that experience. Thus, reliable and valid self-report scales designed to measure meaningful psychological states, especially when combined with psychophysiological measures of embodied cognitive and emotional processing, have tremendous value to the media psychology researcher.

A host of potentially valuable self-report scales exist. Rubin and colleagues have compiled a collection of validated scales for communication research (Rubin, Palmgreen, & Sypher, 1994). This book is a great source for the media psychology researcher looking for validated scales measuring potentially meaningful states that possess a high degree of theoretical relevance to understanding mediated message processing. Many of the measures in Rubin et al. (1994) could be combined with psychophysiological measures of mediated message processing with exciting results. Those interested in the impact of persuasive communications—such as advertisements and PSAs—might also find Bruner, Hensel, and James (2005) applicable. A discussion of each potential self-report scale that could be fruitfully combined with psychophysiological measures is far beyond the scope of this section. Rather, the purpose here is to list a few specific examples of self-report measures that represent distinct analytical directions a media researcher can take when connecting self-report measures to psychophysiological measures of mediated message processing.

Prior to this discussion, however, it is important to note two methodological issues that the researcher must be aware of when combining the collection of self-report and psychophysiological data in the same experiment. The first concerns the potential for collection of the self-report measure to introduce noise into the psychophysiological signal. A very simple form of noise that can significantly contaminate psychophysiological data comes from the motor movements required to fill out the self-report questionnaires themselves. Motor movements required to circle a number on a paper survey or even indicate a response with the click of a computer mouse can, for instance, contaminate the ECG signal. Similarly, movements such as these result in noticeable increases in skin conductance level recorded from the palm. The protocol for an experiment involving collection of psychophysiological data should instruct participants to sit as still as possible, while remaining comfortable, during exposure to stimulus messages. This is obviously not the case when they are completing self-report measures; therefore it is usually of little value to record psychophysiological data while participants complete them. A typical research protocol may have participants respond to self-report measures prior to the presentation of any stimuli, in between exposure to each stimulus message in the experiment itself, and then again after exposure to the last stimulus message.

The second general methodological consideration that researchers need to keep in mind is that completing a self-report measure is a cognitive and emotional task which will have some impact on psychophysiological measures being recorded. The act of completing questions that might be emotionally sensitive, or require a significant level of reflection on the part of the participants, is likely to engage cognitive and emotional processes which will then be reflected in psychophysio-logical data. It is important to design data collection protocols so that any psychophysiological responses evoked by either the motor or cognitive/emotional effort associated with the self-report measures dissipate and activity returns to a resting baseline level prior to exposure to the next message during which psycho-physiological data is being recorded. This can generally be easily accomplished by building in time in the experimental protocol where participants are simply instructed to sit and relax between completion of self-report measures and exposure to the next media message.

With these being the only two serious methodological considerations associated with combining self-report and psychophysiological measures, it is no wonder that they have often been used together to obtain data leading to theoretical insights into mediated message processing. The different ways self-report and psycho-physiological measures have been combined in experiments on mediated message processing reflect distinct approaches to using data from these different forms of measurement to understand mediated message processing. There are three general ways self-report measures can be used in combination with psychophysiological measures of embodied mediated message processing that we believe have tremendous potential—based on existing research—to yield great insight. Self-report measures can be used to index psychological states that are conceptually related to the embodied mental processes psychophysiological measures index. Researchers can also collect self-report measures of psychological states that are believed to either moderate or emerge from variation in embodied mental pro-cesses recorded with psychophysiological measures. Finally, self-report measures can be used to index significant individual differences that might influence embodied mental processing of mediated messages. Each of these is addressed separately below, although they could also be used in combination within the same experimental design.

Self-report measures as indices conceptually related to embodied mental processes

One approach to combining self-report and psychophysiological measures is to include self-report measures of attention and dimensions of emotion in an experi-ment in order to gain insight into the participant's perception of the degree to which messages engage the embodied cognitive and emotional processes indexed with psychophysiological measures. As mentioned earlier, it is important to remember that the insight gained by combining self-report and psychophysiological measures in this way goes beyond the degree to which these measures may or may not be correlated with each other. Experiments in which psychophysiological measures of emotional processing have been combined with conceptually related self-report measures of arousal and valence are more common than experiments combining psychophysiological measures of cognitive processing with self-report measures of attention; however, there are established self-report scales worth discussing that enable the media psychology researcher to conduct both kinds of research.

One of the most common self-report scales used to assess the arousal and valence dimensions of human emotion is the **Self Assessment Manikin scale**, also known as the SAM scale (Bradley & Lang, 1994; Lang, 1980). The SAM scale is a nine-point pictorial scale consistent with the dimensional theory of human emotion (Lang, 1995). Participants are instructed to rate arousal on a continuum ranging from calm to extremely excited and valence on a continuum ranging from unpleasant to pleasant (see Figure 7.3).

Of particular interest to the media psychology researcher, the SAM scale has been extensively validated on and used to study individuals' responses to emotional pictures (Bradley, Cuthbert, & Lang, 1996; Codispoti, Ferrari, & Bradley, 2006; Lang, Greenwald, Bradley, & Hamm, 1993). The scale was used to produce and validate what has become known as the **International Affective Picture System (IAPS)**—a large collection of pictures with normed arousal and valence ratings (Bradley & Lang, 2007b). Selections from the IAPS have frequently been used in emotion research to elicit emotion using stimuli of a known emotional level of arousal and valence. This line of research has enabled psychophysiologists to study how stimuli of a given level of arousal and valence impact psycho-physiological measures. Research in which individuals have viewed pictures from the IAPS has demonstrated that in the context of viewing emotional pictures, arousal ratings on the SAM scale are positively related to skin conductance and

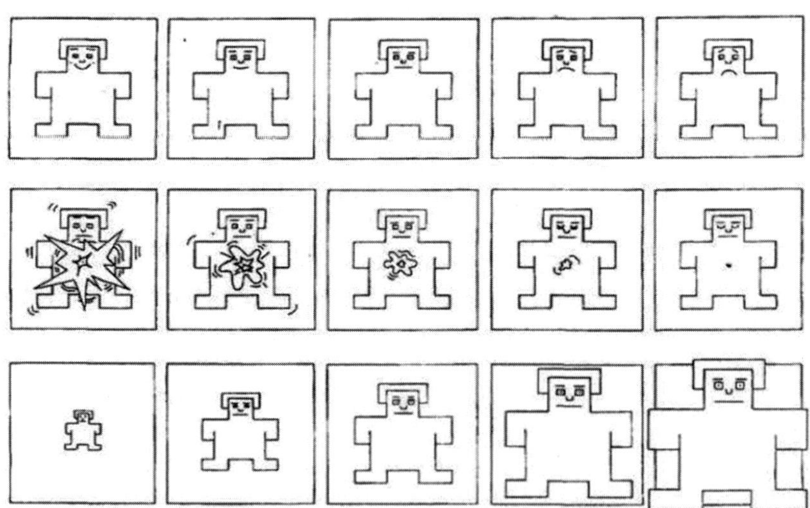

FIGURE 7.3 The Self Assessment Manikin (SAM) scale. The top row measures self-reported valence and the middle row self-reported arousal. The bottom row is a measure of dominance, a dimension of emotion that has proven to be less predictive across many fields and is not often used in media psychology research.

Source: Bradley & Lang, 1994, with permission from Elsevier.

valence ratings on the SAM scale are significantly related to patterns of positive and negative emotional responding in facial EMG (McManis, Bradley, Berg, Cuthbert, & Lang, 2003).

The SAM scale has proven to be extremely valuable in experiments on mediated message processing. It has been used in experiments where psychophysiological data has been combined with SAM scale ratings to study processing of features of media including the visual complexity of websites (Tuch, Bargas-Avila, Opwis, & Wilhelm, 2009), negative political advertising (Bradley, Angelini, & Lee, 2007), and avatar choice in multi-player computer games (Lim & Reeves, 2009). For instance, in a recent experiment on television advertisements, Morris and colleagues found distinct patterns of brain activation as revealed by fMRI that correlated well with the valence and arousal dimensions of the SAM scale (Morris et al., 2009). Research into cognitive emotional processing of audio messages has combined psychophysiological measures with the SAM scale to demonstrate that increasing the structural complexity of audio content increases skin conductance as well as perceived arousal (Potter & Choi, 2006). Lee and Lang (2009) combined psychophysiological data with self-report ratings of arousal and valence on the SAM scale in order to attempt to identify specific patterns of motivational activation underlying the experience of discrete feelings while viewing televised PSAs. They adapted the SAM scale by having participants separately rate pleasantness and unpleasantness in order to separately index appetitive and aversive activation evoked by the televised messages. The predicted pattern of appetitive and aversive activation for messages produced to evoke joy was only found in the self-reported ratings; however, the predicted pattern of appetitive and aversive activation for messages produced to evoke sadness was observed in both self-report and psychophysiological data.

The previous review barely scratches the surface of how media psychology researchers have used the SAM scale in combination with psychophysiological data to better understand emotional processing of mediated messages. However, from this brief review of recent research it should be clear that the SAM scale has become the most widely accepted, valid, and reliable scale for measuring perceptions of the arousal and valence related to emotional processing of mediated messages. This scale is easy to obtain and implement into experiments; therefore it is likely to remain a frequently used scale to provide insight into dimensions of emotional experience elicited during media use.

A significant amount of research has also been conducted utilizing self-report measures of attention to understand cognitive processing of mediated messages. Studies in this area contribute insight into understanding individuals' perception of their own mental effort allocated to perceiving, attending to, and making sense of media content. It is important to keep in mind, however, the limitations of self-report measures of attention when drawing conclusions about how individuals cognitively process media content. In addition to the fact that they are sometimes used in an attempt to measure concepts reflecting unconscious mental processes, self-report measures of attention can often gloss over the functioning of distinct cognitive processes engaged during media use. That is why self-report measures of attention are likely best viewed as measuring the conscious perception of a very broad allocation of mental effort to processing mediated messages. That is not at all to say that insight into the conscious perception of mental effort invested in processing media messages lacks theoretical value. Data obtained from self-report measures of attention—despite the noted limitations—can add tremendous value to data obtained from psychophysiological measures of cognitive and emotional processing. For example, greater theoretical insight into how individuals process highly aversive health messages could be gained by exploring how extremely arousing and unpleasant images impact both actual cognitive resources allocated to encoding—as measured by heart rate or HRV—and conscious perception of mental effort invested in processing such messages indexed with a self-report measure of attention. It is possible that despite the fact that highly unpleasant and arousing images result in defensive withdrawal of resources from processing these kinds of messages, individuals still consciously perceive that they allocate a lot of mental effort to them. Such an interesting pattern of results would obviously only be obtained through the dual use of psychophysiological and self-report measures of cognitive processing.

Fortunately, for media psychology researchers who wish to wrestle with potentially very interesting patterns of results there are some established ways of obtaining a self-report measure of attention that can usefully be combined with psychophysiological measures. Involvement is a concept that has been extensively applied in research on cognitive processing of mediated messages and reflects levels of attention paid to different messages (Greenwald & Leavitt, 1984). Unfortunately, this concept has been defined and operationalized in many different ways (Roser, 1990), only some of which are useful for our purposes here. The concept of involvement has been extensively applied in the study of persuasion (Johnson & Eagly, 1990). Recognized as a multi-dimensional concept that includes two distinct categories, product/issue involvement and message involvement (Zaichkowsky, 1985), self-report scales of involvement can be easily found in the advertising literature (Andrews, Durvasula, & Akhter, 1990). The items from established involvement scales, however, that are clearly most relevant to investigating the direct relationship between conscious perception of mental effort allocated to a message and the embodied process of allocating cognitive resources to processing it are those that directly measure an individual's conscious perception of the level of attention or mental effort. For instance, Andrews and Shimp (1990) developed an index of message involvement that includes items assessing the amount of attention, degree of concentration, level of thought, degree of focus, and level of effort allocated to a message.

Several experiments have included self-report measures of attention that mirror established scales of message involvement to varying degrees while simultaneously including psychophysiological measures of cognitive processing. In an experiment on structural complexity in radio messages, Potter and Choi (2006) measured attention allocated to processing the messages by recording heart rate during exposure to the content and by having participants reflectively self-report their perceived level of attention to each message. The items used on their self-report scale of attention are similar to message involvement scale items in that they asked participants to indicate how much they paid attention to, concentrated on, and thought about each message, as well as how interesting they perceived messages to be. Analysis of the individual items on their self-report attention scale indicated that participants perceived that they paid more attention and had to concentrate more while listening to radio messages with high structural complexity compared to low structural complexity. Interestingly, Potter and Choi observed significantly greater cardiac deceleration during exposure to low complexity radio messages indicating that—contrary to their perceptions—participants actually allocated more cognitive resources to encoding low complexity messages compared to high complexity messages. This study by Potter and Choi, once again, illustrates the theoretical value of combining both self-report and psychophysiological measures of cognitive processing in the same experiment, in that tremendous insight can be gained even when results from these different measures contradict each other.

Another interesting example of the combination of self-report measures of attention with psychophysiological data comes from Smith and Gevins (2004) who measured self-reported attention by asking participants how interesting they perceived television advertisements to be. They also collected EEG—a psychophysiological measure of cognitive processing discussed in Chapter 4—during exposure to the ads. The results indicated a significant relationship between alpha-wave blocking at prefrontal cortex and self-reported interest. This pattern of results led them to conclude that subjective interest in a television ad results in greater cortical activation associated with the control of attention and working memory.

Self-report measures as moderating or emerging from embodied mental processes

A second approach to combining self-report and psychophysiological measures is to obtain self-report measures of meaningful psychological states that might moderate or emerge from cognitive and emotional processing of messages. The ability to use psychophysiological measures to probe inside the black box of the human mind and study cognitive and emotional processes engaged by media use does not decrease the importance of also measuring pre-existing and/or emerging psychological states that may be both theoretically and practically important to truly understanding how the specific form of mediated messages being studied is processed. This brings us back full circle to exploring various kinds of perceptions, attitudes, and behaviors that would be considered "message effects" under a traditional media effects research paradigm but that the media psychology researcher today conceptualizes as psychological states occurring through the dynamic, across time interaction between media messages and message receivers.

There are numerous perceptions, attitudes, and behaviors measured through validated self-report scales that could be potentially relevant to the processing of mediated messages. For instance one can easily find published studies on concepts such as perceived credibility of media messages, attitude toward advertisements, and frequency of various patterns of media use. Significant theoretical advancement in understanding mediated message processing, however, is to be gained by media psychology researchers combining psychophysiological measures with self-report measures to examine the interaction between these concepts and embodied motivated processing of mediated messages.

In designing experiments to investigate the interaction between psychological states and embodied motivated processing of mediated messages it is important for the media psychology researcher to consider how such states might both moderate and emerge from processing of a message. In the study of health campaign messages, for instance, it is likely both theoretically and practically important to consider how current health behaviors and beliefs impact processing of health messages as well as how processing of health messages leads to emerging patterns of health beliefs and behavioral intentions. Fortunately for the media psychology researcher who wishes to study health communication, well-established validated scales of important health concepts such as beliefs, efficacy, and behavioral intentions are found in the published literature. The same state of affairs exists for concepts representative of psychological states that are likely important to other areas of mediated message processing. Validated scales of such concepts—like perceived news credibility, aggressiveness, and perceived realism— are not only found in published articles but can also be located in handbooks such as Rubin et al. (1994).

Media psychology researchers have recently began to conduct more experiments on mediated message processing that utilize psychophysiological measures of cognitive and emotional processing along with self-report measures of relevant psychological states. In an interesting study on the impact of media content delivered over portable versus traditional television platforms Ivory and Magee (2009) measured skin conductance along with a self-reported index of media **flow experience**—a concept that is believed to be associated with a challenging yet entertaining media experience. Participants in their study experienced lower levels of arousal and less perceived flow experience for content delivered over portable handheld devices, leading Ivory and Magee to conclude that the convenience of portable media technology potentially results in a less entertaining mediated experience.

The area of health communication is arguably one of the most fascinating mediated message processing contexts in which to combine psychophysiological measures of cognitive and emotional processing with self-report measures of relevant psychological states. Researchers working in this area have developed self-report measures of psychological states that seem likely to be significantly related to cognitive and emotional processing of a message like perceived threat, efficacy, and behavioral intentions (Witte, 1994). Ordonana, Gonzalez-Javier, Espin-Lopez, and Gomez-Amor (2009) examined the relationship between embodied motivated processing of a fear-appeal based message promoting the tetanus vaccine and psychological states particularly relevant to health persuasion. During the message they recorded heart rate and skin conductance as measures of attention and arousal respectively. After the message, participants completed self-report measures of perceived threat, perceived efficacy, and behavioral intention. The pattern of results obtained through their psychophysiological and self-report measures suggested that participants exposed to a high threat/high efficacy message displayed a pattern of autonomic responding reflective of more effective cognitive/emotional message processing and higher levels of self-reported intention to engage in the recommended behavior.

This discussion represents only a small fraction of the host of important psychological states that media researchers need to study in conjunction with embodied motivated processing of mediated messages. We hope that these brief examples spark research that combines psychophysiological and self-report measures in fascinating ways. Media psychology researchers who engage in this line of research are going to move beyond using psychophysiological and self-report measures to simply validate the existence of cognitive and emotional processes and develop rich theoretical models of mediated message processing that more fully describe the constellation of interacting processes and states underlying media influence.

Self-report measures of individual differences impacting embodied mental processes

A third approach to combining psychophysiological and self-report measures involves using the latter to index individual differences that might impact embodied motivated processing of mediated messages. The embodied human mind is anatomically structured such that individual differences on a host of variables representative of meaningful psychological states and traits could quite easily moderate embodied processes indexed by psychophysiological measures. Recall from the discussion in Chapter 4 that the human brain is biologically structured to process stimuli in both a bottom-up and top-down fashion. It seems plausible that individual differences in certain psychological traits could exert a top-down influence on embodied motivated processing of mediated messages.

Researchers who study the influence of media use on individuals have clearly moved beyond the simplistic powerful effects model to much more extensively considering individual differences in media use and effects (Krcmar, 2009). A theoretical approach to understanding individual differences in media effects that has been suggested categorizes individual differences into needs, readiness to respond, and traits (Oliver & Krakowiak, 2009). Variables examined in media effects research that reflect individual differences in needs include sensation seeking (Zuckerman, 1979) and need for cognition (Cacioppo & Petty, 1982). Readiness to respond reflects an individual difference in the likely intensity of emotional responding to media content. Variables associated with traits traditionally reflect individual differences in established personality characteristics. Media psychology researchers can easily go to the research literature their colleagues studying media effects have generated in order to find validated scales that measure individual differences with a high probability of impacting how the human mind processes mediated messages. The following paragraphs provide examples of potentially interesting individual differences that could lead to different patterns of embodied motivated processing of mediated messages.

There are likely numerous personality traits that, dependent upon the nature of mediated messages being studied, could significantly impact cognitive and emotional processing of a message. The psychology literature contains examples of validated personality measures. Some predominant scales include the NEO Personality Inventory (Costa & McCrae, 2008), the Zuckerman-Kuhlman Personality Questionnaire (Zuckerman, 2008) and the Eysenck Personality Questionnaire (Furnham, Eysenck, & Saklofske, 2008). Some researchers have focused on a specific dimension of the Eysenck Personality Questionnaire—**psychoticism**—as a potential moderator of embodied motivated processing of mediated messages. Individuals who score high on this factor are generally described as aggressive and lacking empathy (Rawlings & Dawe, 2008). Bruggemann and Barry (2002) examined psychoticism as a possible moderator of how individuals emotionally respond to violent media content. They exposed participants to video clips of violence and comedy—measuring skin conductance level over a period of 10 presentations of each kind of video. High psychoticism participants self-reported higher levels of enjoyment and displayed a faster pattern of desensitization of skin conductance level in response to violent video clips in comparison to low psychoticism participants. In an interesting expansion on this study, Ravaja and colleagues examined how psychoticism might modulate psychophysiological measures of cognitive/emotional processing during specific violent video game events (Ravaja, Turpeinen, Saari, Puttonen, & Keitlkangas-Jarvinen, 2008). They concluded that high psychoticism participants appear to be less bothered by the killing and wounding of a video game opponent as evidenced by higher levels of zygomatic and orbicularis oculi muscle activity, indicative of positive emotion, in comparison to low psychoticism participants.

Another personality trait that has received substantial attention in media research is **sensation seeking**. Sensation seeking is believed to be a personality trait reflective of the degree to which an individual purposefully seeks out high-sensation experiences (Zuckerman, 1979). It makes sense to consider sensation seeking as an individual difference that could impact embodied motivated processing of mediated messages because this personality trait is manifested in specific patterns of physiological activity. High sensation seekers have been found to display lower levels of resting physiological arousal in comparison to low sensation seekers (Zuckerman, 1990). It has also been reported that high sensation seekers exhibit lower levels of physiological arousal in comparison to low sensation seekers during exposure to televised substance-abuse public service announcements (Lang, Chung, Lee, Schwartz, & Shin, 2005).

A comparatively recent self-report measure of individual differences that arguably has an extremely strong theoretical connection to embodied motivated processing of mediated messages is known as the **Motivation Activation Measure** (MAM). The MAM has recently been developed and continues to be refined by Annie Lang and colleagues as a reliable and parsimonious measure of individual differences in resting level of activation within the appetitive and aversive motivational systems (Lang, Bradley, Sparks, & Lee, 2007a; Lang, Kurita, Rubenking, & Potter, in press; Lang, Shin, & Lee, 2005). This measure directly draws on the embodied motivated cognition theoretical perspective described in Chapters 4 and 5. In brief, this theoretical perspective proposes that human emotional response consists of activation in underlying appetitive and aversive motivational systems that determine how motivationally relevant stimuli— including mediated messages—are processed and evaluated. It is believed that there are significant individual differences in both the resting level of activation and the responsiveness of these systems to motivationally relevant stimuli (Ito & Cacioppo, 2005). This individual difference is likely rooted in the embodied nature of our motivational system that responds to motivationally relevant stimuli and supports cognitive/emotional processing leading to highly adaptive responses to appetitive and aversive stimuli (Berntson & Cacioppo, 2008). The MAM has been established to index these individual differences in responding to motivationally relevant information. Given this embodied connection between motivation activation and cognitive/emotional processing, there is a strong theoretical rationale for expecting individual differences in motivation activation—as indexed by the MAM—to moderate cognitive and emotional processing of mediated messages—as indexed by psychophysiological measures.

The MAM is a brief self-report measure that can easily be included in experiments on mediated message processing. Administering this measure to participants involves presenting a collection of specific images—of known arousal and valence ratings—selected from the IAPS (Bradley & Lang, 2007b) in a random order. The original MAM scale consists of 90 images—with an abbreviated version developed for children and adolescents. However, a shorter version consisting of 41 images has been developed and validated, allowing MAM to be more easily used in combination with other procedures (such as processing media messages) within a single experimental session (Lang, et al., in press). When taking the MAM, participants are instructed to view each image for as long as they would like and then rate how aroused, positive, negative, each makes them feel. Ratings are given on a modified version of the SAM scale, one that separates out positive and negative ratings on two different valence scales. Participants' ratings of the pictures are used to calculate what A. Lang terms ***appetitive system activation (ASA)*** and ***defensive system activation (DSA)***. Participants' ASA and DSA scores—depending upon the research question being investigated—can be analyzed independently or crossed to create a typology of motivation activation. For instance, media psychology researchers might be interested only in how individual differences in DSA moderate embodied motivated processing of highly emotional media content; alternatively, the nature of the research question might lead to an analysis of how participants high on DSA and low on ASA process emotional media content differently than participants low on DSA and high on ASA.

Research using the MAM to index individual differences in motivation activation suggests that this is a very significant individual difference that moderates media selection as well as embodied motivated processing of mediated messages. Individuals who score high on ASA exhibit patterns of heart rate and skin conductance level indicating that they generally pay more attention to and are less aroused by media content compared to individuals low on ASA (Lang et al., 2007a). Further, it appears that DSA moderates processing of negative emotional media content in that individuals who score high on DSA exhibit patterns of heart rate and skin conductance level that suggests they pay less attention to and are more aroused by negative mediated messages (Lang et al., 2007a). Potter and colleagues have found MAM to be predictive of patterns of media use (Potter, Koruth, Bea, Weaver, Lee, Rubenking, & Kim, 2008). In their study, DSA was positively correlated with a preference for news and information. Given this finding, it would be particularly interesting for media psychology researchers interested in studying processing of news to combine the MAM and psychophysiological measures to examine how DSA might moderate embodied motivated processing evoked by specific message features involving the presentation of highly emotional news stories. The bottom line is that there is a growing body of knowledge indicating that researchers can develop fascinating hypotheses concerning how motivation activation—measured by MAM—might moderate embodied motivated processing of mediated messages.

MAM, SAM, psychoticism, need for cognition, and involvement are only a few of the multitude of self-report scales that can be found in the literature and we encourage you to contemplate the many interesting hypotheses and research questions that can result from using each in tandem with psychophysiological measures. The number of fascinating predictions increases exponentially when you consider that each of the self-reported scales mentioned up to this point measure a research subject's experiential response at a single point in time, and that perhaps there may be a way to more dynamically capture the self-reported experience. We now turn to a discussion of a measure which does just that. Continuous response measurement is an alternative way to index psychological states on a moment-by-moment basis and provides another way to connect experiential measures to psychophysiological ones.

Continuous Response Measurement: a dynamic alternative for measuring psychological states

Continuous Response Measurement (CRM) is a measure of mediated message processing that has not only been used by media psychology researchers to study mental processing of messages but has also achieved a high degree of visibility for its practical applications. Television news coverage of presidential candidate debates in the United States often includes CRM as a way of portraying to viewers how distinct groups of voters evaluate the performance of candidates during the debate. There are even specialized public opinion websites (www. mediacurves.com) that present online CRM data collected from large panel samples in response to various kinds of media content ranging from Super Bowl advertisements to celebrity news conferences and political speeches.

Biocca, David, and West (1994) provide a substantial discussion of methodological and technical considerations in using CRM to study mental processing of mediated messages. Therefore, in this section we will gloss over the specific methodological details in implementing continuous response measurement in experiments on mediated message processing and will instead focus on broader methodological and theoretical connections between CRM and psychophysiological measures.

Continuous response measurement is in essence a moment-by-moment electronic form of self-report measurement (Biocca et al., 1994). Usually subjects use a handheld dial or slider to continuously report their response along a scale of some sort. Scales usually take the form of semantic differentials (e.g., agree/ disagree, calm/arousing, etc.) or numeric ratings of a single concept (e.g., "On a scale of 0–100, how funny is this message right now?") Nearly any concept that can be measured with traditional self-report measures can be indexed through CRM and doing so yields data reflective of momentary fluctuations in the psychological state being measured. Two primary areas of media psychology research in which CRM has been applied to study mental processing of mediated messages are advertising and political communication. This measure has been extensively used to study consumer reactions to advertisements, becoming a solidly established method of copy testing in the advertising industry in the early 1990s (Fenwick & Rice, 1991). Stayman and Aaker (1993) used data obtained from CRM during exposure to advertisements to tease out distinct dimensions of emotion from specific feelings evoked by ads. More recently CRM has been used to examine issue perception in order to study the degree to which individuals can be misled while viewing political candidate debates (Maurer & Reinemann, 2006).

Capturing moment-by-moment change in a higher-level psychological state reflective of mental interpretation of a message is the true strength of CRM. Traditional self-report measures, as discussed in the previous section, reflect a summative evaluation of the perception of a psychological state evoked by messages in an experiment. Given that mental processing of mediated messages unfolds over time, it can be argued that the best measures of relevant psychological states should be sensitive to temporal fluctuation in the state being measured. CRM and psychophysiological measures share this distinct methodological strength, making it worthwhile to consider the conceptual and operational connections between these two measures. Furthermore, it is clear that the extensive application of this measure in the media industry potentially makes CRM a measure that media psychology researchers can use to bridge what are sometimes viewed as wide chasms between the theoretical and practical ramifications of their research on the media–mind interaction. It seems that there may be some unique theoretical and practical benefits to combining CRM with psychophysiological measures of cognitive/emotional processing of mediated messages. These two measures of mediated message processing share a common strength yet tap unique concepts that are important to how messages are mentally processed.

In considering how to productively combine continuous response measurement with psychophysiological measures, media psychology researchers must consider what CRM can be used to reliably index. We have already extensively discussed what psychophysiological measures describe in terms of embodied cognitive/emotional processing. It is possible to use CRM to index perceptions of arousal, emotional valence, and attention during exposure to mediated messages—similarly to what is done with psychophysiological measures. One potentially useful application of combining CRM with psychophysiological measures in this way would be to use CRM in pretesting stimulus messages for an experiment (Bradley, 2007a; Lee & Lang, 2009; Sparks & Lang, 2010). If messages to be included in an experiment are being selected by the researcher on the basis of presumed levels of evoked arousal, emotional valence, required attention, or any other psychological concept, then CRM can provide researchers an indication of the moment-by-moment fluctuation in these psychological processes from real subjects as a way of providing confirmatory data. The use of CRM to pretest messages in this manner represents a wise and efficient use of resources because it is less intrusive and expensive than psychophysiological measurement. The most meaningful difference in what can be validly measured through CRM compared to psychophysiological measures is that—similar to traditional self-report measures—CRM can be used to index higher-level mental states for which a reliable specific autonomic footprint has not been discovered.

Continuous response measurement engages a participant in introspective analysis of their mental states in order to report dynamic variation while they are exposed to a mediated message. Psychophysiological measures clearly do not require such introspection on the part of participants in an experiment. This is a significant difference in the measures in terms of the nature of real-time responses recorded. This also has implications for what mental states a researcher can expect CRM to validly index. Participants should easily be able to validly introspect and report dynamic variation in very simple psychological evaluations of mediated messages, such as level of interest or simple favorable/unfavorable feelings. The more deliberative participants need to be in their introspection in order to report variation in the psychological state being measured the less valid CRM data is likely to be. Researchers need to keep in mind that the task of having to consciously evaluate and report variation in their mental state while simultaneously watching a message takes away cognitive resources from processing the message itself. This fact has significant implications for the selection of variables a media researcher should attempt to index with CRM and thereby places constraints on the kinds of higher-level interpretive states that could be usefully studied with CRM in conjunction with psychophysiological measures of embodied cognitive/emotional processing.

The fact that continuous response measurement and psychophysiological measures possess the strength of being able to index psychological processes and states in real time does not mean that there are not significant differences between these measures that must be kept in mind if data from these two measures are to be productively combined. The timescale on which these measures operate significantly varies. Specific evoked response potentials in the EEG signal, discussed in Chapter 4, have been found to be sensitive to general evaluative processes occurring within 300ms of the onset of a stimulus (Bartholow & Amodio, 2009). The process of a participant in an experiment consciously interpreting message content and then executing a motor response to dial in their reaction in completing a continuous response measure certainly operates on a much longer timescale. This means that the temporal mapping of psychological process or state to the continuous stream of sensory information in mediated messages is significantly tighter for psychophysiological measures than CRM. This temporal difference should be kept in mind, particularly when researchers are studying mental processes and states evoked by specific content or features occurring within mediated messages.

Researchers who use psychophysiological measures to study embodied motivated processing of mediated messages can combine psychophysiological data with data obtained from CRM to study the real time, moment-by-moment connection between embodied processes and emerging higher-level mental interpretation of mediated messages. The ability to do this has tremendous potential to significantly expand insights offered by media psychology researchers who have previously relied on the combination of psychophysiological measures and traditional self-report measures to make this link. For example, Wang, Lang, and Busemeyer (2011, p. 79) combined CRM ratings of positivity, negativity, and arousal with psychophysiological measures to study cognitive/emotional processing of video clips selected for their valence and arousal. One of the drawbacks of CRM is that only one dependent variable can be measured at a time, so each clip used in this experiment was rated for positivity, negativity, and arousal by multiple participants. Then, plotting the results against time, the final experimental stimuli were selected such that:

> [t]he 12 clips that were rated highest on the Positivity scale (means > 5) and stayed below 3 on the Negativity scale (means < 3) were selected as positive clips; the 12 that were rated highest on the Negativity scales (means > 5) but stayed below 3 on Positivity (means < 3) were defined as negative clips. Then within valence categories the 12 clips were ranked on Arousing Content and divided into three levels (arousing, moderately arousing, and calm), with 4 messages in each level.

Later, these 24 messages were systematically arranged across four different TV "channels" and viewed by another set of research subjects who could switch between each channel at will. Participants' heart rate, skin conductance, corrugator and zygomatic psychophysiological data were simultaneously collected and then *combined* with the CRM data to develop a mathematical model which mapped the dynamic relationships between the different variables. This study presents an indication of ways in which CRM and psychophysiological data can be combined beyond a more traditional pretest selection basis.

As all the examples provided where CRM and psychophysiology have been used in tandem suggest, it is complicated and likely invalid to collect both psychophysiological measures and CRM simultaneously within a single experiment. Motor movements required to input responses on a CRM interface will likely introduce significant artifact into physiological signals, not to mention the fact that this task takes away cognitive resources from the processing of a message being indexed with psychophysiological measures. A solution to this problem that could enable the collection of CRM and psychophysiological measures in the same experiment is to collect only psychophysiological measures or CRM during exposure to stimulus messages and vary the specific messages each measure is being collected for. This way, when data is averaged across participants, both forms of data have been collected for every message. Random assignment of participants to data collection conditions is obviously critical to this solution. It also may require a greater number of participants in the study because in essence two experiments are being combined into one. The other solution is to actually conduct two separate experiments, collecting psychophysiological measures in one and continuous response measurement in the other. The two separate experiments—to truly represent a combination of CRM and psycho-physiological measures—should then be written up in one manuscript where the researcher draws general conclusions about mediated message processing by concurrently considering the results obtained from each measure in the two experiments. This is the kind of work that is presently missing in the published literature on mediated message processing. Our overall discussion of CRM as an alternative way to index psychological states should indicate several exciting ways that data from this measure can be combined with psychophysiological data with important implications for understanding mediated message processing.

Thought listing: capturing the qualitative experience of mediated message processing

Thought listing—often referred to as the think aloud procedure—is a measure that gives researchers a glimpse into the mental contents of individuals' minds including specific thoughts, feelings, ideas, expectations, appraisals, or mental images (Cacioppo, von Hippel, & Ernst, 1997; Shapiro, 1994b). Thought listing involves prompting participants to recall and then verbally state any thoughts brought to mind by specific stimuli in an experiment. Thought listing data obtained from participants in experiments on mediated message processing can give researchers a rich qualitative description of the mental experience of consuming media. Thought listing data can also be quantitatively coded for statistical analyses of specific categories of mental contents brought to mind by specific features of mediated messages. Researchers have used the thought listing technique to capture aspects of mental processing of media messages that cannot be richly described by purely quantitative measures. The data obtained by the thought listing technique is truly reflective of participants' phenomenological mental experience of consuming mediated messages as there is a high degree of correspondence between mental experiences and conscious thoughts.

Thought listing has been extensively used to study mental processing of persuasive media messages. Thoughts evoked by a persuasive message have been termed cognitive responses—a concept several researchers believe is highly relevant to attitude change that might result from exposure to a message (Chattopadhyay & Alba, 1988; Petty & Cacioppo, 1986). More recently persuasion researchers have used thought listing to study how the degree of confidence one has in specific thoughts evoked by a persuasive message impacts the influence of emotional appeals on evaluative judgments (Brinol, Petty, & Barden, 2007). Thought listing has also been used recently to study how humor might reduce critical scrutiny of arguments in a political message (Young, 2008). Outside of the context of persuasion, thought listing has been used to explore how exposure to verbally aggressive television sitcoms impacts the presence of aggressive thoughts (Chory-Assad, 2004). The extensive presence of this measure in the communication research literature is likely due to the appeal of being able to measure, in experiments, a more qualitative aspect of the mental experience of consuming media. Thought listing, however, has several unique considerations that researchers would do well to keep in mind in implementing and interpreting this measure of mediated message processing.

One methodological consideration has to do with what researchers can realistically expect individuals to validly report when they reflect on thoughts that might have been evoked by specific messages in a given experiment. Researchers should primarily rely on this measure to simply gain access to the content of thoughts and not have individuals attempt to explain, for instance, why they engaged in certain thought patterns. Research in social psychology has demonstrated that individuals cannot be expected to explain why or how specific mental contents may have been produced by a stimulus (Wilson & Brekke, 1994). Thus, researchers should not rely on thought listing as a way to directly index the functioning of cognitive and emotional processes engaged by mediated messages. The mental contents captured through the thought listing technique describe the *output* of mental processes, or more specifically, reflect what has been described in this chapter as emerging psychological states. It therefore seems best to give participants as general a prompt as possible in instructing them to recall and state any thoughts that may have been evoked by a message (Shapiro, 1994b). A good prompt for thought listing could be as general and simple as "please describe any thoughts that came to mind during this message."

A second methodological concern in using thought listing data to study mediated message processing concerns sources of potential noise in the data. One such source has to do with the accuracy with which individuals can verbally describe relevant thoughts. The thought listing technique engages subjects in an introspective process where they attempt to recall the content of any thoughts they had. The validity of this data rests on the degree to which subjects in an experiment can accurately recall thoughts evoked during exposure to a message. A related issue is whether subjects are able to adequately describe their thoughts in such a manner as to provide the researcher with the insights they are looking for. For example, Stephens and Russo (1997) report that when subjects were asked to categorize their own thoughts as positive, neutral, or negative their results were significantly different from having trained coders categorize the same thought statements later. This would suggest that the subjects know something about the valence associated with their thoughts that they are unable to communicate to impartial readers of the data.

A couple of factors may impact subjects' ability to accurately recall thoughts they had during exposure to a message. One of the most obvious factors is the exact time that they are asked to recall and state their thoughts. Thoughts could be reported online while an individual is consuming media or in between mediated messages included in an experiment. Clearly, if participants are instructed to verbally state their thoughts as they are consuming media in an experiment then thoughts are being recorded nearly immediately as they are activated in working memory during mediated message processing. The accuracy of recorded thoughts under this instruction is not as dependent on memory retrieval processes as is the case when participants recall thoughts after exposure to a message. The weakness in this approach, however, is that the task of reporting one's thoughts while simultaneously processing mediated messages takes cognitive resources away from processing messages in a highly detailed manner—possibly causing participants to not thoroughly process a potentially important characteristic of mediated messages being studied in an experiment.

A second factor that could impact the accuracy of recall in completing a thought listing task is the repeated nature of the task in experiments that involve the presentation of multiple messages. In an experiment that involves thought listing in response to several mediated stimuli, participants probably become increasingly diligent in consciously attempting to recall thoughts due to the anticipation of needing this information at the conclusion of a message. The likelihood of this happening not only points out the importance of randomizing the presentation of stimulus messages used in the study but also brings up the concern that simply instructing participants to recall their thoughts could change the way messages are cognitively and emotionally processed. This not only has implications for the level of noise in thought listing data but could also introduce noise in psychophysiological measures of cognitive and emotional processing. Researchers need to be aware that any part of an experimental protocol that shifts or changes the way individuals allocate cognitive resources to processing stimulus messages— such as informing participants that they are going to be prompted to recall their thoughts—has the potential to impact psychophysiological measures of cognitive and emotional processing that are also being collected in the study.

An additional source of noise in thought listing data is **social response bias**. Social response bias has the potential to contaminate many different measures of mediated message processing but it arguably deserves special consideration here. In asking an individual to describe their thoughts researchers are asking for disclosure of what can be considered one of the most private and personal aspects of an individual. It seems plausible that participants could even reasonably consider having to verbally describe potentially sensitive thoughts an even more invasive intrusion into their private mental life than having to complete quantitative self-report measures that index similarly sensitive attitudes and beliefs. It is therefore all the more critical for researchers to take specific steps to help make participants feel comfortable responding in a completely honest manner. This could include adding emphasis in instructions to subjects on the fact that their responses are generally anonymous and confidential, and perhaps even taking extra steps to increase the privacy of the environment in which thought listing data is collected.

The thought listing technique has been used to gain intriguing insight into mental processing of mediated messages. This qualitatively based measure of mediated message processing when combined with psychophysiological measures of mediated message processing seems likely to have tremendous potential to yield new insight. No study to date has purposefully drawn conclusions about mediated message processing by concurrently interpreting data obtained from psychophysiological measures of embodied motivated processing and thought listing. This could be due to the labor-intensive nature of data analysis for both kinds of measures. The thoughts expressed by subjects in an experiment have to be sorted and coded, with attention being paid to issues such as **inter–coder reliability**. Researchers who are willing to invest this level of work in data analysis could possibly gain the ability to simultaneously observe embodied motivated processing and the phenomenological mental experience of consuming media in theoretically valuable ways. For instance, media psychology researchers could investigate how the degree to which cognitive resources are allocated to encoding a persuasive message—as indexed by heart rate—impacts the presence of thoughts in thought listing data reflective of message counter-arguing or discounting. Alternatively in the arena of new media, researchers might investigate how features of interactivity evoke differential patterns of arousal—indicated by skin conductance—and thoughts reflective of an entertaining and satisfying mediated experience. Thought listing could be combined with psychophysiological data in a slightly less labor-intensive manner by having the subjects themselves categorize their thoughts along a pre-determined typology (Stephens & Russo, 1997). The combination of these measures in experiments on mediated message processing will certainly involve work on the part of researchers and a high degree of attention to methodological considerations, but as should be clear from the above discussion, can also be used to tremendously enrich theoretical understanding of this phenomenon.

Secondary task reaction time: a behavioral measure of cognitive resources

Secondary task reaction time (STRT) is a measure of cognitive processing that has a rich history of being used by cognitive psychologists to study human attention. This measure is conceptually grounded in limited capacity theories of human attention that propose individuals have limited cognitive resources for performing the mental tasks involved in processing multiple sources of information in their environment (Kahneman, 1973; Shiffrin & Schneider, 1977). Operationally, STRT is grounded in a dual task processing research paradigm under which scholars working in cognitive psychology realized that they could operationally study human attention by having research participants engage in two separate mental tasks and assess the degree to which one task affects performance on the other (Pashler, 1998).

The collection of STRT data in an experiment involves instructing participants to pay the most attention to a primary task (e.g. reading a story) but to also behaviorally respond—typically by pressing a button—to a secondary task cue. The amount of time it takes a participant to respond to the secondary task cue (usually a brief audio tone or visual character) is the secondary task reaction time. This data, recorded in milliseconds, is submitted to statistical analysis in order to draw conclusions about cognitive resources. Researchers in cognitive psychology have utilized secondary task reaction time data to help them build basic models of human attention (Posner, 1978) as well as, more recently, in combination with brain imaging, to study the neural underpinnings of processes related to attention (e.g., Britta et al., 2008). Thus, STRT continues to be considered a useful measure in studying how the human mind attends to information.

Communication researchers working in the 1980s, when attention was just beginning to become widely studied in the field, adopted STRT as a useful measure of this concept (Thorson, Reeves, & Schleuder, 1987). Secondary task reaction time data has appeared with growing frequency in the published communication literature since that time. Basil (1994a) described a basic theoretical foundation for applying STRT to the study of cognitive processing of mediated messages. He suggested that consuming media requires the allocation of limited cognitive resources; therefore, STRT ought to be just as useful to the study of attention paid to mediated messages as it had been for basic research on human attention in cognitive psychology. Initially the application of this measure to studying how the mind processes mediated messages produced some puzzling results that ran counter to the traditional interpretation in cognitive psychology of what STRT measures.

The traditional interpretation of STRT data is that as a primary task consumes more attention or mental effort, secondary task reaction time gets slower. Applied to mediated message processing, this interpretation leads to the general hypothesis that more complex messages should result in slower secondary task reaction time than messages that are less complex. Researchers who have used secondary task reaction time to study cognitive processing of mediated messages have noted how several of the early experiments incorporating STRT produced results that failed to support this general hypothesis (Fox, Park, & Lang, 2007; Reeves & Thorson, 1986). For instance, Thorson and colleagues manipulated the audio and visual complexity of commercials and found STRT to be faster when participants were exposed to high complexity compared to low complexity messages (Thorson, Reeves, & Schleuder, 1985). Counterintuitive findings have extended to the relationship between STRT and memory for message content. If, under the traditional interpretation, secondary task reaction time directly measures attention paid to a message, then slower secondary task reaction time—or higher levels of attention paid to a message—should be associated with better memory for message content. This has not always been the case. For example, experiments on the impact of news teasers (Cameron, Schleuder, & Thorson, 1991) and narrative structure (Lang, Sias, Chantrill, & Burek, 1995) in televised messages produced results where faster secondary task reaction time was associated with better memory for the messages being studied.

Counterintuitive results appeared with enough frequency in the published literature by the mid-1990s to lead some scholars to begin questioning exactly what secondary task reaction time measures (Basil, 1994b; Grimes & Meadowcroft, 1995). Lang and Basil (1998) offered a theoretical reinterpretation of the measure, arguing that conceptualizing secondary task reaction time data as directly indexing cognitive resources consumed in processing a mediated message is incorrect and overly simplistic when describing cognitive processing of mediated messages. They suggested that a distinction needs to be drawn between cognitive resources allocated to processing a message and cognitive resources required to process a message. Cognitive resources—as was discussed in Chapter 4—are allocated to processing messages through both controlled and automatic processes. Cognitive resources required to process a mediated message are determined by the content and structural features of the message. Lang and Basil (1998) termed the difference between resources allocated and resources required as cognitive resources available for encoding and suggested that the latter is what STRT actually indexes. This represented a very specific conceptual definition of STRT, distinct from the other ways it had been conceptualized as an indicator of attention.

A real strength of this theoretical interpretation of STRT is that it reflects more accurately the nuanced and complex nature of the mental task of attending to and processing mediated messages. Conceptualizing secondary task reaction time as measuring cognitive resources available for encoding establishes a strong connection between this measure and what is presently the dominant theory of how the mind processes media, LC4MP (Lang, 2009). Recall from our discussion of LC4MP in Chapter 4 that encoding is one of the specific subprocesses involved in attending to and remembering mediated messages. Further, this theoretical model explicitly draws a distinction between cognitive resources allocated to encoding and cognitive resources required to encode a message. This distinction means that cognitive resources allocated to encoding a message can run the gamut from being too few resources to more resources than are actually required to process the message depending on both resources that are actually allocated to encoding by an individual and the degree to which content and structural features of messages require resources for encoding. Lang and Basil (1998) suggested that secondary task reaction time recorded during exposure to mediated messages will vary according to the difference between cognitive resources allocated to encoding and cognitive resources required by the message—in other words, cognitive resources available for encoding.

Recent experiments on cognitive processing of mediated messages have supported conceptualizing secondary task reaction time as measuring cognitive resources available for encoding (Fox et al., 2007; Lang, Bradley, Park, Shin, & Chung, 2006; Lang, Park, Sanders-Jackson, Wilson, & Wang, 2007b). This support has come through a combination of both secondary task reaction time and message recognition data. Lang and colleagues have proposed that faster secondary task reaction time and decreased message recognition indicates that cognitive processing of the primary task has become overloaded due to significantly fewer resources being allocated to a message than are actually required to encode the message (Lang et al., 2006; Lang et al., 2007b). As a result of this overload, the research subject disengages from the primary task of watching the mediated message. This causes recognition memory for content of the message to go down while leaving plenty of resources available for encoding for more rapid response to the secondary task probe and faster STRTs.

Armed with a much clearer conceptualization of the precise aspect of mediated message processing secondary task reaction time indexes, media psychology researchers can proceed to productively combine this measure with psychophysiological measures of mediated message processing. There are, however, significant obstacles to collecting secondary task reaction time and psychophysiological data simultaneously during exposure to mediated messages. The STRT cue is a stimulus that will evoke specific psychophysiological responses in addition to patterns of physiological responding evoked by a message. These additional responses are noise in the data a media psychology researcher is typically most interested in—psychophysiological responses evoked by the message. The motor responses required to respond to the secondary task reaction time cue have the potential to introduce even more noise into psychophysiological measures. Thus—as was the case with continuous response measures—media psychology researchers who wish to combine STRT with psychophysiological measures of mediated message processing should either vary which measure is collected during exposure to each message in an experiment or conduct two entirely separate protocols on the same messages.

It is difficult to find published studies that enable conclusions to be drawn about mediated message processing based on the collection of secondary task reaction time and psychophysiological measures on the same messages. This represents yet another interesting line of future research for media psychology researchers to pursue. Leshner and colleagues studied the impact of fear appeal and disgust-related visual images in televised anti-tobacco ads on cognitive processing by collecting heart rate and secondary task reaction time data for the same messages in two different experiments (Leshner, Bolls, & Thomas, 2009; Leshner, Vultee, Bolls, & Moore, 2010). They found that the addition of disgusting images in fear appeal messages resulted in faster secondary task reaction time, momentary cardiac acceleration, and slightly decreased recognition. Leshner and colleagues interpreted this pattern of results as indicating that the combination of threatening, fear appeal-based content and disgust-related visual images in anti-tobacco messages creates emotionally intense messages capable of overloading cognitive processing. Again in this work, overload was indicated by the combination of faster reaction times and decreased recognition memory for the primary task. This not only illustrates insights to be gained by interpreting data from both STRT and psychophysiological measures but also points out the importance of yet another measure of cognitive processing of mediated messages—measures of memory.

Measures of memory: performance indicators of mediated message processing

Real-time measures of mediated message processing like heart rate and secondary task reaction time are clearly valuable but ultimately in-depth insight into mediated message processing also requires data that describes the impact of features of mediated messages on the content of memory. In the early days of research on attention paid to mediated messages, researchers made the mistaken assumption that memory for message content indicates levels of attention paid to a message (Lang et al., 2009). However, a more current and informed theoretical perspective recognizes that cognitive resources allocated to processing a message and the memory for a message are completely distinct concepts. As mentioned in our discussion of this issue in Chapter 4, an increase in cognitive resources allocated to encoding a message doesn't automatically translate into better recognition of message content (Bolls et al., 2001). Memory for mediated messages seems to be driven by a dynamic interaction between cognitive resource allocation and specific characteristics of messages. It is therefore vitally important for media psychology researchers to measure both cognitive resource allocation and memory in order to draw valid conclusions about how specific forms of mediated messages are processed.

Given that cognitive processing of mediated messages involves the allocation of resources to the subprocesses of encoding, retrieval, and storage, performance at each of these subprocesses needs to be indexed through the use of distinct memory tests. Message **recognition** indexes performance at encoding, **cued recall** measures how well content was stored, and **free recall** indicates how easily message content is retrieved (Craik & Lockhart, 1972). A free recall test involves instructing participants to simply list or describe the messages they can remember being exposed to during an experiment. Testing cued recall involves giving participants a cue for each specific message (e.g., during this study you viewed a message about puppies) and asking them to describe all that they can remember from that specific message. Multiple-choice tests are a common way of testing recognition. Recognition can also be examined in a more nuanced way through speeded recognition tests. These involve the presentation of brief target snippets from messages in an experiment as well as foil snippets from media content that participants were not exposed to during the study. The instruction to participants is for them to indicate as quickly as possible whether or not they believe the snippet is from one of the messages they were exposed to during the study. Speeded recognition tests yield data that enables a signal detection analysis of recognition memory. This more detailed analysis of recognition data produces two parameters—**recognition sensitivity** and **criterion bias**—that allow much more detailed insight into message recognition than recognition accuracy. Recognition sensitivity is an index of a research subject's ability to discriminate between the targets and foils. Criterion bias quantifies how conservative or liberal the subject is when responding that they had been exposed to the snippet during the experiment. Shapiro (1994a) describes these in more detail, plus further discusses the application of signal detection analysis in experiments on mediated message processing.

The implementation of memory tests in experiments on mediated message processing typically involves the inclusion of a distraction task prior to the actual memory test. This is to clear the contents of short-term memory after exposure to the last message and activate neural memory networks corresponding to topics unrelated to the stimulus messages and independent variables of interest. Sometimes distraction tasks consist of watching an unrelated message. Another possibility is to create distraction as part of a research protocol by removing all electrodes that were placed on participants prior to testing memory.

It is not only theoretically important but also methodologically convenient to collect psychophysiological and memory data for all messages in a single experiment. Many of the published studies involving the use of psychophysiological measures of mediated message processing also include memory data. A review of that published literature is beyond the scope of this chapter. Suffice it to say that strong theoretical models like the LC4MP could never have been built without an extensive amount of data obtained from both psychophysiological measures and memory tests.

Summary

This chapter has established the unique roles that various forms of measurement play in observing the mental experience of processing mediated messages. Several measures that can be productively combined with psychophysiological measures in the study of mediated message processing were also covered. It should be clear that psychophysiological measures—or any other measure for that matter—cannot provide meaningful insight into the highly complex and dynamic interaction between the human mind and mediated messages if used alone. Researchers, however, need to be diligent in addressing several unique methodological challenges in combining the collection of psychophysiological data with data obtained from other forms of measurement in the same experiment. We hope that this chapter has not only provided media psychology researchers with a better understanding of measures of mediated message processing but has also sparked ideas for future research in which multiple measures will be combined in exciting ways, to truly advance knowledge.

8

ON YOUR OWN

Setting up a media psychophysiology lab and conducting experiments

If you are still reading this book, you likely don't have a mere passing interest in psychophysiological measures of mediated message processing. Instead, you actually want to *use* them yourself but may not know how to begin doing so. Furthermore, the prospect of setting up your own laboratory may seem particularly daunting psychologically; you may feel as if you need to "know more" or be more of an "expert" to even contemplate such a venture. We understand those feelings and have experienced them ourselves . . . each time we have taken a job at a new university or designed a new lab space. However, we found hope in reading that this petrifying phenomenon has a name: **labophobia** (Lang, 1994a). We were comforted to know we weren't alone in our feelings of inferiority and we gained determination when we read about the two-step cure for labophobia. The two steps are so simple, in fact, that you will be able to complete them right after finishing this chapter. The first is to realize that every media psychophysiology researcher—even the most seemingly brilliant, insightful, and well-published— started by simply claiming a lab space where they could test their hypotheses and move the scientific endeavor forward. The second step is even easier . . . so easy that it may at first seem both silly and unnecessary. It's neither. You need to make a sign. That's right; the first tangible thing to do when setting up a psychophysiological media lab is to make a sign that reads "Laboratory." Your lab can have a fancier name of course, and acronyms abound. We know of *The PRIME Lab, The ICR Lab, The CAP Lab, The CEC Lab* and *The DICE Lab* (see Figure 8.1). Each acronym represents the particular interests of the lab's director and you may want to begin thinking about something catchy. But don't get hung up and petrified over that task, too. Even if the only thing you can think up now is *Professor X's Lab*, make the sign. If you can only afford to print the sign on standard-sized paper using a borrowed laser printer . . . make the sign. The moment

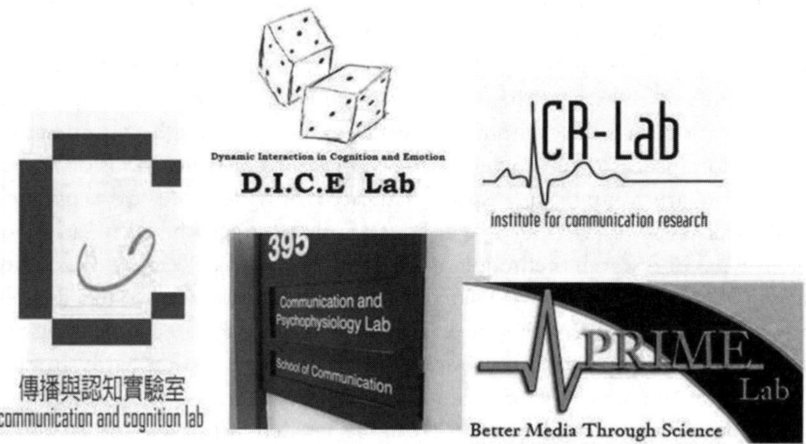

FIGURE 8.1 Signs from some of the labs we've been associated with.

you have made your sign, pause a moment and realize you have accomplished your first goal as director of your own lab. Congratulations! Now, your next goal is to find a place to hang it!

Finding the space

Physical space is perhaps the only thing more rare on a university campus than undergraduates who complete their assigned textbook readings. And, if you are going to have a psychophysiological lab you will need a location to house it in. Luckily, compared to the early 1990s when psychophysiological measures reappeared in communication scholarship, university administrators have become more accustomed to having media psychology researchers ask for permanent lab space in which to conduct their studies. However, if you are reading this chapter prior to going on the job market you should prepare to be specific about what sort of space requirements you will need. You should refrain from telling your prospective Dean *"I need a place to hang my sign . . ."*; nevertheless, you will want to have some ideas of exactly what type of space you will need prior to signing an employment contract.

For most of the measures described in this book—heart rate, skin conductance, facial EMG, eye-blink startle—you don't actually need a lot of physical space. In a very useful chapter on setting up a psychophysiological lab, Curtin, Lozano, and Allen (2007) suggest that the minimum size for a lab is six-foot square. Academic departments often have storage spaces this size, in fact, the first lab one of us worked in was a converted janitor's closet. Although they base their recommendation on the possibility of claustrophobic subjects participating in clinical psychology experiments, these dimensions seem to be a reasonable minimum for media psychology work as well. Whatever space you get will eventually be divided into a minimum of two general areas: the "subject-space" where the media messages will be viewed by research participants and the "experimenter-space" where the bioamplifiers and data collection computer will be. When considering the sectioning of space, and envisioning how to describe your *need* for space to the powers-that-be, make a conscious decision about whether you are asking for a space dedicated only to your own psycho-physiological work or whether it will be space that can also house a variety of different types of research methodologies for you and your colleagues. Flexibility is likely preferable here (Lang, 1994a) and dividing the physical space in a flexible manner is not as daunting as it seems. This is especially the case considering the portability of much of today's psychophysiological data collection hardware that can be transported between your office and the lab space if necessary. A temporary experimenter-space and subject-space can be created using anything from a curtain on a rod stretched across the room to furniture (see Figure 8.2) or temporary and flexible office dividers.

If you are in a position to design a lab from "the ground up" or inherit a space where the experimenter and subject are located in two rooms separated by a permanent wall, remember electrode leads attached to the subject's body in one room will need to reach the input connection of the bioamplifiers in the other. Most equipment vendors do not make leads long enough to wind along walls and through existing doorways. Cable pass-throughs must therefore be installed in the walls. Curtin et al. (2007) describe how two-inch PVC pipes placed in the walls

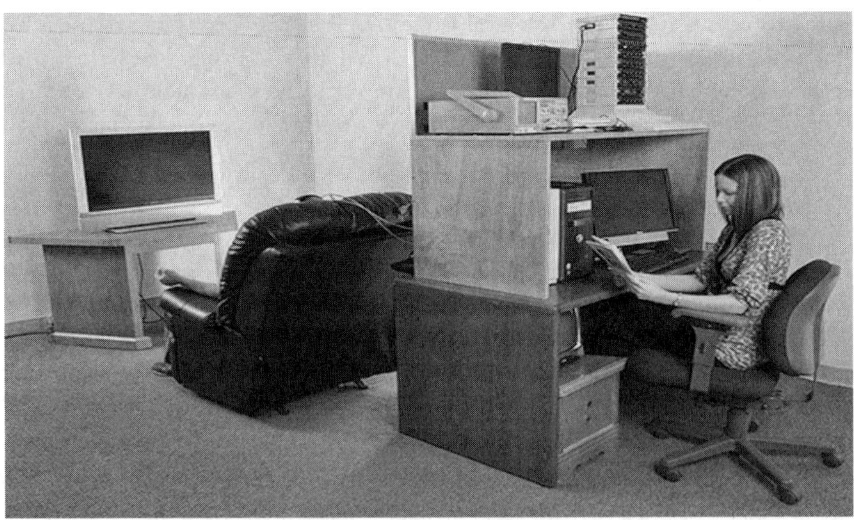

FIGURE 8.2 Simple office dividers create temporary yet obvious experimenter-space and subject-space.

just above the floor surface can serve nicely in this capacity. After running your cables through the pass-through, foam insulation should be placed in each side of the opening to cut down on noise traveling between the two rooms.

Auditory noise should also not be underestimated as a consideration when identifying lab space. While you may think that delivering the audio from your media stimuli via headphones will prevent any need to worry about noises in the hallway outside your lab, you'd be surprised. Finding a location that is somewhat off the beaten path may be preferable to one right in the middle of the main floor of the student union building. However, like with any design decision—building *or* experimental—there are trade-offs. If you locate your lab in a place that is isolated in order to eliminate all possible hallway noises you may find that no one knows where to find you . . . including your experimental subject who has a scheduled appointment to participate in a study at 3:30 this afternoon. If you find that external room noise becomes a problem in the future, many companies make reasonably priced noise dampening foam padding that can be easily adhered to the walls of the subject-space.

Another type of noise is also important to consider when selecting or designing lab space—the ambient electrical noise in the atmosphere at that particular location in the building. While you can't afford to be too picky if you are inheriting an existing space, one stipulation that is paramount is that the location must be away from large sources of extraneous electrical signal in the air. As mentioned throughout this book, the bioelectrical signals that you are trying to measure at the skin surface are extremely small. You will spend a substantial amount of money on bioamplifiers and even more time and effort trying to boost the tiny signals to levels that can be detected by your psychophysiological software programs. This money and time will be spent in vain if boosting those signals simultaneously increases the stray electrical signals coming from an elevator operating right next to the storage room you have converted to your lab space. You also want to avoid close proximity to radio or television studios, which unfortunately is precisely the likely location of spare storage spaces in communication and media departments (Lang, 1994a). Still, being adamant from the beginning about the distance of your assigned space from large pieces of electrical equipment will save you many headaches in the future. Another place to avoid is near the heating, ventilation, and air-conditioning (HVAC) control panels for the building (Curtin et al., 2007).

When you are worrying about the space having too much of the *wrong* kind of electricity don't forget that your lab will also need to have an adequate supply of the *right* kind. At minimum there should be two electrical outlets in the space: one to power the stimulus delivery TV/computer in the subject room and one for the psychophysiology instrumentation in the experimenter space. As a safety precaution it is recommended that all electrical outlets which experimenters or subjects might come in contact with have a ground-fault current interrupter (GFCI) installed by a professional electrician (see Figure 8.3). When a piece of

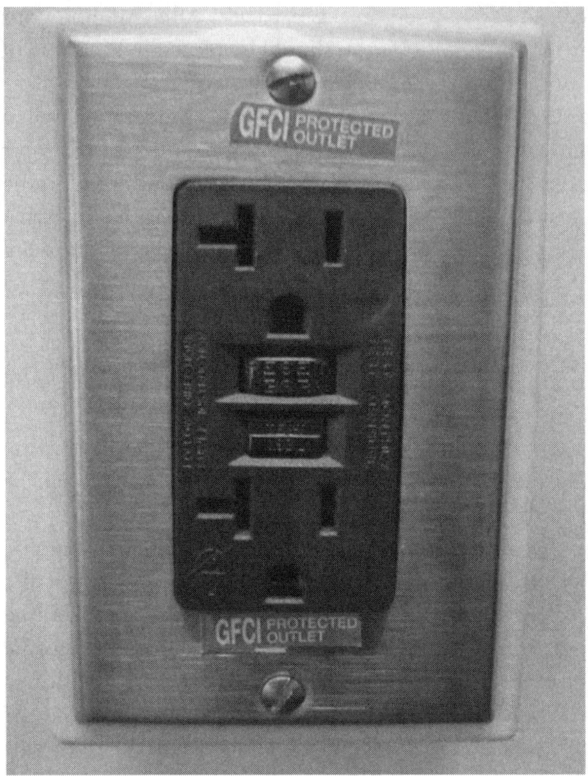

FIGURE 8.3 A ground fault current interrupt (GFCI) is an important tool in ensuring the safety of your research participants and colleagues.

equipment is plugged into a GFCI—which is also known internationally as a Residual Current Device (RCD) or trip switch—the amount of current leaving the outlet is compared to the amount returning from the powered piece of equipment. If there is a difference between the two levels the likely reason is that current is escaping through a faulty connection to ground in the building itself. Discrepancies as small as five milliamps trip the GFCI, preventing further current from leaving the outlet (Greene, Turetsky, & Kohler, 2000). This is a good thing because the electrodes attached to your subject present a low impedance connection between the outlet and the subject. If the subject touches something—say a computer keyboard or a television monitor—which is plugged into an outlet with a broken connection to ground, the current may run through the subject in order to travel to ground. Without the GFCI there to shut off the current at the outlet, dangerous levels of electricity would continue passing through the subject on the way to ground resulting in serious burns, injury, or death. Although most buildings in which your lab might be located will have modern electrical wiring and ground faults are unlikely, the GFCI is an effective form of injury prevention in case of the rare occurrence. Insisting that money be spent by your department, college, or university to have them installed communicates both an understanding of your research craft and the priority you place on subject safety to administrators and is highly recommended. There are other precautions that will become part of your regular research protocol once you have your lab up and running; these are discussed below. But, when you are acquiring space don't forget you will need properly safeguarded sources of electricity to do your work. Other safety concerns that you will want to keep in mind when selecting your lab space include the presence of adequate fire extinguishers and sprinklers, easy access to exits, and a nearby landline phone connection for easy access to emergency support services.

When assessing existing space for locating your lab, also be sure to maximize your ability to control the environment. If there are windows in the subject-space you will want to be able to block them either with blackout film or blinds/curtains if you want to retain the ability to let in sunlight when you aren't collecting data. Electric light sources should also be under your control rather than permanently on or connected to energy saving motion detectors. This allows you to determine the lighting conditions best suited for stimulus delivery in each experiment you conduct. The heating and cooling of the subject room should also be adjustable, "as peripheral psychophysiological response systems may adaptively respond to keep participants cool or warm, potentially confounding the recording of the signals of interest" (Curtin et al., 2007, p. 400).

Let's suppose you are lucky enough to have several places from which you can choose to hang your sign and begin creating your own lab space. Each location meets the "minimum requirements" spelled out above. There are other things that you may want to keep in mind as potential tie-breakers. Is the space close to a supply of running water? Remember, unless you are committed to the periodic costs associated with disposable electrodes you will need to have access to water to clean the used gel out of the reusable ones. Also consider how close the space is to bathroom facilities for the future comfort of both you and your subjects. Are there Internet jacks already installed in the space? What about a wireless Internet signal? If one location has a stronger wireless signal than the other, for example, that may prove important for uploading data to storage servers or downloading future stimulus messages from YouTube.

Furnishing the space

After you have your lab space (and put the sign on the door!) you will need to fill it with the things necessary to conduct research. First you'll need furniture and the most important piece in the whole lab is the chair you have the subjects sit in. Why is it so significant? Consider the amount of use it will get—a typical psychophysiological within-subjects experimental design calls for about 40 people to flop down in that chair. And you may conduct several different studies in a single year. Each of your subjects will sit in that chair for up to 75 minutes watching media messages that they might not *choose* to expose themself to if given the chance. The subject chair therefore needs to be well-built and comfortable. Plus, it should be made out of a material that will minimize the amount of static electricity generated when the subject moves around in it during the experimental session. Artificial leather, in other words, would be preferable to fabric.

After you have spent some money on a new chair for the subjects to sit in, it's time to have the first frank assessment of your research budget. It is a fair bet that you will not have as much money available as you would like to . . . researchers never do. Yet, out of that limited amount of funds you must buy three categories of things: psychophysiological data collection equipment, stimulus presentation equipment, and furniture. For us, this is presented in the order of budgetary priority. With a limited budget, the importance of new and matching furniture for you and your colleagues to use is not very high. You need sturdy desks to set the important electrical equipment on, but they can be obtained from anywhere, really. Most universities have surplus stores where the "hand-me-down" furniture goes when someone with a $1 million grant buys new stuff. Until you get your own $1 million grant, save your budget by getting the used lab furniture. Second-hand stores and garage sales are also great places to look for things of lesser importance and you'd be surprised how far this can help stretch your beginning research budget. Keep in mind, though, if you are outfitting a single-room as your lab space getting used furniture that squeaks may prove to be obnoxiously distracting to research subjects (Curtin et al., 2007). Use all your senses—including your ears—when shopping for the furniture bargains to outfit your lab.

Purchasing and understanding your lab equipment

After you have a place to sit and a desk to work at in your new lab space, the place will become a home-away-from-home because, as Lang (1994a) says, "setting up a lab is a time sink" (p. 230). In fact, our research budgets would be flush for the foreseeable future if we had $5 for every time a graduate student told us, in effect, "Wow, doing a psychophysiological experiment is *a lot of* work!" Experimentation is hard work, and it takes lots of time. So does initially setting up the lab. It takes time to investigate the different types of equipment available and decide which options will allow you to best pursue your particular research interests. It takes even more time to set up the equipment, learn how each individual component works and integrate them into a smoothly functioning whole. It takes time to learn the many software programs you must master: software for stimulus presentation, data collection, data cleaning, data processing and analysis. Each program and equipment manual will initially seem like they are written in a foreign language. Unfortunately, there is no way this or any other book can substitute for the experience and insight you will gain by spending time in your lab learning the intricacies and capabilities of your hardware and your software. At first it will seem very daunting. That's why graduate students reading this book are encouraged to begin familiarizing themselves with the ins and outs of the lab you are currently working in at a technical level beyond simply what is required to collect and analyze data. The sooner you begin investing time in developing technical expertise in both lab hardware and software the better. But, whoever you are—grad student or tenured professor—if you are reading this chapter because you are thinking about starting your own lab, don't let the warnings of the necessary time investment propel you into a relapse of *labophobia*. Instead, remember this:

> [I]n the beginning, the new lab is a lot like a new baby: A whole lot of time, money, and effort are spent on it, and there is not much to show for it. The best defense against the inevitable frustration involved is to remember the time spent getting the lab right means that, in the future, the lab will run smoothly and efficiently, and if you are not careful, it will completely swamp you in data, which you will never have time to write up.
>
> (Lang, 1994a, pp. 230–231)

So, what sort of equipment do you need to buy? An easy way to organize your thinking is to once again consider the concept of the signal chain mentioned in Chapter 3. When building your lab you should think about the signal chain of both independent and dependent variables within your lab. On the independent variable side you will need to deliver to your research subjects media messages that represent a manipulation of features you are studying. How will you do that? Again, much has changed since the early 1990s when most video messages were played back on VHS videotape through standard color television sets. Today many media psychology labs store their stimuli as digitized signals on computer hard drives and use research software packages to play them back for subjects over LCD or Plasma monitors capable of accepting computer signals. So, there are the first three things you need to devote time to researching: a stimulus computer, a monitor, and a stimulus-control software package. Computer and monitor specifications change so rapidly that committing too many parameters to paper here would be futile. Still, when considering the type of computer to store stimuli and load stimulus presentation control software on, make sure it has plenty of hard drive storage capacity, video RAM, and a high-end video card. If investigating the cognitive and emotional processing of audio or music is a part of your research interests then making sure the stimulus computer has a high quality sound card is paramount, as is a good set of headphones. If you plan on measuring eye-blink startle it is recommended that the headphones *not* be noise-cancelling as this tends to impact the instantaneous rise-time in the white noise probe burst that is key to startle elicitation.

In terms of monitor choice, consider your research interests and issues of external validity. If you are investigating the processing of television messages, the trends in terms of home viewing are toward larger—and unfortunately for you, more expensive—liquid crystal display (LCD) monitors rather than more traditional cathode ray tube (CRT) televisions. Nevertheless, bigger may not always be better. If the room in which your experimental subject will sit is small then getting the widest big-screen TV may not provide them with the best possible viewing angle. If you are interested in web browsing behaviors, your monitor should represent the situations you want to test. If you are interested in processing of computer games you'll need to buy a game console that can interface with the monitor you purchase and, ideally, also with the stimulus presentation control software. Finally, remember that as a researcher you will want to be able to see what the research subject is experiencing on whatever monitor you buy. There are a variety of ways to do this. Some researchers rely on video cameras mounted in the subject-space that deliver images of the subject and what's on the screen to a separate monitor in the experimenter-space. Others use a video splitter to replicate the signal being delivered from the stimulus computer onto a second monitor that the experimenter watches. Some researchers send signals from multiple different video streams (the stimulus computer, the psychophysiological recording monitor screen, and different camera angles of the subject experience) to a quad-screen picture-in-picture recording device. This allows for future analysis of subject behaviors, such as "leaning in" or "sitting back" behaviors that change distance to the screen (Bellman, Schweda, & Varan, 2009), as well as easy recognition of movement artifact in the psychophysiological signals during the data cleaning process. Of course, the decision of how elaborate to make your mechanisms for keeping track of the subject and the stimuli delivered will be influenced by budgetary issues—we know of single-room labs that function quite well by having the experimenter occasionally peak through a gap in the curtain separating them from the subject to make sure that everything is still on track.

When it comes to stimulus-presentation software packages there are several to choose from. Most not only play back stimuli in systematic or randomized orders, they also have the capability to collect data from subjects using a variety of methods including many mentioned in Chapter 7 such as STRT, CRM, and self-report questionnaires. If you are interested in recording response time (e.g., response latencies involved in studying attitude accessibility) you will want to be familiar with how accurately the software records key presses on a keyboard. There can be a delay of as much as approximately 300 milliseconds in the recording of key presses by data collection programs and this can significantly impact the validity of response latency data for some measures. Some vendors manufacture special keyboards that are designed to specifically address this issue. Many stimulus software programs can also generate digital signals from external ports of the stimulus computer at times specified by the researcher. This capability provides an important way to synchronize the stimulus being presented with the physiological signals being recorded. Being able to time-lock these allows for the precise representation of the dynamic nature of the cognitive and emotional processing of the message evidenced by the physiological data. Table 8.1 lists several software vendors we are familiar with and Curtin et al. (2007) give a more comprehensive list including several providing the more specialized software required for presenting stimuli in fMRI, EEG, and ERP experiments.

There is an important caveat concerning software in the media psychophysiology lab that should be mentioned here. The closer you can get to the source of the programming language the more flexibility you will have. This is the case for stimulus presentation software as well as physiological data collection and data analysis software. Those who have learned a software language (e.g., Matlab, Java, etc.)—or those who are willing to—will have the ultimate in control over what is shown to a subject along with what physiological responses are recorded and when. But, learning these languages takes time and may not be your cup of tea. If that's the case (it *is* for at least one of the authors of this book!) then you will have to sacrifice a certain amount of flexibility in exchange for the time you will save using an off-the-shelf software program.

Another consideration on the independent variable side of things concerns how you will edit the media stimuli you want to use. It is unlikely that you will want to show your subjects a whole episode of a sitcom. Instead you will need to find examples of different scenes from different programs which vary according to your independent variable of interest. As another example, suppose you want to manipulate television news stories so that images of political candidates are added or removed. These types of concerns raise two related issues. The first is how to import the sitcom, news story, or video stimulus into your computer as a digital signal. The second is how to edit it. Importing video is sometimes a hardware-related issue and you may need to consider the purchase of an analog-to-digital video converter. This device essentially does the same thing to a video signal that the AD/DA board in your psychophysiology data collection computer does for biosignals: it samples the continuous analog signal at a consistent rate and turns those samples into digital representations that the computer can store. A video converter is particularly necessary if you foresee a need to digitize pieces from VHS analog tape or copy-protected digital formats. If, however, your source video is in a digital format to begin with (e.g., it was recorded using a DVR or DVD recorder/player) then importing it directly into a computer for editing is fairly straightforward. Editing of your visual stimuli can be done using a variety of programs ranging from simple shareware to full digital production packages. Like most of these decisions, selecting the digital program best for you is driven by your research interests weighed against available budget.

A final piece of advice about setting up the independent-variable side of your lab: if your space is to be shared by you and your colleagues, be sure to include them in the decision-making processes surrounding stimulus creation and presentation regardless of whether they will be collecting psychophysiological

TABLE 8.1 Name and URLs for major vendors of interest

Vendor name	Product name(s)	Website address
Stimulus presentation software vendors		
Cedrus Corporation	SuperLab	www.superlab.com
Empirisoft Corportation	Media Lab/Direct RT	www.empirisoft.com
The Mathworks, Inc.	MATLAB	www.mathworks.com
Neurobehavioral Systems	Presentation	www.neurobs.com/presentation
Psychology Software Tools, Inc.	E-Prime	www.pstnet.com
Qualtrics, Inc.	Online Survey Software	www.qualtrics.com
Psychophysiological hardware vendors		
Biopac Systems, Inc.	Biopac MP36R/MP100/MP150	www.biopac.com/Research.asp
Contact Precision Instruments	Psychlab	www.psychlab.com
Coulbourn Instruments	Lablinc V	www.coulbourn.com
MindWare Technologies	Mind Ware complete systems	www.mindwaretech.com
Thought Technology, Ltd	Procomp/Flexcomp Infinity	www.thoughttechnology.com
AD/DA board component vendors		
Scientific Solutions, Inc.	Lab Master	www.labmaster.com

dependent measures or not. This approach results in tremendous goodwill plus getting more people involved in ways to utilize the space helps ensure it will rarely be sitting idle. This turns what used to be an old storage room into a more vibrant and active area of scientific enquiry in your department, college, and university.

When it comes to measuring psychophysiological variables as dependent measures, there are four primary purchase points: the bioamplifiers, software, the AD/DA board, and the computer to run it all and store the data on. Table 8.1 lists several of the more commonly used equipment vendors and URLs for their websites. For those who want to "one-stop-shop" several vendors provide you with 75 percent of what you need to get started (not 100 percent, as most vendors leave the purchase of a data collection computer up to you). For those of you still not sure whether psychophysiological measures are for you, both Biopac Systems and Thought Technology sell relatively inexpensive and smaller systems where 4–5 channels will accept a variety of different bioelectrical signal inputs and allow you to analyse them using proprietary software packages. This allows you to experience collecting a wide variety of dependent measures, but understand that the "general use" data collection systems tend to limit the amount of freedom researchers have over things like boosting signal strength gains, high- and low-pass filtering, sampling rates and data analysis over different time courses.

Those who want to retain control over these things will want to choose from systems that are more modular in nature and provide dedicated units designed to measure specific bioelectrical signals. All of the vendors listed in Table 8.1 provide such systems and several allow for even more flexibility by letting the researcher purchase either branded software and AD/DA boards from the system manufacturer or integrate their modular measurement devices with software and computer interfaces from third-party companies. The particular measurement modules that you purchase should be driven by the research questions you are interested in. As mentioned in earlier chapters, the primary measures in the field to date have been skin conductance, facial EMG, and heart rate. It is arguable that the skin conductance coupler becomes less necessary as an index of sympathetic nervous system activation for a researcher devoted to moving HRV measures forward in the field of media psychology, as the relative influence of both branches of the ANS can be ascertained through either frequency- or time-based variability measures. However, the lack of current published work in the area prevents us from making a firm recommendation on this issue. It is good to keep in mind that some vendors sell components labelled as dedicated to particular measures (e.g., *specifically* as EMG bioamplifiers) and others sell more generic bioamplifiers that can be used to collect several different types of signals depending upon the particular hypothesis or research question at the time. In other words, purchasing a generic and flexible bioamplifier would allow you to use it to measure corrugator EMG in one experiment where emotion is the primary focus and heart rate in another study where attention is the dependent concept of interest.

Along with flexibility, it is a good suggestion to design your psychophysiological measurement system to be expandable so that you can add capabilities to your system in the future (Lang, 1994a). Getting a component system that allows you to, for example, add a $500 module to measure another channel of EMG or perhaps something you've always wondered about but never tried (say, skin temperature or breathing rate) allows for exciting new possibilities if an administrator at your university ever finds extra funds at the end of a fiscal year that they want to spread around . . . hey, it *could* happen and you'll want to be prepared if it does!

When it comes to the dependent-variable signal chain, the software used tends to be the same during data collection and data processing. The trade-offs associated with stimulus-control software apply here as well—if you want to have software that is more intuitive and similar to a "point-and-click" system you are going to be up and running quicker than if you take the time to learn a more code-based software language. However, this may be coupled by a lack of flexibility in things like variable sampling rates for specific measures within the same experiment (as discussed with the eye-blink startle response in Chapter 6), the ability to manually explore and clean movement artifact out of IBI data, and different durations of output segmentation during data processing. Although software packages are becoming more powerful and more flexible all the time, and many of the psychophysiological software vendors have outstanding customer support responsive to inquiries and suggestions, some researchers feel there is no substitute to being able to get to the programming code itself.

The purchase of the data collection computer, the stimulus-presentation computer, and the AD/DA board should be done simultaneously in order to make sure that the three systems can communicate with each other. In order to understand why this is important, let's start with a more in-depth discussion of what an AD/DA board does. First, realize that an AD/DA board has two important "halves" to it. The first is an interface between the bioamplifiers/couplers and the board itself. This tends to happen through cabling that comes from the "output" side of the bioamplifier to the "input" side of the AD/DA board. On the board itself you will find analog and digital inputs. The one you use depends upon the type of signal you are dealing with. Remember from Chapter 4 that heart rate is often measured using a dual comparator/window-discriminator where a single pulse is sent whenever a voltage threshold is crossed by the QRS-complex in the heart rate signal. This single pulse is digital—usually the channel is off, but when the voltage threshold is reached and the trigger tripped, a very brief "on" signal is sent before turning the channel off again. Therefore a cable would run from the output of the dual-comparator to the *digital* input of the AD/DA board into the channel which your software program has designated for heart rate. For EMG, skin conductance, or if you wanted an actual analog recording of the ECG signal rather than merely the duration of the inter-beat interval, these would run from the output of these bioamps/couplers to the *analog* input channel corresponding to that signal as dictated by the measurement software.

Again, thinking in terms of signal chain, we now have information from the bioamplifier/coupler travelling to the AD/DA board—but it needs to get to the data collection computer to be saved to the hard drive. This is the second "half" of the AD/DA board arrangement. The board communicates with the computer through a card that gets plugged into the back of the computer—usually through a pin connector similar (but not exactly) like those used to plug in printers in the days before USB connections. The pin connector on the back of the data collection computer is actually the receiving end of the second half of the AD/DA board which is plugged into an Input/Output (I/O) slot on the mother board of the computer. Now, you may not know this—we didn't when we first started—but there are different types of I/O slots on mother boards. And *this* is why you should consider buying your AD/DA board and your data collection computer at the same time. You want to make sure that second "half" of the AD/DA board that you buy can find a place to plug into on your data collection computer. If the correct I/O slot isn't built in, it can be a real headache.

Let's now turn to the communication between the stimulus-presentation computer and the psychophysiological data collection computer. Remember that many stimulus-presentation software programs can also send signals to the data collection computer. Usually this is done as a digital pulse at the onset of an important event like the beginning of a stimulus message. There are a few ways to get this signal into the data collection computer. The easiest, perhaps, is through one of the digital input channels on the AD/DA board itself. However, as Curtin et al. (2007) mention, many stimulus-presentation software packages rely on the delivery of a signal via a parallel printer port input on the data collection computer. Unfortunately, the parallel port is not included on many off-the-shelf models of modern computers. Be sure to know what the parameters of your presentation software and your data collection computer are so you can ease their ability to communicate with each other.

The storage capacity of your psychophysiological data collection computer depends upon the types of signals you are recording. For example, your file sizes for each subject will be quite small if you are only recording IBI data from heart rate because you'll only be storing a single 3–4 digit value about 70 times a minute. If, however, you are recording multi-channel EEG data sampled at 80 Hz you will need substantially more storage space. The psychophysiological equipment vendors should be able to guide you on the recommended size of the hard drive for your storage computer. However, it is also suggested that you look at the recommendations provided by Curtin et al. (2007) concerning the redundant backup of your data on hard drives and/or server space independent of the data collection computer drive. Backing up of data should be a regular protocol for you and your colleagues during any psychophysiological study—you (and your subjects) have gone through plenty in order to provide the data . . . you want to make sure that it was worth it.

A final thought about the issues surrounding the selection of the right equipment for your lab: don't forget the valuable resources available in the community of scholars also interested in psychophysiological research. The Society for Psychophysiological Research has a round table lunch discussion *every year* devoted to assisting new investigators as they set up their laboratories. Those of us who have done it before know what it's like to be in your position on the learning curve and we want to help if we can. We might not be able to, due to the time pressures of our own lab schedules, academic and personal responsibilities. But if you are aware of someone who does the type of work you are interested in, contact them with your questions. Not everyone will be approachable and friendly, but many are. They won't come and set up your lab out of the goodness of their heart, but chances are they will answer a solicitation for advice or input if it is obvious that you have done the intellectual work required to make it a thoughtful and intelligent inquiry.

This provides a nice transition into the next section of this chapter: ways that *you* can pass on all that you know about your lab to students and others in your research group.

Passing on your understanding: lab training

Once you have invested all the time and effort necessary to understand how your lab works you need to pass those details on to others. After all, for many of you reading this chapter teaching is an important reason you do what you do. Having collaborators around your lab not only keeps you from being the only one who collects data from all those subjects who will sit in the comfy chair, it makes the lab environment more vibrant and fun. Plus, as colleagues and students take a larger role in the lab they will begin to learn tricks of the trade that you don't know about and then the transmission of knowledge flows both ways. There are four different mechanisms that can be used to pass on details about the lab to those interested in using it: Lab Manuals, Lab Meetings, Training Days, and Study Notebooks.

Lab manuals—in a university community students and colleagues come and go. Each has a particular skill set and each becomes aware of different idiosyncrasies surrounding hardware, software, research design, research organizations, etc. One of the best things you can do to make your lab as productive as possible is to begin writing down the "things that work" in a lab manual so that they can be remembered and referred to. Make the lab manual user-friendly and cultivate an understanding within your lab that the *first* place people should go when they have a question is the lab manual. This culture does two things. First, it keeps you from having to answer the same questions repeatedly. Second, it subtly encourages the practice of searching for answers in the literature. There are at least two ways to administer lab manuals. The more modern viewpoint is to set up the lab manual as a wiki, updatable and editable by every member of the lab group. Our experience is more centralized, with the lab manual being kept by one person—either the lab director or a designated lab manager. If you decide to administer a lab manual in a manner which allows people other than yourself to input information, make sure that you read your lab manual regularly so that you know what details and instructions are being passed on.

Even if you decide against a wiki approach, there is no reason not to have the manual be an electronic document that anyone in the lab can read. The first thing discussed at the inaugural lab meeting of every semester should be instructions for how to access the lab manual. A slightly-edited version of the Table of Contents from one of our lab manuals appears in the appendix to this chapter. You'll notice that the contents range from mundane issues of housekeeping (phone numbers, maps, inventory) to the philosophical ("Thoughts on Being a Colleague") and practical ("Cleaning Electrodes").

Lab meetings—one of the most effective ways to get people in your department to know about the new place you have created for social scientific data collection is to hold weekly lab meetings. Announce them to the faculty and interested students. If the research space is shared between faculty colleagues, make sure that you express to them how important it is that everyone who has an interest in the space meet regularly to share information about the lab and ways of improving how it functions. Lab meetings should begin with informational announcements about the space itself: details about a planned fire alarm later that afternoon, a new trick that was learned about how to get better audio from the stimulus presentation computer and where it will be put in the lab manual, etc. After that, an effective meeting format that we have used at several institutions is to progress through a list of ongoing studies and have the Principle Investigator give everyone an update. This makes sure that everyone knows just how busy the space actually is, helps communicate research interests between people who may otherwise have no clue what each other does, and helps to motivate and increase productivity as researchers work toward conference paper deadlines, manuscript submissions, and publications, not to mention student theses and dissertations.

Other times during lab meetings questions about particularly troublesome issues surrounding physiological data collection and processing, experimental design, and statistical analysis can be brought up and discussed. Preliminary data can be presented and sample job talks given by advanced graduate students. And, when there is nothing else to do (which is rare), the weekly lab meeting can be used as a journal club to discuss the latest publications in the field of media psychology research (Valentini & Daniels, 1997).

Develop a lab email distribution list and send out a summary following each meeting to ensure that the information is distributed to those who were unable to attend and archived for future reference.

Training days—those of you who have taught media production (or any other skills-based course) know nothing can reinforce information in a textbook like actually seeing, touching, and *experiencing* what is described in texts. Many believe that the way to accomplish this is by getting interested students involved with studies immediately and "letting them get their feet wet." While we practice this approach too, it is not the most effective way of passing along knowledge in the lab (Barker, 2002). This is especially true as the lab and your career develop and must rely almost exclusively on advanced students to pass on knowledge to beginners. Like the old campfire game of "telephone" where the original message ends up quite distorted after being whispered through many different channels, the techniques and protocols actually being practiced in your lab may end up having little resemblance to your ideals unless you gather all the investigators together occasionally and lead face-to-face training sessions. Find out from new members of the lab what procedures they would like tutorials on. Or, better yet, develop a rotating list yourself and set up a periodic training day for your lab group.

Study notebooks—every study that you conduct should have a notebook . . . or two . . . or three . . . into which every detail about that study is placed. The original doodling of an experimental design made during a coffee discussion with a collaborator . . . it goes in the notebook. The list of pretest stimuli . . . it goes in the notebook. The sample of the questionnaire used during the pretest. Printouts of the statistical analyses. The original copy of the approved informed consent document. All in the notebook. Everything should be kept in one place so that whenever a question arises about a particular study the first place you go is to the notebook.

We must admit that this is the lab communication mechanism we struggle with the most in the modern manifestations of our labs. When we were trained as graduate students it was drummed into us that anything (*anything!*) to do with a study was printed off, three-hole punched, and put in one of the study notebooks; with the most recent documents placed at the front for easy retrieval. But in today's paperless environment this strategy has become more difficult in practicality. Instead, the *concept* of the study notebook has evolved into an electronic form. This is fine, except when you take "pages" out of the electronic notebook, work on them, and either forget to put them back in the electronic notebook for others to access or save over the top of the previous page thereby losing the historical trace of the study's progression. Collaboration document delivery programs may be the way that you solve this problem. Or, perhaps you develop a system for naming computer directories and individual documents on your lab server in such a way that old versions remain archived but not confused with the "current thinking" of the study itself. Whatever version of the modern-day study notebook you come up with, it is an important tool for saving all things related to a particular experiment. Then, once you have a particular study notebook protocol in place, be sure to pass it on to all the members working on that study. In fact, it wouldn't be a bad idea to develop a lab-wide protocol for naming and archiving electronic files, using it for the electronic notebooks for all your studies. Where would you keep a generalized description of such a file-naming protocol? That's *right*—the Lab Manual.

Designing experiments

It is impractical to discuss all the intricacies associated with experimental design in this small section of a single chapter when many excellent books have been written on the topic (Cochran & Cox, 1957; Kirk, 1995). Furthermore, perhaps the best advice to media psychology researchers considering designing experiments utilizing psychophysiological dependent measures is to read examples from both the media psychology research and psychophysiological literature which we highlight in this book. They provide good illustrations of how to design experiments to maximize the likelihood of finding significant differences in physiological signals based on independent variable differences. Furthermore, an outstanding source of basic experimental design advice—for any media psychology researcher, not just those using psychophysiology—is a book chapter by Reeves and Geiger (1994) entitled "Designing experiments that assess psychological responses to media messages." Specifically in the area of psychophysiological research, Jennings and Gianaros (2007) also provide important guidance surrounding design issues. The general suggestions given below rely heavily on these two sources.

There are generally two types of experimental designs to choose from: within-subjects and between-subjects designs. While most readers are likely more conceptually familiar with the latter, most psychophysiological researchers use a within-subjects design in their work (Jennings & Gianaros, 2007). In a within-subjects design each individual is exposed to all levels of the independent variable and their responses to each compared for statistically significant differences. In a between-subjects design, on the other hand, participants are randomly assigned to the different levels of the independent variable and experience only one of the levels. The responses from the two groups are then compared for significant differences. In many experimental designs in media psychology research it is assumed that random assignment to treatment groups will adequately address issues of individual differences in confounding variables which may inadvertently affect the outcome. However, the baseline levels of all the major psychophysiological indices differ widely among individuals and for that reason it is a better strategy to compare each subject to themselves using a repeated measures within-subject design. A further benefit to using a within-subjects design for media psychology experiments is that "for many treatments in communication research, all levels of the treatment do in fact exist within the context of a single individual's experiences" (Reeves & Geiger, 1994, p. 175).

So, a general recommendation is to use within-subjects design if the stimuli and hypotheses will allow. However, the issue of carryover effects must also be addressed in the presentation of stimuli via a within-subjects design. Carryover effects are "created when our participants behave differently depending upon the condition they initially (or previously) received" (Jennings & Gianaros, 2007, p. 814). So, consider the simple hypothesis that subjects' zygomatic and orbicularis oculi muscles will be more activated during commercials using cartoon characters than those using real human actors. Suppose that you conducted an experiment and found that the EMG data confirmed this hypothesis but your design always presented the ad with the human actors first and the cartoon ad second. The carryover threat to validity in this within-subjects design is that the activation of the zygomatic and the orbicularis oculi could be due to a *comparison* of the emotional affect generated by the first commercial carried over to the second. If the stimuli were instead reversed, with the cartoon message played first followed by the message using human actors, the effect may disappear. One way around this would be to either randomly present the commercials using your stimulus presentation software or ensure that each of the messages are presented first to half of the subjects.

You likely have enough experience with basic experimental design to notice another threat to the validity of the human-versus-cartoon example. It could be that the commercial containing the human spokesperson has some other feature— besides the fact that it is not populated by cartoon characters—which leads to the significant difference in EMG activation. Perhaps it's for a product that many subjects had a bad experience with. Or the human spokesperson has a particularly irritating voice. Or the ad features a song in a minor key. The list of differences between the single ads chosen to represent the two levels of the independent variable in this hypothetical example is likely quite long. So, here is another general recommendation for experimental design: use more than one message as an exemplar of the different levels of your independent variable. This, in fact, is a good recommendation for studies using either a within- or between-subjects design since the presence of confounding variables would influence the outcome of either.

So, how many messages should you choose to represent each of your levels? This depends upon the amount of variance between the different levels of the independent variable and the amount of variance between the different messages you choose to represent each of these levels (Reeves & Geiger, 1994). In other words, if there is a subtle difference between the different levels of the independent variable then you'll need more messages rather than fewer in order to find a significant effect. Similarly, if there are a lot of differences between the messages *within* a single treatment level you'll need more messages rather than fewer to offset the impact of these on the variance found for your statistical comparisons across levels of the independent variable.

Eventually, the number of messages you pick will depend upon their duration and the amount of time you have available with each subject. If your stimuli are advertisements they are short and you can get a lot of different repetitions in. If instead you are testing some independent variable associated with "suspenseful scenes" in movies, they may take a little longer and you may not be able to have as many message repetitions as if you were studying ads. A researcher interested in exploring the impact of a variable on the processing of an entire episode of a primetime drama would likely have their number of messages limited to one because a general guideline is that a subject's visit to the psychophysiological lab should last no more than 90 minutes. That's *not* 90 minutes of stimulus presentation. The 90 minutes includes filling out of all necessary paperwork, applying the electrodes, conducting impedance checks, presenting stimuli, removing electrodes, and obtaining any post-message self-report measures.

The 90-minute time window sometimes presents another challenge in the media lab. Occasionally an experiment can be designed using an adequate number of stimuli in each level of the independent variable but still the anticipated overall duration of the experiment is quite short—say, less than an hour. When this is the case, consider asking around your lab group to see if there are two experimental protocols that can be combined. Be sure to make design choices which address the carryover effect issue discussed previously. That caution aside, it is our experience that one experiment can often serve as a distraction task to clear short-term memory between the stimulus presentation and the memory-related self-report data collection for another. This seems more respectful of the subject as it acknowledges the fact that they will have had to sit through the monotonous (and perhaps embarrassing and somewhat anxiety-inducing) skin preparation and electrode application procedures and might be somewhat put off if, having gone through all that, they only are shown a very limited number of stimulus messages.

Besides the number of messages to show subjects, experimental design requires an understanding of the number of subjects you will need to expose to your protocol. This is an issue of statistical power, that is the probability that the null hypothesis—the one that states there is *no* impact of your independent variable on the psychophysiological measure—will be rejected if it is in fact false (Faul, Erdfelder, Lang, & Buchner, 2007). Here again, within-subjects design is preferable if possible for reasons explained by Reeves and Geiger (1994):

> the same power in experiments can be achieved with substantially fewer subjects. A group of twenty subjects participating in a within-subject study has the equivalent power of 40 subjects if the treatment factor has two levels, and 60 subjects if there are three levels.

(p. 175)

But still, the question remains how many will be enough since you want to have enough participants to find a significant effect if it is there, but no more than you need (Jennings & Gianaros, 2007). There are several software programs available to allow researchers to input their general design parameters (number of independent variables, number of levels of each, etc.) and calculate the number of participants necessary to reach sufficient statistical power for a range of expected effect sizes. One that is available as shareware is G★Power which can be downloaded directly from the web (www.psycho.uni-duesseldorf.de/abteilungen/aap/gpower3; Faul et al., 2007).

Conducting experiments

After the lab is built, the study designed, the stimuli found, you'll be ready to run your first experiment. But, before you do there is one more important thing to do. You need to make sure that your planned research protects the three cornerstones of ethical treatment of human subjects: respect for persons, beneficence, and justice (Ryan et al., 1979). In a nutshell this means:

1. that you have to obtain informed consent from all the subjects that participate in your experiment;
2. you must ensure your subjects are not harmed and furthermore that the research design maximizes the benefits obtained by the research while minimizing possible harms; and
3. that you are fair in the selection of participants.

Since 1991 the United States Code of Federal Regulations has required that Primary Investigators submit their research plans to an Institutional Review Board (IRB) which ensures these three criteria are being met. This applies to you . . . even if you think it doesn't. If you are getting ready to attach electrodes to a human participant and have not consulted with your university's IRB . . . stop. You have some paperwork to fill out, and official approval to receive, before you continue with your work.

Although filling out that paperwork and waiting to receive approval may seem arduous, it is important to many different people. The first is to your subjects, as it is good to have several pairs of "outside eyes" take a look at your research plan and lab set-up to make sure that the human beings going through your research protocols are protected. And writing out all the things you do to keep your lab safe is a good refresher for you and your students, reminding you what is necessary each time you step in the lab. For example, you should regularly check for both ground faults in your lab's building and current leakage in your lab's electrical equipment using a multimeter. You should be sure that all electrical equipment which will make direct connection to a human subject is fitted with a GFCI and that unused plugs are covered with safety caps. You should *not* run subjects through psychophysiological data collection protocols during thunderstorms and you should not allow subjects to get out of their nice comfortable fake-leather chair while they have electrodes still attached. You will need to spell out all of these precautions when preparing your IRB submission. Furthermore, most IRBs will also require you to explicitly describe your protocol. What happens first in the experiment? What next? Will the electrodes be removed before or after the recognition memory test? All these things will need to be spelled out anyway—in a written protocol—for you and your co-investigators to follow in order to make sure that the data-collection procedure is standardized across all scheduled participants. So it actually benefits you to complete the IRB paperwork, spelling out the sequential steps of the experiment, and then move directly to creating a research checklist or protocol for internal lab use.

A final group of people who benefit from your IRB compliance is one that you would never think of . . . your colleagues across the entire campus. Any university that receives federal funding in the form of research grants is required to keep institutional oversight upon all the research conducted by anyone on its campus—not just research that is grant funded, but *all* research—to ensure that human subjects are protected from harm. If you think that you can fly under the radar you are not only putting your subjects at risk, but the academic endeavours of your colleagues. So, fill out the paperwork, get your study approved, and then you are ready to go.

When the first subject arrives you may be as nervous as, or perhaps more than, they are. The key here is to remember that as with anything, the more times you do it the more comfortable you get. Be professional and courteous, but not overly solemn and serious. You want to set the subject at ease, answering all their questions about what the protocol entails before they sign their informed consent form. Sometimes subjects want to know *specifically* what it is you are studying. If telling them is expected to impact how they process the media message, politely explain that to them and tell them you will gladly discuss the particular experimental design with them after the session or, if necessary, invite them to email you their questions at a later time.

It is best, when going through skin preparations and electrode attachment, to explain each step *prior* to doing it. "Now this is a paper towel that I'm dampening with distilled water . . . Can I just use it to wipe the palm of your hand with?" It is a good habit to get into to begin applying electrodes at the furthest extremity first and work toward the face. In other words, start with putting on skin conductance and heart rate electrodes first and then work on the facial EMG sites. Although this may seem counterintuitive given that obtaining low impedance is of greatest importance for the facial measures and more time and effort may be required there, application to the face is the most intrusive by far. Use the time spent applying the peripheral electrodes to establish rapport with the subject. This will allow them to relax and make you (literally) getting all up in their face less of a big deal. Oh, and along those lines, remember that as a general rule it is best to avoid using the words like *electrodes* or *syringe* or *impedance* or *ground* with subjects. Although this can be difficult, because you use the terms freely with your co-investigators and in your IRB forms and written protocols, it is possible that they will just make your subjects uneasy.

After the physiological data collection is finished, remove the electrodes. If you are using reusable electrodes, be particularly careful to avoid removing them by pulling on the delicate solder point where the electrode lead attaches to the cup. Instead, remove the electrode by pulling the "grab tab" on the adhesive collar. Do so quickly, as you would remove an adhesive bandage. Be sure to thank the subject for participating and escort them to the door of the lab.

After you've done a few data collection sessions you'll be thinking of ways to improve the experience based on the particular circumstances of your own lab . . . just be sure to write those suggested improvements in your Lab Manual. Over time you will find yourself gaining more confidence in customizing the lab—in equipment, procedures, as well as working atmosphere—to make it an exciting, collegial, productive environment for your students, colleagues, and yourself.

Summary

This chapter has covered considerations in setting up a media psychophysiology lab. We have presented suggestions for thinking about physical space needs as well as details to consider when ordering both the hardware and software required for conducting experiments. A productive, functioning media psychophysiology lab is an exciting place to collaborate for researchers ranging from undergraduate students to senior faculty. But conducting media psychology research takes a lot of planning and organization of lab resources. We believe that attention to lab management (maintenance of the lab manual, training, lab meetings, etc.) is every bit as important as attention to technical details of lab operations (equipment, supplies, etc.). In the years that we have been engaged in media psychophysiology research we have discovered that it is really a community of colleagues made up of both students and faculty that create "the lab"—more so than having luxurious lab space and the latest, most expensive research equipment. This chapter has hopefully served to give you both knowledge and enthusiasm that will motivate you as you become or continue to be a part of the scholarly community that uses psychophysiological measures to study mediated message processing.

Appendix—sample table of contents for lab manual

Table of Contents—Professor X Lab

Experiments
Lab General
Lab Library
Lab Rats
Photos
Standard Programs
The Archive
Other Resources on the X-Lab Server
How to Access the X-Lab Server
Instructions/Manuals
    Data Collection Software Manual
    Stimulus Presentation Software Manual
Interface Instructions
    How to Use Label Maker
How to Use the Impedance Meter
How to Use the Multimeter
How to Digitize VHS Tapes
    How to Burn CDs and DVDs
    How to Use Audio Recording Software (document in progress)
How to Connect to the X-Lab Server
How to Set-up Xbox
    How to Use Unified Message Phone System
X-Lab Training Series
    Stimulus Presentation Software
    Safety in the Lab
    X-Lab Server Overview
    Use of Psychophysio Equipment
How to do Physio Prep of Human Subjects
    Physiology Data Collection Programming
    Data Cleaning
    Video Editing
    Audio Editing
    Statistics Programs
    Making Figures for Presentations

Other Resources/Supplies
    Inventory of X-Lab Computers and Equipment
    Software on Lab Computers
    Installing Software—see Admin section below
Checking Out X-Lab Resources
Lab Manager Administration
    Working with Computer Tech Office
Lab System Admin Tasks

9

PSYCHOPHYSIOLOGICAL MEASURES AND MEANING

Implications of current research and a peek at the future

The scientific pursuit of an understanding of the dynamic, socially complex interaction between the human mind and media is arguably at an all-time high. The number of media research labs at universities where scholars include psychophysiological measures in their investigations of mediated message processing has substantially increased in the past two decades. We hope that many of those who read this book contribute to this trend by starting their own labs at universities or by becoming productive researchers in existing ones. It is important to note, however, that the exciting scientific environment for understanding the human mind "on" media is certainly not confined to academia. Many private media research companies are investing in psychophysiological measures as a way to provide more scientifically rigorous data—in comparison to traditional surveys and focus groups—for clients whose business is substantially tied to how consumers process all forms of media content. Nowhere is this industry trend as obvious as in advertising, where the term **neuromarketing** has emerged to identify the explicit pursuit of an understanding of how the human brain processes brand messages (Plassman, Ambler, Braeutigam, & Kenning, 2007). This shift in the advertising industry has been characterized as a redirection from an emphasis on the process of creating and delivering ad campaigns to one of understanding the processor of campaign messages—the human mind (Du Plessis, 2008). We have truly entered a new phase in the history of media research that could be considered an age of aggressive scientific pursuit of media psychological science— the study of the embodied mind "on" media.

The previous chapters have provided a look at how the application of psychophysiological measures to studying how the embodied human mind processes mediated messages emerged as a result of a significant paradigm shift in media research, bursting open the supposed "black box" of the human brain to provide rich theoretical insight into mental processes underlying media consumption and influence. Along with a growth in media psychology research, the years since the work of the first true media psychophysiologists in the 1980s (e.g., Byron Reeves, Esther Thorson, and Annie Lang) have seen a tremendous increase in the amount of available intellectual and technical support for the use of psychophysiological measures in media psychology research. All of these developments have created an intellectually exciting and supportive environment for researchers to continue the pursuit of a scientific understanding of the media–mind interaction with an expanding toolbox of measures stocked with all the psychophysiological indices we have discussed. As we conclude, it is useful to reflect on the research environment that exists for researchers who will use psychophysiological measures to move media psychology forward by increasing our understanding of media consumption, processing, and influence. We will briefly describe the current environment as we see it and review some recent work which illustrates the tremendous value of psychophysiological data in media research. This chapter will conclude with a look to the future—considering opportunities and challenges media psychology researchers face in applying psychophysiological measures to the study of mediated message processing.

At no other point in the history of media research has there been such a fertile and supportive environment for media psychology researchers—with the stars aligning, so to speak, for them to play a dominant role in how the use and influence of media are understood. The value of research designed to peer into the mind as it consumes media and gain an in-depth understanding of the process of media influence is widely recognized. Sherry (2004) notes how in the past 20 years, advances in neurophysiology that have been widely embraced by psychology researchers have provided the foundation for media researchers to study "media effects" from a neuropsychological perspective. In 2006, the journal *Media Psychology* published a special issue devoted to using brain-imaging techniques to study mediated message processing. In it was noted that the ability to observe the brain at work processing mediated messages is likely to provide more insightful biological explanations of historical media effects (Anderson et al., 2006). Media psychology researchers—as scholars who are aware of the most current knowledge of the embodied human brain—are uniquely prepared to lead the way in revolutionizing the way "media effects" are conceptualized and studied. Our discussion of psychophysiological measures of mediated message processing throughout this book should make it clear that today's media psychology researcher has access to methodological tools, technology, and published expertise that researchers working in the late 1980s and early 1990s lacked. The current intellectual environment for media psychology researchers is clearly one that supports a theoretically rigorous and operationally expansive application of psychophysiological measures—in combination with other measures of mediated message processing—to the task of meeting the challenge of understanding the role and influence of media messages in the lives of individuals.

As noted in Chapter 1, concern over the role and influence of media in the lives of individuals is what gave birth to media effects research. The continued investigation of this phenomenon by media psychology researchers clearly has implications for the well-being of individuals in society as well as for the media industry. The production of knowledge that improves communication processes ought to be a primary goal of all communication scientists (Chaffee & Berger, 1987) and it is increasingly recognized that psychophysiological data can play a significant part in that quest. Researchers working over the past two decades—since the re-emergence and acceptance of psychophysiology as a method for studying mediated message processing—have produced a growing body of published research that demonstrates the critical role psychophysiology plays in understanding the human mind as it consumes media and the influence this consumption has on individuals. The knowledge that psychophysiological research provides has important implications because the extent to which we understand the media's influence on individuals determines the extent to which we can minimize negative outcomes of media message processing and maximize positive ones. The important implications of psychophysiological research results prove that this approach should not be dismissed as an *overly* reductionistic one, as some critics might suggest. Rather, this *admittedly* reductionistic approach to studying media influence needs to be embraced as providing foundational knowledge useful to improving the process of mediated communication.

Practically every experiment utilizing psychophysiological measures to study mediated message processing has important implications for specific areas of mediated communication. Studies in which psychophysiological data were collected exist for each major area of media research (e.g., news and politics, sex, violence, and persuasion). An extensive review of all the studies that have used psychophysiological measures to produce important knowledge for society and the media industry would result in a book unto itself. In the following paragraphs we take a brief glimpse at how psychophysiological measures have recently produced data yielding knowledge with important implications for both society and the media industry. We will review recent experiments conducted in three well-established areas of media research, ones historically viewed as having important societal implications: Violence, News, and Persuasion.

Violent media, violent minds? Insights from psychophysiological measures

The impact of mediated portrayals of violence has concerned researchers and members of society for decades. The impact of media violence on individuals has recently been proposed to occur along three lines of primary effects—the *aggressor effect* where exposure to mediated violence leads to higher levels of aggression, the *fear of victimization effect* where mediated violence increases estimates of falling prey to violence, and the *conscience-numbing effect* where exposure to violence leads to the desensitization of natural negative emotional reactions (Bushman, Huesmann, & Whitaker, 2009). Research conducted over the last 50 years has built a substantial body of evidence supporting the occurrence of each of these noted effects of mediated violence (see Bushman et al., 2009 for a brief review). Each category of effect ought to be concerning for researchers and society at large, as each has tremendous potential to impact the way individuals view and interact with each other in "real life." That being said, the connection between psychophysiological measures and the study of the impact of media violence may seem more intuitive for the aggressor and conscience-numbing effects because it is easier to conceptualize them as involving processes identifiable through psychophysiological response patterns. However, there is a case to be made that psychophysiological measures have a significant place in studying psychological processes underlying any theory of the impact of mediated violence on individuals. Psychophysiological measures, after all, index embodied processes evoked during exposure to mediated messages, processes which are foundational for any potential emerging "effect" of media content.

Traditional media effects research, focused on documenting observable outcomes rather than understanding psychological processes, has clearly dominated the study of mediated violence. Studies designed to investigate this issue have primarily involved the use of self-report and behavioral measures in order to demonstrate the so-called "effect" of exposure to violent media content. Bandura's "Bobo-doll" experiments described in Chapter 1 provide a good example of this type of research. The systematic study of psychological processes underlying the effects of violent media content is a fairly recent development. In a recent meta-analysis, Bushman and Huesmann (2006) reported that out of their sample of 431 published experiments only 27 included psychophysiological measures. Throughout this book we have proposed that such measures are critical to the study of psychological processes because, unlike traditional measures of media effects, they index mental activity over time. Clearly then, there is tremendous opportunity for media psychology researchers to utilize psychophysiological measures of dynamic, embodied cognitive and emotional processes engaged during exposure to violent media content to increase understanding of its impact on individuals. This can be made clear by briefly reviewing how some researchers working in this area have applied psychophysiological measures in studying media violence.

Those who have applied psychophysiological measures to study media violence have primarily used them to examine how various types of exposure impacts emotional arousal. For instance, in one early study it was found that individuals who live in an inner-city area display higher levels of arousal—as evidenced by skin conductance—while viewing film portrayals of violence when compared to college students living outside the urban area (Frost & Stauffer, 1987). In another experiment in which physiological arousal was a primary dependent variable, results indicated that viewing violent content on a large screen evokes higher levels of skin conductance compared to medium and small screens (Reeves, Lang, Kim, & Tatar, 1999). An emphasis on studying arousal evoked by violent media content makes theoretical sense given that two of the primary negative effects of exposure to violent content—aggression and desensitization—clearly involve changes in excitatory processes.

Early in the history of research on mediated violence, arousal was theorized to play an extremely important role in the observed positive relationship between exposure to violent media content and both aggression and desensitization. Zillmann developed Excitation Transfer Theory to explain how arousal evoked by viewing violent media content could result in higher levels of aggression in response to "real life" encounters—occurring shortly after the exposure—due to residual arousal evoked by the violent content (Zillmann & Johnson, 1973). Early evidence of desensitization to the portrayal of violence was reported by Linz, Donnerstein, and Adams (1989) who found that young adult males who viewed a sexually violent film displayed lower levels of arousal—as evidenced by heart rate—during subsequent exposure to a scene of a male behaving violently towards a female.

Arousal has remained an important concept in recent media psychology research on the impact of media violence on individuals. A major change in the study of media violence—beyond the inclusion of psychophysiological measures—has been a shift from studying violent content in film and television to a focus on studying the impact of violent content in video games. Research on violent video games has clear implications for society at large. Discussion of the potential harmful effects of this form of mediated content often occurs during coverage of horrible tragedies like school shootings. There are also interesting theoretical reasons for media psychology researchers to focus on studying psychological processes engaged in violent video game play. It has been argued that the interactive and particularly engaging virtual environment of violent video games may serve to amplify the effects of exposure to violent content (Bushman et al., 2009). Further, recent research has indicated that adolescent boys may find it easier to identify with characters in violent video games (Konijn, Nije, & Bushman, 2007). The experiments that media psychology researchers have conducted on violent video games in which psychophysiological measures have been used to index arousal have shed light on this extremely important context of media exposure. This is one area in which psychophysiological measures have clearly built on the foundation of traditional media effects research and amplified the implications of media research. Psychophysiological measures of arousal recorded while individuals play violent video games provide a glimpse into the dynamic psychological processes that underlie the potential negative effects of a mediated entertainment activity that is clearly growing in popularity among both youth and adults. Here we summarize some of the more current experiments where psychophysiological measures have been used to index variation in arousal while individuals play violent video games.

Recall that desensitization to the portrayal of supposedly "real life" violence was one of the effects of exposure to violent films noted in earlier research. Recently researchers have collected evidence that the same effect may occur as a result of playing violent video games. Carnagey and colleagues found that participants who played a violent video game displayed lower levels of galvanic skin response during subsequent exposure to a video containing scenes of real-life violence compared to individuals who played a nonviolent game (Carnagey, Anderson, & Bushman, 2007). This particular study provides evidence that playing violent video games may indeed momentarily dampen the intensity of negative emotional response to violence in society. The immediate, physiological desensitization to violence suggested by this study might not at face value appear all that important; however, future research should investigate whether there are levels of violent video game play that lead to more chronic desensitization to real-life violent events for, if there are, this presents important implications for peaceful societies. For example, it seems plausible that individuals whose physiological, negative emotional responses to violence have been dampened could potentially adopt attitudes that are more tolerant of violence in society, and as a result, become less motivated to participate in promoting peaceful communities. Psychophysiological research in this area has and should clearly continue to clarify this implication of research on playing violent video games by providing the foundational knowledge necessary to evaluate whether this is a genuine societal concern.

Media psychology researchers who have used psychophysiological measures to study arousal evoked by playing violent video games have also explored the impact of specific features of games. It is arguable that in no other form of mediated message have technological developments played such a huge role in the user experience. Games are often reviewed and marketed based on how engaging and "real" the experience within the game seems. Both of these broad areas of features of video games can easily be theorized to significantly impact embodied cognitive and emotional processes involved when playing the game—processes which can be illuminated by psychophysiological measures. In one basic experiment higher quality graphics and auditory elements in newer versions of violent video games were found to intensify arousal—as measured by skin conductance—experienced by individuals playing the game (Ivory & Kalyanaraman, 2007).

An additional feature of video games has been the development of online, multi-player games, where individuals can either collaborate or compete in a virtual online game environment. Recent research on this feature has illustrated the importance of social context in the impact of playing a violent game on arousal. Lower levels of skin conductance have been measured in individuals when they play a collaborative, multi-player violent video game compared to playing a violent game by themselves (Lim & Lee, 2009).

The recent research utilizing psychophysiological measures of mediated message processing to study the impact of violent media content on individuals not only provides insight into embodied cognitive/emotional processing of violent content but has also shed light on features of media and characteristics of individuals that may impact how violent content is processed. Further exploration of the interaction of distinct features of media with characteristics of individuals in the emergence of psychological states resulting from exposure to violent media content appears to represent a critical way that psychophysiological measures can be used to clarify and increase the importance of research on mediated violence. Research into how the embodied mind processes and makes sense of violent media content is likely the most promising path forward if we hope to gain an understanding of all three of the broad forms of "effects" of violent media content noted above. Only such deep understanding will allow us to produce a rich theoretical description of the impact of violent content, one which covers the myriad of ways exposure to violent media content dynamically shapes the functioning of the embodied mind. It is, after all, the embodied mind that guides an individual as they interact and cope with the challenges of surviving in society where the potential for real-life violence is a real possibility. This level of understanding of the impact of violent content can only be gained through a rigorous combination of psychophysiological, self-report, and behavioral measures in experiments on this phenomenon. Researchers who approach the study of violent media content in this way are most likely to provide scientific insight that can arm parents with knowledge to help minimize a potentially negative impact of media on their children and that ought to be the foundation of any policy decisions directed at the media industry.

News and the curious mind: knowledge gained through psychophysiological measurement

News is a form of media content that millions of people use to obtain an understanding of the world. For that reason it is not surprising that researchers have investigated "the news" for decades—producing insights with important implications for both society and the media industry (see Price & Feldman, 2009 for a brief review). It is often argued that on a societal level news is one of the most important forms of media content due to its implications for citizen engagement in democratic societies (Cappella & Jamieson, 1997). Much of the media research on news content has been conducted from a sociological or psychological theoretical perspective focusing on outcomes of news exposure rather than mental processes engaged during news consumption. Particularly absent in all but the most recent work is theory surrounding embodied cognitive and emotional processes involved in news consumption. Arguably, the ideal purpose of news is to make people more knowledgeable about the world they live in, an ideal that theoretically promotes a better society. Further, the business of growing and maintaining an audience for news depends on the production and delivery of content that individuals are motivated to seek out and process, particularly given the vast array of options that characterize the current media environment. An individual's motivation to find and consume news and, as a result, become "smarter" about the world, completely hinges on mental processes engaged by characteristics of news content and the media platforms used to deliver it. Thus, research that uses psychophysiological measures to study cognitive/emotional processing of news content not only provides in-depth theoretical insight into the interaction of media messages and media recipients but has critical implications for helping promote the ideal purpose of news.

In this section we explore how the use of psychophysiological measures helps clarify the mental process of gaining knowledge from exposure to news and therefore increases both the theoretical and practical importance of research in this area. We will provide a general discussion of a theoretical context for research on news conducted from a psychological perspective. This provides the background for understanding precisely how research that includes psychophysiological measures of mediated message processing has expanded an understanding of the impact and function of news. We will then briefly review how media psychology researchers have used psychophysiology to study how specific features of news evoke patterns of embodied cognitive and emotional processing leading to emerging psychological states. This discussion will point out the importance of the continued application of psychophysiological measurement in research on news.

The psychological function of news—as a form of media content—is to provide factual information we can use to form our mental conception of aspects of the world we cannot directly experience. This notion seems to be implicitly built into two well-established approaches applied to studying news—**Uses and Gratifications** and **Agenda Setting**. Scholars working under a uses and gratifications framework have proposed that a primary motive for news consumption is surveillance—a need to learn about potential threats to our well-being in an often uncertain and dangerous world (Rubin, 2009). News content can clue us into potential threats without our having to directly experience them. Researchers who developed agenda setting theory proposed that the selection and coverage of specific topics in news content shapes our perception of the importance of specific issues confronting society (Shah, McLeod, Gotlieb, & Lee, 2009). Thankfully, the impact of news content often occurs outside of the context of most individuals' direct experience, existing instead as topical priorities generated through introspection.

The mental experiences provided by news content can ultimately impact how our embodied mind navigates us through our daily life. News content can mobilize individuals to help others in need—as was the case with news coverage of the 2010 earthquake in Haiti. Information supplied by news helps us make decisions ranging from what clothes we should wear due to the weather forecast to who to vote for in the next election based on our learning and evaluation of political facts. Research conducted under **Cultivation Theory** points to the potential for news content to impact our judgments of how safe or dangerous our world is and, therefore, how we should interact and behave (Morgan, 2009). The very foundation of any potential impact of news on our daily life is the mental conception of our world that develops from embodied cognitive/emotional processing of news content. This is the entry point for research on news that includes psychophysiological measures of mediated message processing. The ability of these measures to index patterns of embodied cognitive/emotional processing of news content allows researchers to glimpse mental experiences.

Considerations of mental experience and the function of news, along with broader theoretical descriptions of the impact of news content, describe how some of today's media psychology researchers investigate how specific features of news stories engage cognitive and emotional processing of information. This work has provided much-needed theoretical insight into the details of mental processes—missing from a majority of the early research on news—and thereby fleshed out the context for understanding the impact of news on individuals. This detailed knowledge of mental processes engaged by specific features of news content has come from rigorous experiments that have combined psychophysiological measures with measures of memory for news content. We will now briefly review some of the recent work in this area.

News content can often contain highly emotional, negatively arousing, images of news events. This is a specific content feature of news that media psychology researchers have investigated. In one of the more recent experiments in this area, Hutchinson and Bradley (2009) investigated how the emotional intensity and valence of images in televised news stories about U.S. involvement in Iraq and Afghanistan impact cognitive and emotional processing of the story. They found that high-intensity visual images in televised news stories evoke greater attention (lower heart rate) and arousal (increased skin conductance) regardless of the emotional valence of the images. Also testing recognition memory for both audio and visual information presented in the televised news stories used in their experiment, they found that negative high-intensity images in television news stories increases visual recognition but decreases audio recognition leading to the conclusion that for negative news footage the increase in cognitive resources allocated to processing high-intensity visual images occurs at the expense of processing audio information in the voiceover of the story. This recent experiment is a great example of how psychophysiological measures of mediated message processing have been used to provide detailed insight into processing of very specific content features of news and of the importance of combining them with other measures of mediated message processing. Given that learning from news can have a significant impact on public opinion related to political issues—such as a government's military involvement in other countries—studies like this have important societal implications.

Production technology enables news departments to include different kinds of textual and animated graphics in television news stories as a way of presenting information. Theoretically this is a specific production feature of news that could significantly impact cognitive processing of information presented in a story. One recent study investigated how the inclusion of graphics in televised news stories impacts cognitive processing of the story for young adult college students compared to older adults, aged 28–80 (Fox et al., 2004). Combining heart rate as a measure of cognitive resource allocation and with cued recall and recognition memory measures, results show that news graphics help both younger and older viewers store and retrieve information presented in the story. Graphics in particular enhanced younger viewers' ability to effectively encode stories about more difficult topic matter. The combination of cardiac and memory results suggested that younger viewers process television news stories in a more automatic fashion whereas older viewers tend to engage in more controlled processing of televised news. This study not only provides valuable insight into learning from television news stories but illustrates the importance of considering distinct news audiences and how they might differentially process features of news. News producers interested in designing news to deliver information to younger viewers should consider using on-screen textual delivery, particularly in stories where the content is more challenging to make sense of.

Arguably one of the most important insights to be gained about mental processing of news from psychophysiological measures concerns the design and production of news stories in a way that is optimally engaging and memorable. One study illustrates the importance of understanding how the design and production of television news stories impacts processing by testing what they termed tabloid versus standard production style (Grabe, Lang, & Zhao, 2003). Tabloid production style involves the use of special effects such as slow-motion, music, flash frames, and an obtrusive reporter voice. The results indicate that tabloid production style increases resources allocated to encoding television news stories as evidenced by cardiac deceleration; however, when combined with arousing story content (e.g., violence and disasters) tabloid production style overloaded cognitive resources resulting in decreased memory for the information in the story.

Another study designed to optimize news processing used psychophysiological measures to evaluate actual television news stories that had been experimentally reproduced to better adhere to theoretical principles of how the human mind processes media (Lang, Potter, & Grabe, 2003). These principles broadly involved intensifying the emotional tone of the story, being conscious of production pacing, and writing the story such that information presented in video matches information presented in the audio. Results showed that the reproduced stories performed better in terms of attention, arousal, and memory in comparison to the originally aired stories. Not only does this study offer important theoretical verification of principles provided by previous research on mediated message processing but also results in specific production guidelines television news producers should use in order to produce engaging and memorable news stories.

Research that has utilized psychophysiological measures of mediated message processing to study cognitive/emotional processes evoked by news consumption has provided tremendous insight into how individuals attend to and potentially learn from news. As stated previously, this is an extremely important area for media psychology researchers to contribute insight into how the mind processes media, due to the substantial implications of news for the growth of informed individuals in democratic societies. The human mind needs to process news effectively in order to be well informed about the world. Research that combines psychophysiological measures of mediated message processing with other measures of memory and learning is arguably the best for improving the ability for news content to effectively deliver information about our world. The few studies we reviewed in this section illustrate the value of this research approach. In a media environment where news sources and delivery systems offer individuals many more options not only in content but also in distinct ways of *telling* news stories, it is even more critical for media psychology researchers to conduct in-depth research on how the mind processes news content. For instance media psychology researchers in the future could explore how features of news content such as embedded text, audio, video, and still images in online news websites interact to impact embodied cognitive/emotional processing of news stories. Some early attempts at this kind of investigation are being conducted (e.g., Wise, Bolls, Myers, & Sternadori, 2009). However, research on new media platforms for delivering news content that utilize multi-sensory forms of information presentation is clearly in its infancy. These kinds of news presentations represent a significant change in format and packaging of news content than what has been investigated by previous research. Thus, there are clearly exciting opportunities for media psychology researchers to use psychophysiological measures in studying the multiple ways news content is produced and delivered.

Persuasion and psychophysiological measures of mediated message processing

The application of psychophysiological measures of mediated message processing to understanding how the human mind processes persuasive messages has an interesting history intersecting academia and the advertising industry. Advertising is the one specific area of media research with an established history of psycho-physiological measures being used by industry practitioners to conduct research for clients. Several intriguing discussions over the use and application of psycho-physiological measures to study and evaluate advertising occurred in articles published in advertising journals during the 1970s and 1980s (Cacioppo & Petty, 1985; Stewart, 1984; Werner, 1979). In his position as manager of corporate public opinion research at General Electric, **Herbert Krugman** authored an article on the advantages of EEG in measuring media involvement (Krugman, 1971). Many of the stimuli the earliest media psychology researchers studied in establishing psychophysiology as a method for studying how the mind processes media were advertisements.

Insight into how the human mind processes persuasive messages remains both practically and theoretically valuable to media psychology researchers and media practitioners alike. As noted at the beginning of this chapter, both have recognized the value of understanding the human mind to better understand how persuasive messages are processed. Academic researchers approach the enterprise with the goal of advancing theory, however, while industry researchers clearly have desired objectives in mind tied to company performance. Billions of dollars are spent each year to produce and deliver advertisements that companies hope will persuade consumers to buy their products. Research that is directed at helping companies do this more effectively has tremendous implications for both companies and consumers. And perhaps that is why no other area of media research has arguably embraced the research paradigm we recommend in this book— combining psychophysiological with other measures of mediated message processing in order to understand the media–mind interaction—more than researchers focused on understanding persuasion.

The published research that has resulted from experiments using psychophysiological measures to study persuasion not only examines traditional product advertising but also areas where persuasion has tremendous implications for the well-being of society. Two major areas in which psychophysiological measures have recently been used to provide insight into cognitive/emotional processing of persuasive messages are political advertising and health communication. Media psychology researchers who conduct experiments in these areas not only provide practical knowledge related to the design of psychologically powerful persuasive messages but are also conducting science relevant to two critically important societal issues—politics and public health. The implications of persuasion research on political landscapes as well as public health, impacting both individuals and society at large, are clear. The published literature on persuasion spans decades of research and does a great job establishing the importance of research in these areas; however, the very small portion of it that has included psychophysiological measures of mediated message processing provides a glimpse into the value of in-depth understanding of how the mind processes persuasive messages.

Researchers who use psychophysiological measures of mediated message processing to study persuasive messages are uniquely positioned to provide specific insight into a form of communication that has tremendous potential for both positive and negative impact on individuals and society. Arguably, this is one of the most important areas of media research in which media psychology researchers study the mind and media interaction. The interaction between specific features of persuasive messages and the minds of targeted individuals is the very foundation for behaviors that any organization engaging in a persuasive campaign hopes to impact. It is only through an in-depth understanding of this interaction—made possible by the combination of psychophysiological measures with measures of psychological states representative of persuasive outcomes—that advertising practitioners can better serve their clients, or that a level of knowledge of the persuasive process that is capable of helping individuals avoid potentially harmful effects can be attained.

Psychophysiological measures of mediated message processing offer the opportunity to directly observe embodied cognitive/emotional processes engaged during mediated exposure to an organization's persuasive message. Such processes are likely to represent the earliest stages of attitude formation that has been extensively studied by persuasion researchers. Despite an established history of psychophysiological measures being used to study processing of persuasive messages, it is still the case that an overwhelming majority of the existing research has relied on self-report measures that cannot be used to uncover the basic cognitive/emotional processes at play during message exposure. Thus, there is tremendous opportunity for media psychology researchers to conduct experiments utilizing psychophysiological measures to index foundational cognitive/emotional processes that lead to the emerging attitudes, memories, and behaviors targeted through persuasive media campaigns. Researchers who do so not only clarify the impact of persuasive messages found in previous research but increase the importance of research in this area by providing insight that can link cognitive/emotional processes evoked by specific features of persuasive messages to the likely outcome of such messages. We will illustrate this point by reviewing some of the recent research that has utilized psychophysiological measures to study cognitive/emotional processing of consumer product advertising, political advertising, and health communication messages.

In the realm of product advertising, numerous specific features of advertisements have been investigated by researchers using psychophysiological measures of mediated message processing. In a study on animated web advertising it was found that the animation speed of a web advertisement significantly impacts arousal levels and resulting psychological evaluations of the brand message (Sundar & Kalyanaraman, 2004). Media psychology researchers have also used psychophysiological measures to study how the emotional tone of radio advertising impacts attention and intensity of emotions evoked (Bolls, Lang, & Potter, 2001). Research on the emotional tone of radio advertising revealed that while listeners pay more attention to negatively-toned radio advertisements, as evidenced by cardiac deceleration, message recognition is primarily impacted by the level of arousal in the radio ad regardless of emotional valence.

A substantial amount of advertising research indicates that the programming environment in which an ad is embedded significantly impacts cognitive and emotional processing of the message. Such was the case in an experiment that found that negative emotion—as indicated by corrugator EMG—evoked by a fear-appeal based advertisement is less intense when the advertisement is placed in a comedy versus sad television programming (Potter, LaTour, Braun-LaTour, & Reichert, 2006). Recent research that utilizes psychophysiological measures to study advertising has not only borne out the importance of advertising context but has also provided a convincing argument for the use of psychophysiological measures in indexing the level of emotional engagement consumers have with advertising messages (Marci, 2006).

These are but a few recent examples of research utilizing psychophysiological measures to gain insight into cognitive/emotional processing of consumer product advertising. This line of research provides critical practical knowledge concerning the design and delivery of effective advertisements for ad agency clients. There is clearly renewed industry enthusiasm for the application of psychophysiological measures in the study of advertising, as media psychology researchers conduct experiments that demonstrate how these measures index critically important cognitive and emotional processing of even fleeting, specific elements of product advertising—even elements that are as minute as specific gestures of a model in a television advertisement (Ohme, Reykowska, Wiener, & Choromanska, 2009). Keep in mind, however, that in an industry where billions of dollars are spent on the combined production, distribution, and placement of persuasive messages any insight is welcomed that can make a persuasive message more likely to be effective.

Political advertising is a specific form of persuasion where effectiveness is ultimately determined by election results. Despite the large literature in the area of political persuasion, a literature which spans many decades, there is very little which utilizes psychophysiological measures during the processing of the persuasive messages. There is some, of course. For example, research utilizing EEG—specifically indexing evoked response potentials as physiological markers of attitudes—has demonstrated that political stimuli elicit strong implicit evaluations in the form of automatically activated attitudes (Morris, Squires, Taber, & Lodge, 2003). This research suggests that political advertising could be an especially motivational stimulus evoking a particularly strong response pattern of embodied cognitive/emotional processing, especially for politically-engaged individuals. In another study, eye-blink startle has recently been used to study aversive activation evoked by negative political advertisements compared to positive ones (Bradley, Angelini, & Lee, 2007). Results show larger magnitude of startle eye-blinks during exposure to negative- compared to positive-toned advertisements. Results also revealed that the negative advertisements in this study were more arousing, as indicated by higher levels of skin conductance, and resulted in better recognition of detailed information presented in the message.

With these two studies leading the way as examples, the gap in the political persuasion literature presents a tremendous opportunity for media psychology researchers to step in and conduct investigations on this specific form of persuasive messages, applying psychophysiological measures of mediated message processing in an area of critical importance to democratic societies. It seems likely that political advertising is a form of persuasion for which the motivational relevance of the content significantly varies across individuals who hold a wide range of political attitudes. If true, this makes it all the more important to conduct research on such messages from an embodied motivated processing theoretical perspective that heavily relies on data obtained with psychophysiological measures. One specific direction such research could take would be to examine how the strength of pre-existing political attitudes moderates embodied motivated processing—indexed through psychophysiological measures—and memory of political advertisements. The bottom line is that political advertising research is an area that is ripe for media psychology researchers to demonstrate both the theoretical and practical importance of applying psychophysiological measures to the study of the interaction between persuasive messages and the minds of targeted individuals.

The final area of persuasion research we will cover in which psychophysiological measures of mediated message processing can be used to provide practical knowledge concerning effective message design is health communication. Arguably this area of persuasion research has tremendous implications for the promotion of healthier lifestyles among individuals. Thus, it is an area of persuasion research in which the application of psychophysiological measures of mediated message processing has the potential to provide both theoretical and practical insight with significant societal value by guiding the design of more effective health campaign messages.

A specific feature of health campaign messages that has been recently studied by media psychology researchers is **message sensation value**—a composite variable having to do with the sensory intensity of audio, visual, and content features of the message (Palmgreen, Stephenson, Everett, Baseheart, & Francies, 2002). In a recent experiment on the message sensation value of televised health public service announcements, data obtained from fMRI scans combined with message recognition tests revealed that PSAs with lower sensation value evoked significantly greater activation in prefrontal and temporal cortex resulting in better message recognition in comparison to high sensation value messages (Langleben et al., 2009).

An extremely relevant feature of health communication campaign messages is the visual portrayal of unhealthy, risky products. The brief visual presentation of such products could evoke meaningful patterns of embodied cognitive/emotional processing yielding insight into effective message design. Indeed, in an experiment designed to test this notion, it was found that simply the visual appearance of risky products in photos evokes stronger orienting responses as revealed by psychophysiological measures (Lang, Chung, Lee, & Zhao, 2005). We have barely scratched the surface of how psychophysiological measures have been applied in this area of persuasion research. There are clearly numerous opportunities for media psychology researchers to study health communication messages, revealing insights into embodied motivated processing of this very important form of media content.

This brief glimpse of some of the more current research in which psycho-physiological measures were used to study mediated messages demonstrates how psychophysiology is now a well-established research method in media psychology research. Further, it is clear that the application of psychophysiological measures to studying mental processes through which specific forms of media content impact individuals increases the theoretical and practical importance of media research. The three general areas of media research we have reviewed here—mediated violence, news, and persuasion—represent a small fraction of exciting areas in which media psychology researchers can investigate mediated message processing with a growing toolbox of methods and measures that now includes both well established and recently developed psychophysiological measures. The future indeed looks very bright for scholars who want to pursue this research endeavor; thus, we now turn to a discussion of trends and considerations in the role psychophysiology will play in the future of mediated message processing research.

The future of psychophysiology in studying mediated message processing

The value of using psychophysiological measures to burst open the black box of the human mind "on" media has become widely accepted among both media psychology researchers and professionals within the media industry. Psychophysiological data adds tremendous depth of insight into how the human mind processes a wide range of media content delivered over an expanding range of technological platforms. Insight in this area goes far beyond basic knowledge provided by the traditional outcome measures that have historically been applied in media research; thus, the value of knowledge gleaned from the application of psychophysiological measures in conjunction with other measures relevant to mediated message processing is likely to only increase in the future. This trend leads us to believe that the future of psychophysiology in the study of mediated message processing is likely to be characterized by tremendous growth in the application of these measures in experiments designed to investigate mediated message processing across a wider range of contexts, contents, and technological platforms.

The continued development of new media platforms over which changing forms of media content are delivered will provide endless opportunities for media psychology researchers to pose practically and theoretically important research questions that will best be answered through direct observation of the mind processing media—as enabled by psychophysiological measurement. The increasingly interactive nature of media content and technological platforms over which it is delivered—enabling shared mediated social experiences—will present new contexts in which to study the human mind interacting with features of media. The technology and expertise to rigorously apply psychophysiological measures of mediated message processing in a constantly changing media environment is more accessible than ever before and will only increase as the application of psychophysiology to studying the mind as it processes media expands.

An expanding range of psychologically meaningful features of mediated messages, technological development of psychophysiological measures, and expanding research expertise will construct the future scientific environment in which psychophysiology is likely to be a dominant part of the research paradigm media psychology researchers use to study the media–mind interaction. The value of any knowledge produced by the application of psychophysiology in studying mediated message processing will hinge, however, on the establishment of a rigorous, biologically based, theoretical view of the human mind. It seems likely that the increased adoption among media scholars of an embodied motivated processing theoretical perspective for understanding how the human mind processes media will be the catalyst for an even more extensive application of psychophysiological measures to studying mediated message processing. This will, in turn, serve to establish this theoretical perspective as a dominant view of the human mind in media psychology research. A theoretical perspective of embodied, motivated cognitive processing has guided the conceptualization, organization, and presentation of information in this book. Such a perspective has been widely adopted in psychology to establish a conceptual connection between the mind and the brain. Communication and media research has a history of adopting strong theoretical perspectives from psychology, making it all the more likely that an embodied motivated processing view of the human mind could become a dominant theoretical perspective in the field. The Limited Capacity Model of Motivated Mediated Message Processing (LC4MP; Lang, 2009) is a specific example of such a perspective and one that is being widely adopted. Such a theoretical perspective of the human mind positions psychophysiological measures as critical tools for researchers to be able to observe the functioning of the mind as it engages in any activity involved in processing complex social stimuli such as media content.

A strong theoretical foundation that substantially relies on psychophysiology is a critical component of the explication of cognitive and emotional processes in a way that ensures the future value of peer-reviewed academic research that uses psychophysiological measures of mediated message processing. The future application of psychophysiological measures to studying how the mind processes media, however, certainly will not be limited to basic research in academic settings. As mentioned, companies specializing in neuromarketing have sprung up utilizing a range of psychophysiological tools including measures of the peripheral (EKG, EMG, EDA) and central (EEG and fMRI) nervous systems. These companies have been contracted by many major advertisers to provide proprietary scientific data concerning the evaluation of specific advertisements. Table 9.1 provides a brief listing of some of these companies along with their websites. The for-profit nature of most neuromarketing companies means that much of their work is unavailable for scrutiny by external trained researchers. These companies do, however, occasionally receive coverage in popular press and at least one company, Sands Research (www.sandsresearch.com), makes some of its data publicly available online. Data displayed online from the Sands Research Super Bowl advertising studies include images of brain activation recorded by EEG. Glimpses into the operations of neuromarketing companies can also be obtained from neuromarketing blogs (e.g., www.neurosciencemarketing.com/blog). Given that the entire media industry is in the business of attracting audience—a business objective that fundamentally relies on motivated mental processes on the part of the sought-after audience—practical research that utilizes psychophysiological measures of mediated message processing to understand the attraction of audiences to various media products is likely to expand beyond advertising and marketing in the future.

All of these trends create a very promising outlook for the application of psychophysiology in the study of mediated message processing. This being said, however, this exciting future will not come to pass unless psychophysiological measures of mediated message processing are applied to the problem of understanding the mind–media interaction in a way that indeed produces truly valuable and generalizable knowledge. The largest consideration in this regard has to do with ensuring that media psychology researchers are well trained in psychophysiology. In some ways, excitement and interest in psychophysiology among media scholars has outpaced training. User-friendly systems for the collection and analysis of psychophysiological data are of great benefit to media psychology researchers but are no substitute for rigorous theoretical training. It is certainly hoped that this book has taken a step forward in providing accessible training material for media psychology researchers in the application of psychophysiological measures to studying mediated message processing. As psychophysiological measures are applied in future research on mediated message processing, it is also advisable that those applying them become active in academic associations dedicated to the continued advancement of psycho-physiology. The key role the **Society for Psychophysiological Research** (www.sprweb.org) played in the advancement of the field was mentioned in Chapter 2. The value of interdisciplinary research for solving complex research problems—like understanding how the human mind processes media—is increasingly being recognized most in the scholarly community. Media psychology researchers housed in communication-related university departments can certainly increase their ability to rigorously apply psychophysiological measures to the study

TABLE 9.1 Select companies that specialize in neuromarketing research

Company name	Company website
EmSense	www.emsense.com
Innerscope Research	www.innerscoperesearch.com
Mindsign Neuromarketing	http://mindsignonline.com
Neurofocus	www.neurofocus.com

of mediated message processing by conducting interdisciplinary research with colleagues from neurology, neuroscience, and psychology. Further, given the tremendous excitement over neuromarketing, media psychology researchers who are well trained in psychophysiology could form interesting industry/academic partnerships in which psychophysiological measures of mediated message processing are applied to understanding the media and mind interaction in ways that increase the quality of both basic and applied research.

Conclusion

This book has provided a survey of the historical development of the application of psychophysiological measures to studying mediated message processing. The conceptual and operational knowledge necessary to collect specific psychophysiological measures of cognitive/emotional processing of media in experiments on mediated message processing was also covered along with issues to consider in setting up a media research lab with psychophysiological capabilities. This is the first book to exclusively focus on the application of psychophysiological measures to studying mediated message processing and therefore provides a resource for media psychology researchers who wish to add them to their methodological toolbox. This book, however, is truly most valuable when read in conjunction with the other tremendously informative volumes written by psychophysiologists, which have been cited throughout this book. Media psychology researchers adopt and then apply psychophysiological measures, whereas, one of the fundamental missions of the psychophysiologist is to conduct the conceptual and operational work necessary for demonstrating the validity and reliability of specific psychophysiological measures. The ability for media psychology researchers to continue and even expand the application of psychophysiological measures to the study of mediated message processing is most likely to come through a strong grounding in conceptual and operational knowledge produced by psychophysiologists that is reviewed at a more in–depth level in other volumes.

Psychophysiological measures of mediated message processing are clearly the best tool available for media psychology researchers to use when peering inside the human mind and observing embodied cognitive and emotional processes engaged by media. In our increasingly media-saturated society knowledge produced in this manner will have significant implications for the media industry and society at large. The research environment for the production of this knowledge has never been better in terms of both support and the range of relevant, fascinating potential research questions. This is truly an exciting time in media research as the field is still somewhat in the process of a paradigm shift from traditional media effects research to a dynamic processes paradigm of studying mediated message processing. We are convinced that media psychology researchers who are equipped with knowledge of how to appropriately use psychophysiological measures—along with other measures of mediated message processing—to thoroughly describe the mind–media interaction will push our field toward a future era of media research characterized by an understanding of media influence informed by rich theoretical models of mediated message processing rather than static descriptions of media "effects." We hope that this book has contributed to that future.

GLOSSARY

Acetylcholine   a neurotransmitter in the autonomic nervous system. It is the neurotransmitter responsible for eccrine sweat gland secretion that results in skin conductance activity.

Action Potential   a change in a cell's electrical membrane potential that sends information down the axon of a neuron in a brief all-or-nothing manner.

AD/DA Board   an Analog to Digital, Digital to Analog Board. The A-D function converts a continuous physiological signal into discrete data points that can be read by a computer. The D-A function takes digital pulses from the computer and transforms them into analog signals like an audio tone.

Afferent Signals   nerve signals traveling along pathways from sense organs receiving external stimuli to the Central Nervous System. These signals propagate in the opposite direction of efferent signals.

Agenda Setting   a communication theory proposed in the early 1970s suggesting that the news media influences which news topics individuals find most pressing or salient, originating the phrase "the media don't tell us what to think, but what to think about."

Aggressor Effect   one of three major theories of violent media effects. The aggressor effect postulates that exposure to media violence leads to greater aggression.

Aliasing   digital misrepresentation of an analog signal due to sampling at a rate slower than the Nyquist frequency, or twice the expected frequency of the physiological signal of interest. Aliasing causes a high frequency signal to appear like a lower frequency one.

Alpha Waves electromagnetic oscillations in the brain falling within the frequency range of 8–12 Hz. Commonly associated with feelings of restful, but not stressful, awakeness. Also referred to as **alpha rhythm**.

Amplitude the increase in voltage exhibited in a physiological measure following an eliciting stimulus. In an isolated physiological measure amplitude is synonymous with magnitude. However, when calculating averages across conditions or subjects mean amplitudes do not include non-responders while mean magnitudes do.

Apocrine Sweat Glands glands which become functional at puberty and are of little psychological interest. Responsible for secreting pheromones, apocrine glands are found primarily in the armpits and pubic regions.

Appetitive System Activation stimulation of the motivational system responsible for approach behaviors. Also referred to as ASA. Under a dimensional theory of emotion, ASA occurs independently of Defensive System Activation (DSA).

Arousal a key component of a dimensional view of emotion. Arousal is thought to measure the intensity of a response to a stimulus, regardless of valence. High arousal can be conceptualized as exciting or stressful, while low arousal as calm, peaceful, or boring.

Atria/Atrium the two smaller, upper chambers of the heart. The right atrium is the location of the SA or pacemaker node responsible for generating the electrical impulse that initiates the cardiac cycle.

Attentional Inertia a phenomenon characterized by the increasingly lower likelihood of breaking attention with a television stimulus the longer one looks at it.

Attitudes relatively stable evaluative judgments about a given item, which may be stored in memory, activated automatically, and measured in direct and indirect ways. Typically conceptualized as separate from behavior or behavioral intentions.

Automatic Processing a type of information processing that is mostly subconscious, uncontrollable, and requiring little cognitive resources to execute, in contrast to controlled processing. Automatic processing is often elicited by motivationally relevant stimuli.

Autonomic Nervous System regulatory branch of the Central Nervous System which helps regulate activity in blood vessels, blood pressure, heart, glands, smooth muscles, respiration, digestion, salivation, perspiration, pupil dilation, and sexual arousal.

Albert F. Ax early psychophysiologist who was a founder of the Society for Psychophysiological Research. He and his wife Beryl wrote and circulated **Psychophysiology Newsletter** for nine years prior to becoming the first editor of **Psychophysiology**.

Bandpass Filter a device containing a circuit that allows only a set range of frequencies to pass or continue in the signal chain.

Albert Bandura widely recognized psychologist who is responsible for social learning theory and the famous Bobo doll experiments, which informed his view that certain conditions must be met in order for behavior to be modeled.

Behaviorism a school of thought in psychology, popular in the early twentieth century, that focused solely on objective, observable behaviors in place of cognition and/or internal processing. Watson and Skinner are widely associated with the paradigm.

Gary Berntson a pioneer in the field of social neuroscience, past president of the Society for Psychophysiological Research and co-editor of the **Handbook of psychophysiology**. Berntson conducts research outlining the functional organization of brain mechanisms related to behavioral and affective processing. His methodological contribution in psychophysiology has included publications addressing multilevel analysis of physiological measures as well as autonomic influences on cardiac activity.

Beta Waves electromagnetic oscillations in the brain falling within the frequency range of 12–30 Hz. Sometimes further classified as High Beta Waves (> 19 Hz), Beta Waves (15–18 Hz), and Low Beta Waves (12–15 Hz). Associated with normal wakeful activity, but can also indicate anxiety or stress.

Bioamplifier device which receives physiological data via electrodes/electrode cables and increases the voltage level of the biopotential of interest. Bioamplifiers often have variable gain (amplification), bandpass filters, and noise-reduction functions.

Biopotential electrical activity at the cellular level, typically low in amplitude, and within a narrow frequency of signals depending upon the point of origin across the body.

Bipolar Recording method which compares electrical signals from two active electrodes without a reference electrode but always with a ground electrode.

BOLD Signal the signal resulting from the Blood Oxygen Level Dependent method common in fMRI studies. The BOLD signal is due to the variations in blood flow, blood volume, and oxygen consumption in specific brain regions during the cognitive and emotional processing of stimuli.

Walter Bradford Cannon physiologist best known for defining homeostasis as a fluid matrix within the body in which the sympathetic and parasympathetic systems were in balanced opposition to one another.

Margaret Bradley   psychophysiologist and past president of the Society for Psychophysiological research, among the most prominent psychologists to examine emotion and attention with psychophysiological tools. Created the International Affective Picture System (IAPS) with Peter Lang.

John Cacioppo   a pioneer in the field of social neuroscience and past president of the Society for Psychophysiological Research. Cacioppo is an editor of the *Handbook of psychophysiology* and has published several methodological papers in the area of psychophysiology including an article that outlines guidelines for the collection of facial EMG.

Cardiac Cycle   the repetitive electrical events, and the accompanying physical contractions and relaxations, which occur in the heart to circulate blood throughout the body.

Cardiac Response Curve   the graphic representation of heart rate or heart period change scores from baseline over time.

Central Nervous System (CNS)   the brain and spinal cord; generally responsible for integrating information received from the Peripheral Nervous System and coordinating activity in the body.

Steven Chaffee   communication scholar who, in the 1970s, bemoaned the discipline's continued use of the two-variable model and advocated instead the use of an information systems approach popular in psychology at the time.

Change Score   a way of representing data that is calculated by subtracting physiological data at each subsequent point in time from a standard baseline. Related to the subtractive method pioneered by Donders.

Classical Conditioning   first posited by Pavlov under the behaviorism paradigm, this type of associative learning pairs a neutral stimulus with one that evokes an automatic behavioral response. Once the association has been learned the neutral stimulus is presented alone and evokes the same response.

Confederate   someone who appears as a subject in an experimental setting, but is actually an experimenter there to ensure specific conditions related to the study goal occur.

Conscience-numbing Effect   one of three major theories of violent media effects. The conscience-numbing effect suggests desensitization of negative reactions following repeated exposure to violent media content.

Continuous Response Measurement (CRM)   an over-time, self-report measurement tool in which subjects move a cursor or turn a dial indicating their level of a variable of interest while being exposed to media stimuli.

Controlled Processing   a conscious, voluntary, intentional allocation of cognitive resources to processing a given stimulus. The focus of controlled processing often depends on the goals of the individual. In contrast to automatic processing.

Corrugator Supercilii   a small facial muscle located just above the medial start of the eyebrow. EMG recording of this muscle generally shows greater activation during negative and lesser activation during positive emotion.

Criterion Bias   a recognition memory variable under the signal detection paradigm, criterion bias indicates how liberal or conservative one is when declaring that they have previously been exposed to the memory stimulus in question.

Cued Recall   a memory measure where a subject is asked to remember and describe all aspects of a cued stimulus. The cue is usually either a single visual image taken from the stimulus or a descriptive phrase. Cued recall indexes the storage subprocess of memory.

Cultivation Theory   a communication theory proposed by George Gerbner and colleagues in the 1970s that posits a passive television audience that views the real world as closer to the TV representation. The original cultivation theory focused on the extent to which individuals were likely to experience violence in their real lives.

Current Density   the density of electrical current occurring within a set cross-section of surface area.

Chester Darrow   early psychophysiologist who was a founder of the Society for Psychophysiological Research and served as the society's first president.

Charles Darwin   famous naturalist who proposed the scientific theory of evolution based on natural selection as an explanation for the diversity of biological life. Also was one of the first modern scientists to examine emotion in relation to bodily responses.

R. C. Davis   early psychophysiologist and founder of the Society for Psycho-physiological Research.

Defensive System Activation   stimulation of the motivational system responsible for avoidance or withdrawal behaviors. Also referred to as DSA. Under a dimensional theory of emotion, DSA occurs independently of Appetitive System Activation (ASA).

Depolarization   a change in the electrical potential across a cell's membrane where the interior becomes more positively charged compared to the exterior.

Rene Descartes   a seventeenth-century French philosopher whose work focused on the nature of emotion, or what at the time was known as the passions. Descartes believed that the mind and body were separate entities, an idea known as Cartesian dualism, that dominated discussion of the mind-body problem for several centuries after Descartes' death.

Franciscus Donders a Dutch ophthalmologist credited with creating the subtractive method.

Edward Donnerstein communication scholar who was part of the second wave of media physiological studies in the 1970s. Applied a Stimulus-Response paradigm and Excitation Transfer Theory to physiological measures such as blood pressure.

Emil Du Bois-Reymond the father of experimental electrophysiology, he invented the nerve galvanometer and used it to show how electrical signals moved across muscle neurons, thus identifying action potentials and resting potentials.

Duchenne Smile indicated by movement in the zygomatic major and orbicularis oculi, it is thought to be a better index of a "genuine" smile than just zygomatic measurement alone. Named after French physiologist Guillaume Duchenne, whose pictures of facial muscle movements appeared in Darwin's **The expression of emotion in man and animals**.

Dynamic System a set of units that interact over time according to fixed rules or parameters that are both known and unknown.

Wendell S. Dysinger a graduate student member of the Payne Fund Study research team whose impressive data collection demonstrated individual differences in physiological responses to film content during real-life settings.

Eccrine Sweat Glands sweat glands innervated solely by the sympathetic nervous system and which secrete in response to emotional stressors and for thermoregulation. The highest density of eccrine glands is on the palms of the hands and the soles of the feet.

Ecological Validity the extent to which experimental conditions mirror those in real life; related to the generalizability, or external validity, of a study.

Efferent Signals nerve signals sent from the Central Nervous System to other parts of the body in a feed forward direction. These signals go in the opposite direction of afferent signals.

Einthoven's Triangle the recommended pattern of electrode placement on the body in order to optimize the different aspects of the ECG waveform. Three different configurations were proposed by Willem Einthoven, who won the Nobel Prize for his work in this area.

Paul Ekman psychologist who pioneered facial "microexpressions" as an indicator of discrete emotion by studying that facial muscles signify different discrete emotions. Achieved popular cultural success as an author and inspiration for the television show **Lie to Me**.

Electrocardiogram (ECG)   the measurement of the electrical activity of the heart via surface electrodes.

Electrode Cable   conducts an electrical signal from the electrode lead to the bioamplifier.

Electrode Lead   a thin cable which transfers the electrical signal measured by the electrode at the skin surface either to an electrode cable or directly into the bioamplifier.

Electrodermal Activity (EDA)   a generalized term referring to the range of measures and analyses used to index differences in the electrical activity on the skin surface due to eccrine sweat gland secretion.

Electrolyte Gel   a jelly-like substance containing free ions making it a good conductor of biopotentials from the skin to the electrode.

Emotions   a response or experience characterized by certain dimensions—such as valence and arousal—or by more discrete labels such as anger, happiness, joy, or disgust. Emotion can be measured by the media psychology researcher via self-report, behavioral observation, and/or psychophysiological responses such as skin conductance and facial EMG. Emotions are usually conceptualized as occurring over a shorter time period than moods or dispositions.

Encoding   one of three parallel memory subprocesses (the others being storage and retrieval) that occur during stimulus processing. The process of encoding is that of selecting further information to process.

Epidermis   the very outer layer of skin. Most electrodes used in the media psychophysiological laboratory are attached to the epidermis using adhesive collars.

Excitation-Transfer Theory   a theory that proposes excitation from one stimulus or interaction can enhance excitatory responses in a second stimulus or interaction, regardless of the valence of the stimuli, first developed by Dolf Zillmann in the late 1960s.

Excitation Voltage   a small amount of voltage (usually 0.5v) delivered to the epidermis of the palm or sole by a skin conductance coupler. The ease with which this voltage is conducted across the bipolar electrodes provides the quantification of electrodermal activity.

External Validity   the extent a study's findings may be generalizable or applied to a larger population.

Fast-Fourier Transform   a mathematical procedure used to deconstruct complex waveforms such as the EEG into component periodic waveforms of specific amplitudes.

Fear of Victimization Effect one of three major theories of violent media effects. The fear of victimization effect postulates that exposure to media violence leads to overestimation of likelihood to fall prey to violence in real life.

Charles Féré an early pioneer in the recording of electrodermal activity, Féré was the first to measure skin conductance using an excitation voltage.

Flow Experience a concept introduced by Mihaly Csikszentmihalyi that entails complete mental immersion in a challenging yet enjoyable activity.

Free Recall a memory measure where a subject is asked to remember a list of stimuli previously exposed to without any further cue. Free recall indexes the retrieval subprocess of memory.

Galen of Pergamon 130–200 AD, a prolific physician and writer of antiquity whose theory on organs and veins in the body employed principles of hydraulics.

Luigi Galvani in the late eighteenth century, serendipitously discovered that muscles are electrical capacitors. Subsequently conducted some of the first studies on bioelectricity.

Ganglion a cluster or mass of nerve cell bodies.

Frances Graham a former president of the Society of Psychophysiological Research and a pioneer in research identifying and distinguishing among the orienting response, defensive response, and startle response.

Habituation the process of decreased physiological response to a repeated presentation of the same stimulus.

William Harvey first to use thought experiments and calculations to correctly describe the systematic circulation patterns of blood through the body.

Heart Period another term for inter-beat interval (IBI) which quantifies the milliseconds between R spikes in the QRS waveform of a cardiac cycle. Heart period is one way of quantifying cardiac activity for analysis, the other being heart rate.

Heart Rate a second way of quantifying cardiac activity for analysis (the other being heart period). Heart rate analysis converts the heart period into the average heartbeats-per-minute for a specific periodic time interval. This is commonly done using beats-per-minute/second.

Heart Time Analysis an analysis of cardiac data using heart period as the measure rather than heart rate.

High-pass Filter a filter which allows signals above a set frequency point to pass and continue on in the signal flow and attenuates frequencies below. Can be used in coordination with a low-pass filter to allow a range of frequencies to pass through unaltered.

Hypodermic Needle Theory   a strong-effects view widely held in the early twentieth-century which suggested that messages powerfully and immediately had direct effects on audiences. Also referred to as the Magic Bullet Theory.

Impedance   resistance that the bioelectrical signal meets at the skin's surface due to dead skin cells, dirt, electrolyte gel, and through the electrode lead. Attempts should be made to reduce it to increase the signal-to-noise ratio.

Inion   the most protruding part of the back of the skull.

Inter-coder Reliability   the extent to which independent coders or experimenters agree on the categorization of data using the same instrument of analysis.

International Affective Picture System (IAPS)   a collection of color images normed for valence, arousal, and dominance created and maintained by Margaret Bradley and Peter Lang at the University of Florida. IAPS images are often used in psychological studies of emotion.

International 10–20 System   a widely recognized way of referring to locations on the skull and/or corresponding electrodes in EEG research. The name of the system refers to the expectation that the distance between each location is either 10 or 20 percent of the actual length of the skull from front-to-back or side-to-side.

William James   considered by many to be the originator of modern psychology, James developed one of the earliest formal theories of emotion with Carl Lange. The James-Lange theory claimed that experienced emotion occurred only after physiological responses to external events were evaluated.

Carl Jung   although best known for his work in dream analysis, Jung was also one of the first to use a galvanometer to measure changes in skin conductance in clinical experiments using word associations.

Herbert Krugman   one of the first to use EEG measures in advertising research. Krugman was a former president of the American Academy of Public Opinion Research and a Manager of Public Opinion for General Electric.

Labophobia   a light-hearted characterization of the anxiety often experienced when contemplating setting up one's own lab.

Annie Lang   a communication scholar active in the third wave of physiology as a dependent variable whose 1993 book on measuring psychological responses to media helped solidify the cognitive processing approach to media psychophysiology. Developed the Limited Capacity Model of Motivated, Mediated Message Processing (LC4MP).

Peter Lang   psychophysiologist and past president of the Society for Psychophysiological research, among the most prominent psychologists to examine emotion, attention, and anxiety with psychophysiological tools. Created the International Affective Picture System (IAPS) with Margaret Bradley.

Latency   the durations between the onset of an evoking stimulus and a subject's behavioral or physiological response.

Law of Initial Values   the idea that the physiological reaction to any stimulus is determined to a certain extent by the initial level of activation within the measured system.

LC4MP   the Limited Capacity Model of Motivated, Mediated Message Processing; a data-driven theoretical model that provides tools for examining the interactions between a message, medium, and user over time. Created by Annie Lang.

Levator Labii superioris   a facial muscle group located between the side of the nostril and the corner of the mouth. Recent EMG measures of this muscle have been conducted in communication research as an index of disgust.

Low-pass Filter   a filter which allows signals below a set frequency point to pass and continue on in the signal flow and attenuates frequencies above. Can be used in coordination with a high-pass filter to allow a range of frequencies to pass through unaltered.

Magnitude   the increase in voltage exhibited in a physiological measure following an eliciting stimulus. In an isolated physiological measure magnitude is synonymous with amplitude. However, when calculating averages across conditions or subjects mean magnitude includes non-responders while mean amplitudes do not.

Message Sensation Value (MSV)   a composite variable indexing the visual change, audio change, and sensational content.

Model   a graphical representation of a phenomenon which attempts to break down larger experiences into their composite parts.

Mood   a relatively long-lasting affective state which most often cannot be tied to a specific eliciting event.

Motivated Attention   the automatic allocation of cognitive resources to processing motivationally or emotionally relevant stimuli.

Motivation Activation Measure (MAM)   a non-invasive measure of trait individual differences in Appetitive System Activation and Defensive System Activation developed by Annie Lang and colleagues.

Motor System   the part of the Central Nervous System largely responsible for regulating and coordinating movement.

Motor Unit   all of the muscle fibers connected to a single motor neuron and innervated by a single motor neuron axon.

Motor Unit Action Potential   also known as MUAPs. The specific name given to the action potential associated with the simultaneous firing of all muscle fibers attached to a single motor neuron. EMG measures the summative signal of many MUAPs from a single muscle group.

Movement Artifact   physiological changes resulting from physical movement unrelated to the response pattern of the physiological concept of importance.

Myocardium   a layer of muscle fibers in the heart, contraction of which results in the pumping of blood.

Nasion   where the top of the nose joins the skull.

Neuromarketing   a recent trend in the advertising/marketing industry where psychophysiological measures are used to provide insights into consumer behavior.

Neuron   a specialized cell whose activity underlies the signal recorded by most psychophysiological measures. Neurons consist of a cell body, dendrites, and axons that interconnect neurons to each other forming neural networks. Activity in neurons is driven by bioelectrical processes created through biochemical reactions in the body. Two specialized forms of neurons, sensory and motor neurons, underlie all sensory processing and motor action in the body.

Non-response Trials   experimental trials where no physiological response can be detected either because one did not occur or when electrical noise or movement artifact obscures it. Also known as flat responses.

Nonspecific Electrodermal Activity   skin conductance responses that are recorded over time and not evaluated as occurring in reaction to a specific stimulus event.

Notch Filter   a combination of high-pass and low-pass filtering that allows a small range of frequencies to continue in the signal chain.

Nyquist Function   a rule that states physiological data should be sampled at twice the highest frequency present in the signal of interest. Doing so prevents aliasing.

Ohm's Law   formulaically represented as $I=V/R$, the electrical law states that current equals the amount of voltage passing a point divided by the resistance it encounters. Named after German physicist George Ohm.

Orbicularis Oculi   the facial muscle responsible for closing the eyelid. EMG measurement occurs on the lower portion of the OO muscle just above the bony structure of the skull forming the eye socket.

Orienting Response   an automatic response to novel stimuli resulting in cognitive resource allocation to encoding. Also known as the "What is It" response or an OR, it can be measured physiologically.

Parasympathetic Nervous System   part of the ANS, it is responsible for regulating activities while the body is at rest. Parasympathetic activation of the heart is controlled by the vagus nerve and often associated with increased cognitive intake.

Parsimony   a goal of scientific theory, it is the simplest explanation of a phenomenon.

Ivan Pavlov   Russian scholar widely known for first introducing the concept of classical conditioning.

Payne Fund Studies   a series of studies in the 1940s headed by Reverend William Harrison Short. Their purpose was to show hypodermic-needle-type effects of media but instead resulted in mixed results and many examples of individual differences.

Peripheral Nervous System   consists of nerves and ganglia outside the brain and spinal cord but connecting the CNS to the limbs and organs. Can be further divided into the somatic and autonomic nervous systems.

Phasic Response   a term to describe physiological activity characterized as relatively short in duration and in response to a specific element of the stimuli.

Photoplethysmograph   a transducer which uses reflected light to detect changes in light absorption as a result of volume of blood flow. Also known as a PPG, this gives an indirect index of the time between heartbeats and can be used to calculate heart rate.

Pinna   the outer part of the ear, attached to the skin on the skull by the post-auricular muscle. Recommended placement of electrodes when measuring PAR is on or near the pinna.

Post-auricular Muscle   muscle behind the ear attaching the pinna to the back of the head which pulls the ear up and back. The reflexive movement of this muscle is a relatively new psychophysiological indicator of appetitive activation.

Pre-pulse Paradigm   experimental paradigm pioneered by Frances Graham to investigate pre-pulse inhibition, the phenomenon where orienting to a moderate stimulus attenuates the blink response to a subsequent startle probe.

Psychophysiological Measures   empirical indices that link psychological concepts to bodily activity.

Psychoticism   one of Eysenck's personality traits believed to be biologically based, and characterized by aggressiveness, proneness to psychosis and lack of agreeableness and empathy.

Real Time Analysis   an analysis of cardiac data where heart period is first transformed into beats-per-minute values over aggregated periodic time periods.

Recognition   an index of the encoding subprocess of memory. Typically recognition tests expose a subject to target stimuli that were seen previously in the experimental protocol and foil stimuli that were not. The subject must then distinguish between them.

Recognition Sensitivity   a recognition memory variable under the signal detection paradigm, sensitivity is a subject's ability to distinguish between what they have seen during the experimental protocol and what they have not.

Rectification   a conversion process where the absolute value of a negative portion of an alternating electrical signal is mirrored on the positive scale.

Byron Reeves   a communication scholar and Fellow of the International Communication Association. Reeves was a co-author on one of the first published studies in which researchers used EEG to study how individuals attend to television content. Reeves is also well known for co-authoring (with Clifford Nass) *The media equation*, a book that has encouraged new growth in the area of media psychology research, particularly on newer forms of media.

Repolarization   a change in the electrical potential across a cell's membrane where the interior becomes more negatively charged compared to the exterior.

Response Pattern   a term used to refer to the temporal and spatial characteristics of physiological activity recorded by psychophysiological measures. Response patterns are typically identifiable as waveforms graphed across time.

Resting Potential   a static, resting voltage found in neurons due to a larger concentration of negative ions on the inside of the cell membrane compared to the outside.

Retrieval   one of three parallel memory subprocesses (the others being encoding and storage) that occur during stimulus processing. Retrieval is the activation of previously stored information into working memory and is indexed with free recall measures. The process of encoding is that of selecting further information to process.

RF Pulse   used in fMRI studies, a magnetic pulse used to propel protons out of their normal magnetic alignment so that recovery can be measured. RF pulses are used in fMRI to illuminate bone, white, and gray matter in and near the brain.

Christian A. Ruckmick   researcher involved with the Payne Fund Studies whose data collection in the lab and the field demonstrated individual differences in physiological responses to film content.

Sampling   the process of representing continuous physiological responses in discrete voltage values. The frequency with which this happens is reported in Hertz (Hz) or the number of samples per second. For example, skin conductance data is often sampled at 20 Hz or 20 times per second.

Schmitt Trigger   an electrical circuit which produces a digital pulse whenever the voltage of the R-wave of the ECG signal crosses a preset threshold level.

Secondary Task Reaction Time (STRT)   a dual-task protocol that measures the speed in which a subject can behaviorally respond to a secondary task cue (e.g., an auditory tone) while engaged in a primary task (e.g., watching a TV show). Shorter response times indicate more resources available to the subprocess of encoding.

Self Assessment Manikin Scale   a set of pictorial self-report scales that measure emotion from a dimensional approach. Created by Margaret Bradley and Peter Lang.

Sensation Seeking   an individual difference first introduced by Marvin Zuckerman with biological and genetic roots. It is characterized by traits such as novelty-seeking and risk-taking and generally shares a positive correlation with substance use.

Sensitization   an increase in the size of a physiological response after repeated exposures to the same stimulus.

Sensory System   the part of the nervous system that processes sensory input, such as visual, auditory, somatic, and olfactory.

Signal Chain   the sequence of steps that an electrical signal takes as it moves from action potential to discrete numerical value in a computer.

Sinoatrial (SA) Node   an electrically active, impulse-generating muscle at the upper tip of the right atrium of the heart. Primary generator of electrical impulses which produce contraction of the heart. Innervated by the right vagus.

Skin Conductance Coupler   an electrical circuit that generates the electrical signal needed of record changes in the electrical properties of the skin. Used in place of a bioamplifier.

B. F. Skinner   primary architect of the behaviorism paradigm who introduced the operant conditioning chamber, his experimental work focused on matching an external stimulus to observable responses.

Smoothing   part of the cleaning process for EMG data, done to the rectified signal with a low-pass filter by selecting a time constant on the integrator/contour follower to capture the waveform. 500 ms is recommended for facial EMG.

Social Learning/Social Cognitive Theory   a theory with behaviorist underpinnings suggesting that people learn from observing the actions of others and the consequences they result in. Created by Albert Bandura.

Social Response Bias   or social desirability bias, is the tendency of subjects to respond in ways that make them appear favorable in others' eyes. A drawback of self-report data.

Society for Psychophysiological Research   international society formed in 1960 devoted to investigations exploring "the interrelationships between the physiological and psychological aspects of behavior" (www.sprweb.org).

Sphericity Assumption   the required assumption of repeated-measures ANOVA that variances will be equal across each point in time. This assumption is often violated by psychophysiological data and statistical corrections such as the Greenhouse-Geisser or Huynh-Feldt must be made.

Stimulus–Response (S–R) Model   based in behaviorism and dismissive of cognition, the two-variable model predicts a direct influence of one independent variable on one dependent variable.

Storage   one of three parallel memory subprocesses (the others being encoding and retrieval) that occur during stimulus processing. Storage is the creation of long-term memory network representations of encoded information. Cued recall is a common measure of storage.

Subdermis   the third or innermost layer of skin.

Subtractive Method   a design and analysis approach originated by Donders who subtracted the duration of a task thought not to require a specific cognitive process from the duration of a task that did. Today, the subtractive method is used when comparing activity of physiological systems during a task thought to require certain cognitive or emotional components with activity of the same system during a task without such a component.

Sympathetic Nervous System (SNS)   part of the ANS which activates and prepares the body for action when under stress, induces fight or flight responses. Complementary to the parasympathetic nervous system.

Louis Tassinary   a leading scholar in the area of psychophysiology of emotion, perception, and cognition, co-editor of the *Handbook of psychophysiology*. Tassinary made significant contribution to psychophysiology through publications outlining methodological guidelines for the recording of muscle activity.

Tonic Response   a term to describe physiological activity characterized as relatively long in duration and in response to a general stimulus condition rather than a discrete event within it.

Transducer   a device which converts one form of energy into another. Electrodes are a common transducer of bioelectrical energy in an electrical signal.

Uses and Gratifications a communication theory developed in the mid–1970s which proposes individuals as active audience members who deliberately use the media to fulfill specific gratifications, such as escapism, or information seeking.

Vagus Nerve controls parasympathetic activation of the heart, it descends from the brain in the carotid sheath. The right vagus innervates the S-A Node.

Valence the intrinsic positivity and/or negativity of a stimulus.

Vasoconstriction/dilation the narrowing/widening of blood vessels.

Ventricles the two larger, lower chambers of the heart. The right ventricle accepts deoxygenated blood from the right atrium and then expels it to the lungs. The left ventricle then accepts the oxygenated blood from the left aorta and pumps it to the body.

Vesalius an anatomist and physician whose books on human anatomy were widely adopted.

Alessandro Volta physicist who (wrongly) believed electrical currents found between metals and biological muscles were a property of the metal, not the muscle, in opposition to his contemporary, Galvani. Also developed the first electric cell.

Hermann von Helmholtz German physicist and physician who was among the first to apply electrical stimulation to motor nerves and measure the time it took for muscles to contract.

Dolf Zillmann part of the second wave of media scholars using physiology. Created the Excitation-Transfer Theory based on S-R models and found limited success with physiological measures.

Zygomaticus Major facial muscle which raises when the corner of the mouth is turned upward in a smile. EMG recording of this muscle is used as an indicator of positivity.

BIBLIOGRAPHY

Akselrod, S., Gordon, D., Madwed, J. B., Snidman, N. C., Shannon, D. C., & Cohen, R. J. (1985). Hemodynamic regulation: Investigation by spectral analysis. *Am J Physiol Heart Circ Physiol, 249*(4), H867–875.

Allen, J. J. B., Chambers, A. S., & Towers, D. N. (2007). The many metrics of cardiac chronotropy: A pragmatic primer and a brief comparison of metrics. *Biological Psychology, 74*(2), 243–262.

Alwitt, L. F., Anderson, D. R., Lorch, E. P., & Levin, S. R. (1980). Preschool children's visual attention to television. *Human Communication Research, 7*, 52–67.

Anderson, D. R., & Bryant, J. (1983). Research on children's television viewing: The state of the art. In J. Bryant & D. R. Anderson (Eds.), *Children's understanding of television: Research on attention and comprehension* (pp. 331–354). New York: Academic Press.

Anderson, D. R., Bryant, J., Murray, J. P., Rich, M., Rivkin, M. J., & Zillmann, D. (2006). Brain imaging—an introduction to a new approach to studying media processes and effects. *Media Psychology, 8*(1), 1–6.

Anderson, D. R., & Burns, J. (1991). Paying attention to television. In J. Bryant & D. Zillmann (Eds.), *Responding to the screen: Reception and reaction processes* (pp. 3–26). Hillsdale, NJ: Lawrence Erlbaum Associates.

Anderson, D. R., & Levin, S. R. (1976). Young children's attention to Sesame Street. *Child Development, 47*, 806–811.

Anderson, D. R., & Lorch, E. P. (1983). Looking at television: Action or reaction? In J. Bryant & D. R. Anderson (Eds.), *Children's understanding of television: Research on attention and comprehension* (pp. 1–34). New York: Academic Press.

Andreassi, J. L. (2000). *Psychophysiology: Human behavior & physiological response* (4th ed.). Hillsdale, NJ: Lawrence Erlbaum Associates.

Andreassi, J. L. (2007). *Psychophysiology: Human behavior & physiological response* (5th ed.). Mahwah, NJ: Lawrence Erlbaum Associates.

Andrews, C. J., Durvasula, S., & Akhter, S. H. (1990). A framework for conceptualizing and measuring the involvement construct in advertising research. *Journal of Advertising, 19*(4), 27–40.

Andrews, C. J., & Shimp, T. A. (1990). Effects of involvement, argument strength, and source characteristics on central and peripheral processing of advertising. *Psychology & Marketing*, 7(3), 195–214.

Anthony, B. J., & Graham, F. K. (1985). Blink reflex modification by selective attention: Evidence for the modulation of "automatic" processing. *Biological Psychology*, 21(1), 43–59.

Anttonen, J., Surakka, V., & Koivuluoma, M. (2009). Ballistocardiographic responses to dynamic facial displays of emotion while sitting on the eMFi chair. *Journal of Media Psychology: Theories, Methods and Applications*, 21(2), 69–84.

Appel, V., Weinstein, S., & Weinstein, C. (1979). Brain activity and recall of TV advertising. *Journal of Advertising Research*, 19(4), 7.

Arnetz, B. B., Edgren, B., Levi, L., & Otto, U. (1985). Behavioural and endocrine reactions in boys scoring high on Sennton neurotic scale viewing an exciting and partly violent movie and the importance of social support. *Social Science & Medicine*, 20(7), 731–736.

Babbie, E. (2010). *The practice of social research*. Belmont, CA: Wadsworth.

Bailey, R., Wise, K., & Bolls, P. (2009). How avatar customizability affects children's arousal and subjective presence during junkfood-sponsored online video games. *Cyber Psychology & Behavior*, 12(3), 277–283.

Balaban, M. T., Losito, B. D. G., Simons, R. F., & Graham, F. K. (1986). Off-line latency and amplitude scoring of the human reflex eyeblink with Fortran IV. *Psychophysiology*, 23(5), 612.

Baldaro, B., Mazzetti, M., Codispoti, M., Tuozzi, G., Bolzani, R., & Trombini, G. (2001). Autonomic reactivity during viewing of an unpleasant film. *Perceptual and Motor Skills*, 93, 797–805.

Bandura, A. (2006). Toward a psychology of human agency. *Perspectives on Psychological Science*, 1(2), 164–180.

Bandura, A. (2009). Social cognitive theory of mass communication. In J. Bryant & M. B. Oliver (Eds.), *Media effects: Advances in theory and research* (pp. 94–124). New York: Routledge.

Bandura, A., Ross, D., & Ross, S. A. (1963). Imitation of film-mediated aggressive models. *The Journal of Abnormal and Social Psychology*, 66(1), 3–11.

Barker, K. (2002). *At the helm: A laboratory navigator*. Cold Spring Harbor, NJ: Cold Spring Harbor Laboratory Press.

Barrett, L. F., & Lindquist, K. A. (2008). The embodiment of emotion. In G. R. Semin & E. R. Smith (Eds.), *Embodied grounding: Social, cognitive, affective, and neuroscientific approaches* (pp. 237–262). New York: Cambridge University Press.

Barrett, L. F., Mesquita, B., Ochsner, K. N., & Gross, J. J. (2007). The experience of emotion. *Annual Review of Psychology*, 58, 373–403.

Barrett, L. F., & Wager, T. D. (2006). The structure of emotion: Evidence from neuroimaging studies. *Current Directions in Psychological Science*, 15(2), 79–83.

Bartholow, B. D., & Amodio, D. M. (2009). Using event-related brain potentials and social psychological research: A brief review and tutorial. In E. Harmon-Jones & J. S. Beer (Eds.), *Methods and social neuroscience*, (pp. 198–232). New York: The Guilford Press.

Basil, M. D. (1994a). Secondary reaction-time measures. In A. Lang (Ed.), *Measuring psychological responses to media* (pp. 85–98), Hillsdale, NJ: Lawrence Erlbaum Associates.

Basil, M. D. (1994b). Multiple resource theory II: Empirical examination of specific attention to television scenes. *Communication Research*, 21, 208–231.

Baumgartner, T., Valko, L., Esslen, M., & Lutz, J. (2006). Neural correlate of spatial presence in an arousing and noninteractive virtual reality: An EEG and psychophysiology study. *CyberPsychology & Behavior, 9*(1), 30–45.

Bear, M. F., Connors, B. W., & Paradiso, M. (2007). *Neuroscience: Exploring the brain* (3rd ed.). Philadelphia: Lippincott, Williams, & Wilkins.

Beaumont, J. G. (2008). *Introduction to neuropsychology* (2nd ed.). New York: Guilford Press.

Bell, C. (1844). *The anatomy of expression in human faces in painting.*

Bellman, S., Schweda, A., & Varan, D. (2009). Viewing angle matters—screen type does not. *Journal of Communication, 59*(3), 609–634.

Benning, S. D., Patrick, C. J., & Lang, A. R. (2004). Emotional modulation of the post-auricular reflex. *Psychophysiology, 41*(3), 426–432.

Berger, H. (1929). Uber das electrenkephalogramm des menschen (On the electroencephalogram of man). *Archiv fur Psychiatrie un Nervenkrankheiten, 87,* 551–553. Reprinted in English in S. W. Porges & M. G. H. Coles (Eds.), *Psychophysiology.* Stroudsburg, PA: Dowden, Hutchinson, & Ross, Inc.

Bernard, C. (1865/1957). *An introduction to the study of experimental medicine.* New York: Dover.

Bernard, C. (1878/1974). *Lectures on the phenomena of life common to animals and plants.* Springfield, IL: Thomas.

Berntson, G. G., & Cacioppo, J. T. (2007). Integrative physiology: Homeostasis, allostasis, and the orchestration of systemic physiology. In J. T. Cacioppo, L. G. Tassinary, & G. G. Berntson (Eds.), *Handbook of psychophysiology* (pp. 433–452). New York: Cambridge University Press.

Berntson, G. G., & Cacioppo, J. T. (2008). The functional neuroarchitecture of evaluative processes. In A. J. Elliot (Ed.), *Handbook of approach and avoidance motivation* (pp. 307–321). New York: Psychology Press, Taylor & Francis Group.

Berntson, G. G., Cacioppo, J. T., & Fieldstone, A. (1996). Illusions, arithmetic, and the bidirectional modulation of vagal control of the heart. *Biological Psychology, 44,* 1–17.

Berntson, G. G., Cacioppo, J. T., & Quigley, K. S. (1993). Cardiac psychophysiology and autonomic space in humans: Empirical perspectives and conceptual implications. *Psychological Bulletin, 114*(2), 296–322.

Berntson, G. G., Cacioppo, J. T., & Quigley, K. S. (1995). The metrics of cardiac chronotropism: Biometric perspectives. *Psychophysiology, 32,* 162–171.

Berntson, G. G., Quigley, K. S., & Lozano, D. (2007). Cardiovascular psychophysiology. In J. T. Cacioppo, L. G. Tassinary, & G. G. Berntson (Eds.), *Handbook of psychophysiology* (3rd ed., pp. 182–210). New York: Cambridge University Press.

Biocca, F., David, P., & West, M. (1994). Continuous response measurement (CRM): A computerized tool for research on the cognitive processing of communication messages. In A. Lang (Ed.), *Measuring psychological responses to media* (pp. 15–64). Hillsdale, NJ: Lawrence Erlbaum Associates.

Black, J. (2002). Darwin in the world of emotions. *Journal of the Royal Society of Medicine, 95,* 311–313.

Blumenthal, T. D., & Berg, W. K. (1986). Stimulus rise time, intensity, and bandwidth effects on acoustic startle amplitude and probability. *Psychophysiology, 23,* 635–641.

Blumenthal, T. D., Cuthbert, B. N., Filion, D. L., Hackley, S., Lipp, O. V., & Van Boxtel, A. (2005). Committee report: Guidelines for human startle electromyographic studies. *Psychophysiology, 42*(1), 1–15.

Blumenthal, T. D., Elden, A., & Flaten, M. A. (2004). A comparison of several methods used to quantify prepulse inhibition of eyeblink responding. *Psychophysiology, 41*(2), 326–332.

Blumenthal, T. D., & Goode, C. T. (1991). The startle eyeblink response to low intensity acoustic stimuli. *Psychophysiology, 28*(3), 296–306.

Bohlin, G., & Graham, F. K. (1977). Cardiac deceleration and reflex blink facilitation. *Psychophysiology, 14*(5), 423–430.

Bolls, P. D. (2002). I can hear you but can I see you? The use of visual cognition during exposure to high-imagery radio advertisements. *Communication Research, 29*, 537–563.

Bolls, P. D. (2007). It is just your imagination: The effect of imagery on product versus non-product information in radio advertisements. *Journal of Radio Studies, 13*(2), 201–213.

Bolls, P. D. (2010). Understanding emotion from a superordinate dimensional perspective: A productive way forward for communication processes and effects studies. *Communication Monographs, 77*(2), 146–152.

Bolls, P. D., & Lang, A. (2003). I saw it on the radio: The allocation of attention to high imagery radio advertisements. *Media Psychology, 5*(1), 49–71.

Bolls, P. D., Lang, A., & Potter, R. F. (2001). The effects of message valence and listener arousal on attention, memory, and facial muscular responses to radio advertisements. *Communication Research, 28*(5), 627–651.

Bolls, P. D., Miles, S., & Zhang, J. (2006). Intense emotions: Developmental differences in cognitive/emotional processing of the visual portrayal of threat and substance abuse prevention messages. *Psychophysiology, 43*, supplement 1, August.

Bolls, P. D., Muehling, D. D., & Yoon, K. (2003). The effects of television commercial pacing on viewers' attention and memory. *Journal of Marketing Communications, 9*(1), 17–28.

Bolls, P. D., & Potter, R. F. (1998). I saw it on the radio: The effects of imagery evoking radio commercials on listeners' allocation of attention and attitude toward the ad. In D. D. Meuhling (Ed.), *Proceedings of the 1998 conference of the American Academy of Advertising* (pp. 123–130). Madison, WI: Omnipress.

Boucsein, W. (1992). *Electrodermal activity.* New York: Plenum Press.

Boylan, M. (2007). Galen: On blood, the pulse, and the arteries. *Journal of the History of Biology, 40*(2), 207–230.

Bradley, M. M., Cuthbert, B. N., & Lang, P. J. (1993). Pictures as prepulse: Attention and emotion in startle modification. *Psychophysiology, 30*(5), 541–545.

Bradley, M. M., Cuthbert, B. N., & Lang, P. J. (1996). Picture media and emotion: Effects of a sustained affective context. *Psychophysiology, 33*, 662–670.

Bradley, M. M., & Lang, P. J. (1994). Measuring emotion: The self-assessment manikin and the semantic differential. *Journal of Behavioral Therapy and Experimental Psychiatry, 25*, 49–59.

Bradley, M. M., & Lang, P. J. (2000). Measuring emotion: Behavior, feeling, and physiology. In R. D. Lane & L. Nadel (Eds.), *Cognitive neuroscience of emotion* (pp. 242–276). New York: Oxford University Press.

Bradley, M. M., & Lang, P. J. (2007a). Emotion and motivation. In J. T. Cacioppo, L. G. Tassinary, & G. G. Berntson (Eds.), *Handbook of psychophysiology* (pp. 581–607). New York: Cambridge University Press.

Bradley, M. M., & Lang, P. J. (2007b). The International Affective Picture System (IAPS) in the study of emotion and attention. In J. A. Coan & J. B. Alan (Eds.), *Handbook of emotion elicitation and assessment* (pp. 29–46). New York: Oxford University Press.

Bradley, S. D. (2007a). Examining the eyeblink startle reflex as a measure of emotion and motivation to television programming. *Communication Methods and Measures, 1*(1), 7–30.

Bradley, S. D. (2007b). Dynamic, embodied, limited capacity attention and memory: Modeling cognitive processing of mediated stimuli. *Media Psychology, 9*(1), 211–239.

Bradley, S. D., Angelini, J. R., & Lee, S. (2007). Psychophysiological and memory effects of negative political ads. *Journal of Advertising, 36*(4), 115–127.

Bradley, S. D., Maxian, W., Wise, W. T., & Freeman, J. D. (2008). Emotion trumps attention: Using prepulse startle probe methodology to assess cognitive processing of television. *Communication Methods and Measures, 2*(4), 313–322.

Brazier, M. A. B. (1959). The historical development of neurophysiology. In J. Field, H. W. Magoun, & V. E. Hall (Eds.), *Handbook of physiology: A critical, comprehensive presentation of physiological knowledge and concepts* (Vol. I, pp. 1–58). Washington, DC: American Physiological Society.

Brinol, P., Petty, R. E., & Barden, J. (2007). Happiness versus sadness as a determinant of thought confidence in persuasion: A self-validation analysis. *Journal of Personality & Social Psychology, 93*(5), 711–727.

Britta, H., Wolkenberg, F. A., Ross, T. J., Myers, C. S., Heishman, S. J., Stein, D. J., Kurup, P. K., & Stein, E. A. (2008). Divided versus selective attention: Evidence for common processing mechanisms. *Brain Research, 1215*, 137–146.

Bromehead, C. E. N. (1942). The early history of water-supply. *The Geographical Journal, 99*(4), 183–193.

Brown, S. L., & Schwartz, G. E. (1980). Relationships between facial electromyography and subjective experience during affective imagery. *Biological Psychology, 11*, 49–62.

Brownley, K. A., Hurwitz, B. E., & Schneiderman, N. (2000). Cardiovascular psychophysiology. In J. T. Cacioppo, L. G. Tassinary, & G. G. Berntson (Eds.), *Handbook of psychophysiology* (2nd ed., pp. 224–264). New York: Cambridge University Press.

Bruggemann, J. M., & Barry, R. J. (2002). Eysenck's P as a modulator of affective and electrodermal responses to violent and comic film. *Personality and Individual Differences, 32*(6), 1029–1048.

Bruner, G. C., Hensel, P. J., & James, K. E. (2005). *Marketing scales handbook.* Mason, OH: Thomson Higher Education.

Bryant, J., & Rockwell, S. C. (1991). Evolving cognitive models and mass communication reception processes. In J. Bryant & D. Zillmann (Eds.), *Responding to the screen: Reception and reaction processes* (pp. 217–228). Hillsdale, NJ: Lawrence Erlbaum Associates.

Burch, G. E., & DePasquale, N. P. (1964). *A history of electrocardiography.* Chicago: Year Book Medical Publishers, Inc.

Bushman, B. J., & Huesmann, L. R. (2006). Short-term and long-term effects of violent media on aggression in children and adults. *Archives of Pediatrics & Adolescent Medicine, 160*, 348–352.

Bushman, B. J., Huesmann, L. R., & Whitaker, J. L. (2009). Violent media effects. In R. L. Nabi & M. B. Oliver (Eds.), *The Sage handbook of media processes and effects* (pp. 361–376). Newbury Park, CA: Sage.

Cacioppo, J. T., Berntson, G. G., & Klein, D. J. (1992). What is an emotion? The role of somatovisceral afference, with special emphasis on somatovisceral illusions. *Review of Personality and Social Psychology, 14*, 63–98.

Cacioppo, J. T., & Decety, J. (2009). What are the brain mechanisms on which psychological processes are based? *Perspectives on Psychological Science, 4*(1), 10–18.

Cacioppo, J. T., & Gardner, W. L. (1999). Emotion. *Annual Review of Psychology, 50*, 191–214.

Cacioppo, J. T., Gardner, W. L., & Berntson, G. G. (1999). The affect system has parallel and integrative processing components: form follows function. *Journal of Personality and Social Psychology, 76*(5), 839–855.

Cacioppo, J. T., Larsen, J. T., Smith, N. K., & Berntson, G. G. (2004). The affect system: What lurks below the surface of feelings? In A. S. R. Manstead, N. H. Frijda, & A. H. Fischer (Eds.), *Feelings and emotions: The Amsterdam conference* (pp. 223–242). New York: Cambridge University Press.

Cacioppo, J. T., & Petty, R. E. (1982). The need for cognition. *Journal of Personality & Social Psychology, 42*, 116–131.

Cacioppo, J. T., & Petty, R. E. (1985). Physiological responses and advertising effects: Is the cup half full or half empty? *Psychology & Marketing, 2*(2), 115–126.

Cacioppo, J. T., Petty, R. E., Losh, M. E., & Kim, H. S. (1986). Electromyographic activity over facial muscle regions can differentiate the valence and intensity of affective reactions. *Journal of Personality and Social Psychology, 50*(2), 260–268.

Cacioppo, J. T., Tassinary, L. G., & Berntson, G. G. (2007a). *Handbook of psychophysiology* (3rd ed.). New York: Cambridge University Press.

Cacioppo, J. T., Tassinary, L. G., & Berntson, G. G. (2007b). Psychophysiological science: Interdisciplinary approaches to classic questions about the mind. In J. T. Cacioppo, L. G. Tassinary, & G. G. Berntson (Eds.), *Handbook of psychophysiology* (pp. 1–18). New York: Cambridge University Press.

Cacioppo, J. G., von Hippel, W., & Ernst, J. M. (1997). Mapping cognitive structures and processes through verbal content: The thought-listing technique. *Journal of Consulting & Clinical Psychology, 65*(6), 928–940.

Cajavilca, C., Varon, J., & Sternbach, G. L. (2009). Luigi Galvani and the foundations of electrophysiology. *Resuscitation, 80*(2), 159–162.

Cameron, G. T., & Frieske, D. A. (1994). Response latency. In A. Lang (Ed.), *Measuring psychological responses to media* (pp. 149–164). Hillsdale, NJ: Lawrence Erlbaum Associates.

Cameron, G. T., Schleuder, J., & Thorsen, E. (1991). The role of news teasers in the processing of news and commercials. *Communication Research, 18*, 667–684.

Cannon, W. B. (1927). The James-Lange theory of emotions: A critical examination and an alternative theory. *American Journal of Psychology, 39*, 106–124.

Cannon, W. B. (1929). Organization for physiological homeostasis. *Physiol. Rev., 9*(3), 399–431.

Cantor, J. R., Zillmann, D., & Bryant, J. (1975). Enhancement of experienced sexual arousal in response to erotic stimuli through misattribution of unrelated residual excitation. *Journal of Personality and Social Psychology, 32*(1), 69–75.

Cantor, J. R., Zillmann, D., & Einsiedel, E. F. (1978). Female responses to provocation after exposure to aggressive and erotic films. *Communication Research, 5*(4), 395–412.

Cantril, H. (1940). *The invasion from Mars*. Princeton, NJ: Princeton University Press.

Cappella, J. N., & Jamieson, K. H. (1997). *Spiral of cynicism: The press and the public good*. New York: Oxford University Press.

Carnagey, N. L., Anderson, C. A., & Bushman, B. J. (2007). The effect of videogame violence on physiological desensitization to real-life violence. *Journal of Experimental Social Psychology, 43*, 489–496.

Carpentier, F. R., Brown, J. D., Bertocci, M., Silk, J. S., Forbes, E. E., & Dahl, R. E. (2008). Sad kids, sad media? Applying mood management theory to depressed adolescents' use of media. *Media Psychology, 11*(1), 143–166.

Chaffee, S. H. (1980). Mass media effects: New research perspectives. In G. C. Wilhoit & H. de Bock (Eds.), *Mass communication review yearbook* (Vol. 1, pp. 77–108). Beverly Hills, CA: Sage.

Chaffee, S. H. (1991). *Explication*. Newbury Park, CA: Sage.

Chaffee, S. H., & Berger, C. R. (1987). What communication scientists do. In C. R. Berger & S. H. Chaffee (Eds.), *Handbook of communication science* (pp. 99–122). Newbury Park, CA: Sage.

Chapman, H. A., Kim, D. A., Susskind, J. M., & Anderson, A. K. (2009). In bad taste: Evidence for the oral origins of moral disgust. *Science, 323*(5918), 1222–1226.

Chattopadhyay, A., & Alba, J. W. (1988). The situation importance of recall and inference and consumer decision-making. *Journal of Consumer Research, 15*, 1–12.

Chen, L., Zhou, S., & Bryant, J. (2007). Temporal changes in mood repair through music consumption: effects of mood, mood salience, and individual differences. *Media Psychology, 9*, 695–713.

Choi, H. P., & Anderson, D. R. (1991). A temporal analysis of toy play and distractibility in young children. *Journal of Experimental Child Psychology, 52*, 41–69.

Chory-Assad, R. M. (2004). Effects of television sitcom exposure on the accessibility of verbally aggressive thoughts. *Western Journal of Communication, 68*(4), 431–453.

Chung, Y. (2007). *Processing web ads: The effects of animation and arousing content*. Youngstown, NY: Cambria Press.

Churchland, P. S., & Sejnowski, T. J. (1992). *The computational brain*. Cambridge, MA: MIT Press.

Clark, A. (1997). *Being there: Putting brain, body, and world together again*. Boston: Massachusetts Institute of Technology.

Cochran, W. G., & Cox, G. M. (1957). *Experimental design* (2nd ed.). New York: John Wiley & Sons.

Codispoti, M., & De Cesarei, A. (2007). Arousal and attention: Picture size and emotional reactions. *Psychophysiology, 44*, 680–686.

Codispoti, M., Ferrari, V., & Bradley, M. M. (2006). Repetitive picture processing: Autonomic and cortical correlates. *Brain Research, 12*, 213–220.

Codispoti, M., Surcinelli, P., & Baldaro, B. (2008). Watching emotional movies: Affective reactions and gender differences. *International Journal of Psychophysiology, 69*(2), 90–95.

Cohen, A. R. (1957). Need for cognition and order of communication as determinants of opinion change. In C. I. Hovland (Ed.), *Order of presentation* (pp. 79–97). New Haven, CT: Yale University Press.

Costa, P. T., & McCrae, R. R. (2008). The revised NEO personality inventory (NEO-PI-R). In G. J. Boyle, G. Matthews, & D. H. Saklofske (Eds.), *The Sage handbook of personality theory and assessment: Volume 2 personality measurement and testing* (pp. 179–198), Los Angeles: Sage.

Craik, F. I. M., & Lockhart, R. S. (1972). Levels of processing: A framework for memory research. *Journal of Verbal Learning and Verbal Behavior, 11*, 671–684.

Cunningham, W. A., Packer, D. J., Kesek, A., & Van Bavel, J. J. (2009). Implicit measurement of attitudes: A physiological approach. In R. E. Petty, R. H. Fazio, & P. Brinol (Eds.), *Attitudes: Insights from the new implicit measures* (pp. 485–512). New York: Taylor & Francis.

Curtin, J. J., Lozano, D. L., & Allen, J. J. B. (2007). The psychophysiological laboratory. In J. B. Coan & J. J. B. Allen (Eds.), *Handbook of emotion elicitation and assessment* (pp. 398–425). New York: Oxford University Press.

Damasio, A. R. (1994). *Descartes' error: Emotion, reason, and the human brain.* New York: Grossett/Putnam.

Damasio, A. (1999). *The feeling of what happens: Body and emotion in the making of consciousness.* San Diego, CA: Harcourt.

Darrow, C. W. (1964). Psychophysiology, yesterday, today, and tomorrow. *Psychophysiology, 1*(1), 4–7.

Darwin, C. (1872/1965). *The expression of the emotions in man and animals.* Chicago: University of Chicago Press.

Darwin, C. (1897). *The expression of the emotions in man and animals.* New York: D. Appleton.

Dawson, M. E., Schell, A. M., & Filion, D. F. (2007). The electrodermal system. In J. T. Cacioppo, L. G. Tassinary, & G. G. Berntson (Eds.), *Handbook of psychophysiology* (3rd ed., pp. 159–181). New York: Cambridge University Press.

De Pascalis, V., Barry, R. J., & Sparita, A. (1995). Decelerative changes in heart rate during recognition of visual stimuli: Effects of psychological stress. *International Journal of Psychophysiology, 20,* 21–31.

Delorme, A., & Makeig, S. (2004). EEGLAB: An open source toolbox for analysis of single-trial EEG dynamics including independent component analysis. *Journal of Neuroscience Methods, 134*(1), 9–21.

Deschaumes-Molinaro, C., Dittmar, A., & Vernet-Maury, E. (1992). Autonomic nervous system response patterns correlate with mental imagery. *Physiology & Behavior, 51*(5), 1021–1027.

Detenber, B. H., Simons, R. F., & Bennett, G. G. (1998). Roll 'em!: The effects of picture motion on emotional responses. *Journal of Broadcasting & Electronic Media, 42*(1), 113–128.

Diao, F., & Sundar, S. S. (2004). Orienting response and memory for web advertisements: Exploring effects of pop-up window and animation. *Communication Research, 31*(5), 537–567.

Dickinson, A., & Dearing, M. F. (1979). Appetitive-aversive interactions and inhibitory processes. In A. Dickinson & R. A. Boakes (Eds.), *Mechanisms of learning and motivation* (pp. 203–231). Hillsdale, NJ: Lawrence Erlbaum Associates.

Dillard, J. P., & Nabi, R. L. (2006). The persuasive influence of emotion and cancer prevention and detection messages. *Journal of Communication, 56,* S123–S139.

Dillard, J. P., & Peck, E. (2001). Persuasion and the structure of affect dual systems and discrete emotions as complementary models. *Human Communication Research, 27*(1), 38–68.

Dillard, J. P., Plotnick, C. A., Godbold, L. C., Freimuth, V. S., & Edgar, T. (1996). The multiple affective outcomes of AIDS PSAs. *Communication Research, 23*(1), 44–72.

Donchin, E. (1979). Event-related brain potentials: A tool in the study of human information processing. In H. Begleiter (Ed.), *Evoked brain potentials and behavior.* New York: Plenum.

Donchin, E. (1981). Surprise! Surprise? *Psychophysiology, 18*(5), 493–513.

Donchin, E., & Israel, J. B. (1980). Event-related potentials and psychological theory. In H. H. Kornhuber & L. Deecke (Eds.), *Motivation, motor, and sensory processes of the brain: Electrical potentials, behavior, and clinical use: Progress in brain research.* North Holland, Amsterdam: Elsevier.

Donders, F. C. (1868/1969). On the speed of mental processes. *Acta Psychologica, 30,* 412–431.

Donnerstein, E., & Barrett, G. (1978). Effects of erotic stimuli on male aggression toward females. *Journal of Personality and Social Psychology, 36*(2), 180–188.

Donnerstein, E., & Hallam, J. (1978). Facilitating effects of erotica on aggression against women. *Journal of Personality and Social Psychology, 36*(11), 1270–1277.

Dormire, S. L., & Carpenter, J. S. (2002). An alternative to Unibase/glycol as an effective non-hydrating electrolyte medium for the measurement of electrodermal activity. *Psychophysiology, 39*, 423–426.

Du Plessis, E. (2008). *The advertised mind: Groundbreaking insights into how our brains respond to advertising.* Philadelphia: Kogan Page.

Duchenne, G.-B. (1862/1990). *The mechanism of human facial expression* (R. A. Cuthbertson, Trans.). New York: Press Syndicate of the University of Cambridge.

Duncan, S., & Barrett, L. F. (2007). Affect as a form of cognition: A neurobiological analysis. *Cognition and Emotion, 21*, 1184–1211.

Dysinger, W. S., & Ruckmick, C. A. (1933). *The emotional responses of children to the motion picture situation.* New York: Macmillan.

Eagly, A. H., & Chaiken, S. (1993). *The psychology of attitudes.* Orlando, FL: Harcourt Brace Jovanovich.

Edelberg, R. (1972). Electrical activity of the skin: Its measurement and uses in psychophysiology. In N. S. Greenfield & R. A. Sternbach (Eds.), *Handbook of psychophysiology* (pp. 367–418). New York: Holt.

Edelberg, R. (1974). For distinguished contribution to psychophysiology: Albert F. Ax. *Psychophysiology, 11*(2), 216–218.

Ekman, P. (1989). The argument and evidence about universals and facial expressions of emotion. In H. Wagner & A. Manstead (Eds.), *Handbook of psychophysiology: The biological psychology of emotions and social processes* (pp. 143–164). London: John Wiley Ltd.

Ekman, P. (1993). Facial expression and emotion. *American Psychologist, 48*(4), 384–392.

Ekman, P., & Friesen, W. V. (1982). Felt, false, and miserable smiles. *Journal of Nonverbal Behavior, 6*, 238–252.

Ekman, P., Davidson, R. J., & Friesen, W. V. (1990). The Duchenne smile: Emotional expression and brain physiology II. *Journal of Personality and Social Psychology, 58*(2), 342–353.

Ekman, P., Friesen, W. V., & Ancoli, S. (1980). Facial signs of emotional experience. *Journal of Personality and Social Psychology, 39*, 1125–1134.

Ekman, P., Levenson, R. W., & Friesen, W. V. (1983). Autonomic nervous system activity distinguishes among emotions. *Science, 221*, 1208–1210.

Ewing, D. J., Borsey, D. Q., Bellavere, F., & Clarke, B. F. (1981). Cardiac autonomic neuropathy in diabetes: Comparison of measures of R-R interval variation. *Diabetologia, 21*, 18–24.

Fabiani, M., Gratton, G., & Federmeier, K. (2007). Event-related brain potentials: Methods, theory, and applications. In J. T. Cacioppo, L. G. Tassinary, & G. G. Berntson (Eds.), *Handbook of psychophysiology* (3rd ed., pp. 85–119). New York: Cambridge University Press.

Faul, F., Erdfelder, E., Lang, A.-G., & Buchner, A. (2007). G★Power 3: A flexible statistical power analysis program for the social, behavioral, and biomedical sciences. *Behavior Research Methods, 39*(2), 175–191.

Fenwick, I., & Rice, M. D. (1991). Reliability of continuous measurement copy-testing methods. *Journal of Advertising Research, 31*(1), 23–29.

Féré, C. (1888). Notes on changes in electrical resistance under the effect of sensory stimulation and emotion. *Comptes Rendus des Seances de la Societe de Biologie, 5*, 217–219. Reprinted in English in S. W. Porges and M. G. H. Coles (Eds.), *Psychophysiology.* Stroudsburg, PA: Dowden, Hutchinson, & Ross, Inc.

Fetzner, J. (1996). Obituary: Albert F. Ax (1913–1994). *International Journal of Psychophysiology, 22*, 133–140.

Fowles, D. C., Christie, M. J., Edelberg, R., Grings, W. W., Lykken, D. T., & Venables, P. H. (1981). Publication recommendations for electrodermal measurements. *Psychophysiology, 18*, 232–239.

Fox, J. R., Lang, A., Chung, Y., Lee, S., Schwartz, N., & Potter, D. (2004). Picture this: Effects of graphics on the processing of television news. *Journal of Broadcasting & Electronic Media, 48*(4), 646–674.

Fox, J. R., Park, B., & Lang, A. (2007). When available resources become negative resources: The effects of cognitive overload on memory sensitivity and criterion bias. *Communication Research, 34*(3), 277–296.

Fridlund, A. J., & Cacioppo, J. T. (1986). Guidelines for human electromyographic research. *Psychophysiology, 23*(5), 567–589.

Friestad, M., & Thorson, E. (1993). Remembering ads: The effects of encoding strategies, retrieval cues, and emotional response. *Journal of Consumer Psychology, 2*(1), 1–23.

Frijda, N. H. (1994). Varieties of affect: Emotions and episodes, moods, and sentiments. In P. Ekman & R. J. Davidson (Eds.), *The nature of emotion* (pp. 59–67). New York: Oxford University Press.

Frost, R., & Stauffer, J. (1987). The effects of social class, gender, and personality on physiological responses to filmed violence. *Journal of Communication, 37*(2), 29–45.

Furnham, A., Eysenck, S. B. G., & Saklofske, D. H. (2008). The Eysenck personality measures: Fifty years of scale development. In G. J. Boyle, G. Matthews, & D. H. Saklofske (Eds.), *The Sage handbook of personality theory and assessment: Volume 2 personality measurement and testing* (pp. 199–218). Los Angeles: Sage.

Gale, A., & Smith, D. (1980). On setting up a psychophysiological laboratory. In I. Martin & P. H. Venables (Eds.), *Techniques in psychophysiology*. New York: John Wiley & Sons.

Gardiner, H. M. s. N., Metcalf, R. C., & Beebe-Center, J. G. (1937/1970). *Feeling and emotion*. Westport, CT: Greenwood Press.

Geenen, R., & Van de Vijver, F. J. R. (1993). A simple test of the Law of Initial Values. *Psychophysiology, 30*(5), 525–530.

Geiger, S., & Newhagen, J. (1993). Revealing the black box: Information processing and media effects. *Journal of Communication, 43*(4), 43–50.

Geiger, S., & Reeves, B. (1993). The effects of scene changes and semantic relatedness on attention to television. *Communication Research, 20*, 155–175.

Gevins, A. S., Zeitlin, G. M., Yingling, C. D., Doyle, J. C., Dedon, M. F., Schaffer, R. E., et al. (1979). EEG patterns during cognitive tasks I. Methodology and analysis of complex behaviors. *Electroencephalography and Clinical Neurophysiology, 47*, 693–703.

Gomez, P., Zimmermann, P., Guttormsen-Schar, S., & Danuser, B. (2005). Respiratory responses associated with affective processing of film stimuli. *Biological Psychology, 68*(3), 223–235.

Goodlett, C. R., & Horn, K. H. (2001). Mechanism of alcohol-induced damage to the developing nervous system. *Alcohol Research & Health, 25*(3), 175–184. Retrieved from http://pubs.niaaa.nih.gov/publications/arh25–3/175–184.pdf.

Grabe, M. E., Lang, A., & Zhao, X. (2003). News content and form: Implications for memory and audience evaluations. *Communication Research, 30*(4), 387–413.

Graham, F. K. (1975). The more or less startling effects of weak prestimulation. *Psychophysiology, 12*(3), 238–248.

Graham, F. K. (1979). Distinguishing among orienting, defense, and startle reflexes. In H. D. Kimmel, E. H. Van Olst, & J. F. Orlebeke (Eds.), *The orienting reflex in humans* (pp. 137–167). Hillsdale, NJ: Lawrence Erlbaum Associates.

Graham, F. K. (1980). Control of reflex blink excitability. In R. F. Thompson, L. H. Hicks, & V. B. Shvyrkov (Eds.), *Neural mechanisms of goal-directed behavior and learning* (pp. 511–519). New York: Academic Press.

Graham, F. K., & Clifton, R. K. (1966). Heart rate change as a component of the orienting response. *Psychological Bulletin, 65*, 305–320.

Graham, F. K., Putnam, L. E., & Leavitt, L. A. (1975). Lead-stimulation effects on human cardiac orienting and blink reflexes. *Journal of Experimental Psychology: Human Perception and Performance, 1*(2), 161–169.

Greene, W. A., Turetsky, B., & Kohler, C. (2000). General laboratory safety. In J. T. Cacioppo, L. G. Tassinary, & G. G. Berntson (Eds.), *Handbook of psychophysiology* (pp. 951–977). New York: Cambridge University Press.

Greenwald, A. G., & Leavitt, C. (1984). Audience involvement in advertising: Four levels. *Journal of Consumer Research, 11*(1), 581–592.

Grewe, O., Nagel, F., Kopiez, R., & Altenmuller, E. (2007). Emotions over time: Synchronicity and the development of subjective, physiological, and facial affective reactions to music. *Emotion, 7*(4), 774–788.

Grimes, T., & Meadowcroft, J. (1995). Attention to television and some methods for its measurement. In B. R. Burleson (Ed.), *Communication yearbook* 18 (pp. 133–161). Thousand Oaks, CA: Sage.

Haidt, J., McCauley, C., & Rozin, P. (1994). Individual differences in sensitivity to disgust: A scale sampling seven domains of disgust elicitors. *Personality and Individual Differences, 16*, 701–713.

Hansen, A. L., Johnsen, B. H., & Thayer, J. F. (2003). Vagal influence on working memory and attention. *International Journal of Psychophysiology, 48*, 263–274.

Harmon-Jones, E., & Peterson, C. K. (2009). Electroencephalographic methods in social and personality psychology. In E. Harmon-Jones & J. S. Beer (Eds.), *Methods and social neuroscience* (pp. 170–197). New York: The Guilford Press.

Harvey, W. (1628/1998). On the motion of the heart and blood in animals (Vol. Modern History Sourcebook). Available from www.fordham.edu/halsall/mod/1628harvey-blood.html.

Hazlett, R. L., & Hazlett, S. Y. (1999). Emotional response to television commercials: Facial EMG vs. self-report. *Journal of Advertising Research, 39*(2), 7–23.

Hess, U. (2009). Facial EMG. In E. Harmon-Jones & J. S. Beer (Eds.), *Methods in social neuroscience* (pp. 70–91). New York: The Guilford Press.

Hess, U., Sabourin, G., & Kleck, R. E. (2007). Postauricular and eyeblink startle responses to facial expressions. *Psychophysiology, 44*(3), 431–435.

Heuttel, S. A., Song, A. W., & McCarthy, G. (2008). *Functional magnetic resonance imaging* (2nd ed.). Sunderland, MA: Sinauer Associates, Inc.

Hopkins, R., & Fletcher, J. E. (1994). Electrodermal measurement: Particularly effective for forecasting message influence on sales appeal. In A. Lang (Ed.), *Measuring psychological responses to media* (pp. 113–132). Hillsdale, NJ: Lawrence Erlbaum Associates.

Hovland, C. I. (1957). *Order of presentation*. New Haven, CT: Yale University Press.

Hovland, C. I., Janis, I. L., & Kelly, H. H. (1953). *Communication and persuasion*. New Haven, CT: Yale University Press.

Hurst, J. W. (1998). Naming of the waves in the ECG, with a brief account of their genesis. *Circulation, 98*(18), 1937–1942.

Huston, A. C., & Wright, J. C. (1983). Children's processing of television: The informative functions of formal features. In J. Bryant & D. R. Anderson (Eds.), *Children's understanding of television: Research on attention and comprehension* (pp. 35–68). New York: Academic Press.

Hutchinson, D., & Bradley, S. D. (2009). Memory for images intense enough to draw an administration's attention: Television and the "war on terror." *Politics and the Life Sciences, 28*(1), 31–47.

Ito, T. A., & Cacioppo, J. T. (2005). Variations on the human universal: Individual differences in positivity offset and negativity bias. *Cognition and Emotion, 19*(1), 1–26.

Ivarsson, M., Anderson, M., Åkerstedt, T., & Lindblad, F. (2009). Playing a violent television game affects heart rate variability. *Acta Pædiatrica, 98*(1), 166–172.

Ivory, J. D., & Kalyanaraman, S. (2007). The effects of technological advancement and violent content in video games on players' feelings of presence, involvement, physiological arousal, and aggression. *Journal of Communication, 57*, 532–555.

Ivory, J. D., & Magee, R. G. (2009). You can't take it with you? Effects of handheld portable media consoles on physiological and psychological responses to video game and movie content. *CyberPsychology & Behavior, 12*(3), 291–297.

Izard, C. E. (1972). *Patterns of emotions: A new analysis of anxiety and depression.* New York: Academic Press.

Izard, C. E. (2009). Emotion theory and research: Highlights, unanswered questions, and emerging issues. *Annual Review of Psychology, 60*, 1–25.

Jacobson, E. (1927). Action currents from muscular contractions during conscious processes. *Science, 66*, 403.

James, K. H., James, T. W., Jobard, G., Wong, A. C. N., & Gauthier, I. (2005). Letter processing in the visual system: Different activation patterns for single letters and strings. *Cognitive Affective & Behavioral Neuroscience, 5*(4), 452–466.

James, W. (1884). What is an emotion? *Mind, 9*, 188–205.

Jansen, D. M., & Fridja, N. H. (1994). Modulation of the acoustic startle response by film-induced fear and sexual arousal. *Psychophysiology, 31*(6), 565–571.

Jansma, J. M., Ramsey, N. F., de Zwart, J. A., van Gelderen, P., & Duyn, J. H. (2007). FMRI study of effort and information processing in a working memory task. *Human Brain Mapping, 28*(5), 431–440.

Jasper, H. H. (1958). The ten-twenty electrode system of the International Federation. *Electroencephalography and Clinical Neurophysiology, 10*, 371–375.

Jennings, J. R. (1992). Is it important that the mind is in a body? Inhibition and the heart. *Psychophysiology, 29*, 369–383.

Jennings, J. R., Berg, W. K., Hutcheson, J. S., Obrist, P., Porges, S., & Turpin, G. (1981). Publication guidelines for heart rate studies in man. *Psychophysiology, 18*(3), 226–231.

Jennings, J. R., & Gianaros, P. J. (2007). Methodology. In J. T. Cacioppo, L. G. Tassinary, & G. G. Berntson (Eds.), *Psychophysiology* (Vol. 3, pp. 812–833). Cambridge, MA: Cambridge University Press.

Johnson, B. T. & Eagly, A. H. (1990). Involvement and persuasion: Types, traditions, and the evidence. *Psychological Bulletin, 107*, 375–384.

Johnstone, T., Kim, M. J., & Whalen, P. J. (2009). Functional magnetic resonance imaging in the affective and social neurosciences. In E. Harmon-Jones & J. S. Beer (Eds.), *Methods in social neuroscience* (pp. 313–336). New York: The Guilford Press.

Jowett, B. (September 15, 2008). The project Gutenberg Ebook of Timaeus, from www.gutenberg.org/files/1572/1572.txt.

Jowett, G., Jarvie, I. C., & Fuller, K. H. (1996). *Children and the movies: Media influence and the Payne Fund controversy*. New York: Cambridge University Press.

Kahneman, D. (1973). *Attention and effort*. Englewood Cliffs, NJ: Prentice Hall.

Kalat, J. W. (2007). *Biological psychology* (9th ed.). Belmont, CA: Thompson Wadsworth.

Kamath, M. V., & Fallen, E. L. (1993). Power spectral analysis of heart rate variability, a noninvasive signature of cardiac autonomic function. *Critical Reviews in Biomedical Engineering, 21*, 245–311.

Kandel, E. R., Schwartz, J. H., & Jessell, T. M. (2000). *Principles of neural science*. New York: McGraw-Hill.

Kaviani, H., Gray, J. A., Checkley, S. A., Kumari, V., & Wilson, G. D. (1999). Modulation of the acoustic startle reflex by emotionally-toned film-clips. *International Journal of Psychophysiology, 32*, 47–55.

Kirk, R. E. (1994). *Experimental design*. Belmont, CA: Wadsworth.

Kirk, R. E. (1995). *Experimental design: Procedures for the behavioral sciences* (3rd ed.). Pacific Grove, CA: Brooks/Cole Publishing Company.

Knobloch, S. (2003). Mood adjustment via mass communication. *Journal of Communication, 53*, 233–250.

Konijn, E. A., Nije, P. M., & Bushman, B. J. (2007). I wish I were a warrior: The role of wishful identification in effects of violent video games on aggression in adolescent boys. *Developmental Psychology, 43*, 1038–1044.

Koruth, J., Potter, R. F., Bolls, P. D., & Lang, A. (2007). An examination of heart rate variability during positive and negative radio messages. *Psychophysiology, 44* (Supplement), S60.

Koruth, K. J. (2010). *Separating attention from arousal during TV viewing: Using heart rate variability to track variations in sympathetic and parasympathetic activation*. Ph.D., Indiana University, Bloomington, IN.

Krcmar, M. (2009). Individual differences in media effects. In R. L. Nabi & M. B. Oliver (Eds.), *The Sage handbook of media processes and effects* (pp. 237–250). Los Angeles: Sage Publications Inc.

Kreibig, S. D., Wilhelm, F. H., Roth, W. T., & Gross, J. J. (2007). Cardiovascular, electrodermal, and respiratory response patterns to fear- and sadness-inducing films. *Psychophysiology, 44*, 787–806.

Krugman, H. E. (1971). Brainwave measures of media involvement. *Journal of Advertising Research, 11*(1), 3–9.

Lacey, B. C., & Lacey, J. I. (1980). Cognitive modulation of time-dependent primary bradycardia. *Psychophysiology, 17*, 209–221.

Lacey, J. I., & Lacey, B. C. (1962). The law of initial value in the longitudinal study of autonomic constitution: Reproducibility of autonomic responses and response patterns over a four-year interval. *Annals of the New York Academy of Sciences, 98*(4), 1257–1290.

Lacey, J. I., & Lacey, B. C. (1974). On heart rate responses and behavior: A reply to Elliott. *Journal of Personality and Social Psychology, 30*, 1–18.

Lachman, R., Lachman, J. L., & Butterfield, E. C. (1979). *Cognitive psychology and information processing: An introduction*. Hillsdale, NJ: Lawrence Erlbaum Associates.

Landis, C., & Hunt, W. A. (1939). *The startle pattern*. New York: Farrar and Reinhart.

Lane, D. R., & Harrington, N. G. (2009). Electromyographic response as a measure of effortful cognitive processing. In M. J. Beatty, J. C. McCroskey, & K. Floyd (Eds.),

Biological dimensions of communication: Perspectives, research, and methods (pp. 117–131). Cresskill, NJ: Hampton Press, Inc.

Lang, A. (1990). Involuntary attention and physiological arousal evoked by structural features and emotional content in TV commercials. *Communication Research, 17*(3), 275–299.

Lang, A. (1994a). Comments on setting up a laboratory. In A. Lang (Ed.), *Measuring psychological responses to media* (pp. 227–232). Hillsdale, NJ: Lawrence Erlbaum Associates.

Lang, A. (1994b). *Measuring psychological responses to media.* Hillsdale, NJ: Lawrence Erlbaum Associates.

Lang, A. (1994c). What can the heart tell us about thinking? In A. Lang (Ed.), *Measuring psychological responses to media* (pp. 99–112). Hillsdale, NJ: Lawrence Erlbaum Associates.

Lang, A. (2009). The limited capacity model of motivated mediated message processing. In R. L. Nabi & M. B. Oliver (Eds.), *The Sage handbook of media processes and effects* (pp. 193–204). Thousand Oaks, CA: Sage Publications.

Lang, A., & Basil, M. D. (1998). Attention, resource allocation, and communication research: What do secondary task reaction times measure, anyway? In M. E. Roloff (Ed.), *Communication yearbook 21* (pp. 443–473). Thousand Oaks, CA: Sage.

Lang, A., Bolls, P., Potter, R. F., & Kawahara, K. (1999). The effects of production pacing and arousing content on the information processing of television messages. *Journal of Broadcasting & Electronic Media, 43*, 451–475.

Lang, A., Borse, J., Wise, K., & David, P. (2002). Captured by the World Wide Web— orienting to structural and content features of computer-presented information. *Communication Research, 29*(3), 215–245.

Lang, A., Bradley, S. D., Chung, Y., & Lee, S. (2003). Where the mind meets the message: Reflections on ten years of measuring psychological responses to media. *Journal of Broadcasting & Electronic Media, 47*(4), 650–655.

Lang, A., Bradley, S. D., Park, B., Shin, M., & Chung, Y. (2006). Parsing the resource pie: Using STRTs to measure attention to mediated messages. *Media Psychology, 8*, 369–394.

Lang, A., Bradley, S. D., Sparks Jr, J. V., & Lee, S. (2007a). The Motivation Activation Measure (MAM): How well does MAM predict individual differences in physiological indicators of appetitive and aversive activation? *Communication Methods and Measures, 1*(2), 113–136.

Lang, A., Chung, Y., Lee, S., & Zhao, X. (2005). It's the product: Do risky products compel attention and elicit arousal in media users? *Health Communication, 17*(3), 283–300.

Lang, A., Chung, Y., Lee, S., Schwartz, N., & Shin, M. (2005). It's an arousing, fast-paced kind of world: The effects of age and sensation seeking on the information processing of substance abuse PSA's. *Media Psychology, 7*(4), 421–454.

Lang, A., Geiger, S., Strickwerda, M., & Sumner, J. (1993). The effects of related and unrelated cuts on television viewers' attention, processing capacity, and memory. *Communication Research, 20*(1), 4–29.

Lang, A., Kurita, S., Rubenking, B., & Potter, R. F. (In press). miniMAM: Validating a short version of the motivation activation measure. *Communication Methods and Measures.*

Lang, A., Newhagen, J., & Reeves, B. (1996). Negative video as structure: Emotion, attention, capacity, and memory. *Journal of Broadcasting & Electronic Media, 39*(2), 313–327.

Lang, A., Park, B., Sanders-Jackson, A. N., Wilson, B. D., & Wang, Z. (2007b). Cognition and emotion in TV message processing: How valence, arousing content, structural complexity, and information density affect the availability of cognitive resources. *Media Psychology, 10*(3), 317–338.

Lang, A., Potter, R. F., & Bolls, P. (1999). Something for nothing: Is visual encoding automatic? *Media Psychology, 1*(2), 145–164.

Lang, A., Potter, R. F., & Bolls, P. D. (2009). Where psychophysiology meets the media: Taking the effects out of media research. In J. Bryant & M. B. Oliver (Eds.), *Media effects: Advances in theory and research* (3rd ed., pp. 185–206). New York: Routledge.

Lang, A., Potter, D., & Grabe, M. E. (2003). Making news memorable: Applying theory to the production of local television news. *Journal of Broadcasting & Electronic Media, 47*(1), 113–123.

Lang, A., Shin, M., & Lee, S. (2005). Sensation seeking, motivation, and substance use: A dual system approach. *Media Psychology, 7*(1), 1–29.

Lang, A., Sias, P., Chantrill, P., & Burek, J. A. (1995). Tell me a story: Narrative structure and memory for television messages. *Communication Reports, 8*, 1–9.

Lang, P. J. (1980). Behavioral treatment and bio behavioral assessment: Computer applications. In J. B. Sadowski, J. H. Johnson, & T. A. Williams (Eds.), *Technology in mental health care delivery systems* (pp. 119–137). Norwood, NJ: Ablex Publishing.

Lang, P. J. (1995). The emotion probe: Studies of motivation and attention. *American Psychologist, 50*, 372–385.

Lang, P. J., & Bradley, M. M. (2008). Appetitive and defensive motivation is the substrate of emotion. In A. J. Elliot (Ed.), *Handbook of approach and avoidance motivation* (pp. 51–66). New York: Psychology Press, Taylor & Francis Group.

Lang, P. J., Bradley, M. M., & Cuthbert, B. N. (1990). Emotion, attention, and the startle reflex. *Psychological Review, 97*(3), 377–395.

Lang, P. J., Bradley, M. M., & Cuthbert, B. N. (1997). Motivated attention: Affect, activation, and action. In P. J. Lang, R. F. Simons, & M. T. Balaban (Eds.), *Attention and orienting: Sensory and motivational processes* (pp. 97–135). Hillsdale, NJ: Lawrence Erlbaum Associates.

Lang, P. J., Greenwald, M. K., Bradley, M. M., & Hamm, A. O. (1993). Looking at pictures: Affective, facial, visceral, and behavioral reactions. *Psychophysiology, 30*, 261–273.

Langleben, D. D., Loughead, J. W., Ruparel, K., Hakun, J. G., Busch-Winokur, S., Holloway, M. B., Strasser, A. A., Cappella, J. N., & Lerman, C. (2009). Reduced prefrontal and temporal processing and recall of high "sensation value" ads. *Neuroimage, 46*(1), 219–225.

Larsen, J. T., Berntson, G. G., Poehlmann, K. M., Ito, T. A., & Cacioppo, J. T. (2008). The psychophysiology of emotion. In R. Lewis, J. M. Haviland-Jones, & L. F. Barrett (Eds.), *The handbook of emotions* (3rd ed., pp. 180–195). New York: Guilford.

Larsen, J. T., Norris, C. J., & Cacioppo, J. T. (2003). Effects of positive and negative affect on electromyographic activity over zygomaticus major and corrugator supercilii. *Psychophysiology, 40*(5), 776–787.

Lasswell, H. D. (1927/1971). *Propaganda technique in World War I.* Cambridge, MA: MIT Press.

LeDoux, J. E. (1995). Emotion: Clues from the brain. *Annual Review of Psychology, 46*, 209–235.

Lee, S., & Lang, A. (2009). Discrete emotion and motivation: Relative activation in the appetitive and aversive motivational systems as a function of anger, sadness, fear, and joy during televised information campaigns. *Media Psychology, 12*, 148–170.

Leshner, G., & Bolls, P. D. (2005). Scare em or disgust em: The effects of disgusting images in anti-smoking advertisements. Paper presented to the Information Systems Division of the International Communication Association, New York.

Leshner, G., Bolls, P. D., & Thomas, E. (2009). Scare 'em or disgust 'em: The effects of graphic health promotion messages. *Health Communication, 24*(5), 447–458.

Leshner, G., Vultee, F., Bolls, P., & Moore, J. (2010). When a fear appeal isn't just a fear appeal: The effects of graphic anti-tobacco messages. *Journal of Broadcasting and Electronic Media, 54*(3), 485–507.

Levy, M. R., & Gurevitch, M. (1993). Editor's note. *Journal of Communication, 43*(3).

Lim, S., & Lee, J. R. (2009). When playing together feels different: Effects of task types and social contexts on physiological arousal and multiplayer online gaming contexts. *Cyber Psychology & Behavior, 12*(1), 59–61.

Lim, S., & Reeves, B. (2009). Being in the game: Effects of avatar choice and point of view on psychophysiological responses during play. *Media Psychology, 12*(4), 348–370.

Linz, D., Donnerstein, E., & Adams, S. M. (1989). Physiological desensitization and judgments about female victims of violence. *Human Communication Research, 15*(4), 509–522.

Lowery, S. A., & DeFleur, M. (1995). *Milestones in Mass Communications Research* (3rd ed.). White Plains, NY: Longman.

Lykken, D. T., & Venables, P. H. (1971). Direct measurement of skin conductance: A proposal for standardization. *Psychophysiology, 8*, 656–671.

Lynn, R. (1966). *Attention, arousal, and the orientation reaction.* Oxford, UK: Pergamon Press.

McCabe, D. P., & Castel, A. D. (2008). Seeing is believing: The effect of brain images on judgments of scientific reasoning. *Cognition, 107*, 343–352.

MacInnis, D. J., & Price, L. L. (1987). The role of imagery information processing: Review and extensions. *Journal of Consumer Research, 13*, 473–491.

McManis, M. H., Bradley, M. M., Berg, W. K., Cuthbert, B. N., & Lang, P. J. (2003). Emotional reactions in children: Verbal, physiological, and behavioral responses to affective pictures. *Psychophysiology, 38*(2), 222–231.

Marci, C. D. (2006). A biologically-based measure of emotional engagement: Context matters. *Journal of Advertising Research, 46*(4), 381–387.

Marshall-Goodell, B. S., Tassinary, L. G., & Cacioppo, J. T. (1990). Principles of bioelectrical measurement. In J. T. Cacioppo & L. G. Tassinary (Eds.), *Principles of psychophysiology: Physical, social, and inferential elements* (pp. 113–148). New York: Cambridge University Press.

Massey, G. J. (1995). Rhetoric and rationality in William Harvey's *De Motu Cordis.* In H. Krips, J. E. McGuire, & T. Melia (Eds.), *Science, reason, and rhetoric* (pp. 13–46). Pittsburgh, PA: University of Pittsburgh Press.

Maurer, M., & Reinemann, C. (2006). Learning versus knowing. *Communication Research, 33*(6), 489–506.

Meltzer, S. J. (1897). Emil Du Bois-Reymond. *Science, 5*(110), 217–219.

Miller, G. A. (2003). The cognitive revolution: A historical perspective. *Trends in Cognitive Sciences, 7*(3), 141–144.

Miller, J. G. (1973). The nature of living systems. *The Quarterly Review of Biology, 48*(1), 63–91.

Morgan, M. (2009). Cultivation analysis and media effects. In R. L. Nabi & M. B. Oliver (Eds.), *The Sage handbook of media processes and effects* (pp. 69–82). Newbury Park, CA: Sage.

Morris, J. D., Klahr, N. J., Shen, F., Villegas, J., Wright, P., He, G., & Liu, Y. (2009). Mapping a multidimensional emotion in response to television commercials. *Human Brain Mapping, 30*(3), 789–796.

Morris, J. P., Squires, N. K., Taber, C. S., & Lodge, M. (2003). Activation of political attitudes: A psychophysiological examination of the hot cognition hypothesis. *Political Psychology, 24*(4), 727–745.

Murray, A., Ewing, D. J., Campbell, I. W., Neilson, M. M., & Clarke, B. F. (1975). R—R interval variations in young male diabetics. *British Heart Journal, 37*, 882–885.

Nabi, R. L. (1999). A cognitive-functional model for the effects of discrete negative emotions on information processing, attitude change, and recall. *Communication Theory, 9*(3), 292–320.

Nabi, R. L. (2002). The theoretical versus the lay meaning of disgust: Implications for emotion research. *Cognition and Emotion, 16*, 695–703.

Nabi, R. L. (2010). The case for emphasizing discrete emotions in communication research. *Communication Monographs, 77*(2), 153–159.

Nabi, R. L. & Wirth, W. (2008). Exploring the role of emotion in media effects: An introduction to the special issue. *Media Psychology, 11*(1), 1–6.

Neumann, R., Hess, M., Schulz, S. M., & Alpers, G. W. (2005). Automatic behavioral responses to valence: Evidence that facial action is facilitated by evaluative processing. *Cognition and Emotion, 19*(4), 499–513.

Newell, A. (1990). *Unified theories of cognition.* Boston: Harvard University Press.

Newhagen, J. E., & Reeves, B. (1992). The evening's bad news: Effects of compelling negative television news images on memory. *The Journal of Communication, 42*(2), 25–41.

Ohme, R., Reykowska, D., Wiener, D., & Choromanska, A. (2009). Analysis of neurophysiological reactions to advertising stimuli by means of EEG and galvanic skin response measures. *Journal of Neuroscience, Psychology, and Economics, 2*(1), 21–31.

Oliver, M. B., & Krakowiak, K. M. (2009). Individual differences in media effects. In J. Bryant & M. B. Oliver (Eds.), *Media effects: Advances in theory and research* (pp. 517–531). New York: Routledge.

Ordonana, J. R., Gonzalez-Javier, F., Espin-Lopez, L., & Gomez-Amor, J. (2009). Self-report and psychophysiological responses to fear appeals. *Human Communication Research, 35*, 195–220.

Paisley, W. (1984). Communication in the communication sciences. In B. Dervin & M. Voight (Eds.), *Progress in communication sciences* (pp. 2–42). Norwood, NJ: Ablex.

Palmgreen, P., Stephenson, M. T., Everett, M. W., Baseheart, J. R., & Francies, R. (2002). Perceived message sensation value (PMSV) into the dimensions and validation of a PMSV scale. *Health Communication, 14*, 403–428.

Pashler, H. (1998). *The psychology of attention.* Cambridge, MA: MIT Press.

Pavlov, I. P. (1927). *Conditioned reflexes: An investigation of the physiological activity of the cerebral cortex.* Oxford, UK: Oxford University Press.

Pearce, J. (2001). Historical note: Emil Heinrich Du Bois-Reymond. *Journal of Neurology, Neurosurgery & Psychiatry, 71*, 620.

Penn, D. (2010). Neuroscience can add insight in complementing classical research. *Admap, 45*, 14–15.

Petty, R. E., & Cacioppo, J. T. (1986). *Communication and persuasion: Central and peripheral routes to attitude change.* New York: Springer.

Pfurtscheller, G., Grabner, R. H., Brunner, C., & Neuper, C. (2007). Phasic heart rate changes during word translation of different difficulties. *Psychophysiology, 44*(5), 807–813.

Phelan, J. J. (1919). *Motion pictures as a phase of commercial amusement in Toledo, Ohio.* Toledo, OH: Little Book Press.

Pivik, R. T., Broughton, R. J., Coppola, R., Davidson, R. J., Fox, N., & Nuwer, M. R. (1993). Guidelines for the recording and quantitative analysis of electroencephalographic activity in research contexts. *Psychophysiology, 30,* 547–558.

Pizzagalli, D. A. (2007). Electroencephalography and high-density electrophysiological source localization. In J. T. Cacioppo, L. G. Tassinary, & G. G. Berntson (Eds.), *Handbook of psychophysiology* (3rd ed., pp. 56–84). New York: Cambridge University Press.

Plassman, H., Ambler, T., Braeutigam, S., & Kenning, P. (2007). What can advertisers learn from neuroscience? *International Journal of Advertising, 26*(2), 151–175.

Plutchik, R. (1980). *Emotion: A psychoevolutionary synthesis.* New York: Harper & Row.

Porges, S. W. (1991). Vagal tone: An autonomic mediator of affect. In J. Garber & K. A. Dodge (Eds.), *The development of emotion regulation and dysregulation* (pp. 111–128). Cambridge, UK: Cambridge University Press.

Porges, S. W. (2007). The polyvagal perspective. [Review]. *Biological Psychology, 74*(2), 116–143.

Porges, S. W., Ackles, P. A., & Truax, S. R. (1983). Psychophysiological measurement: Methodological constraints. In A. Gale & J. A. Edwards (Eds.), *Physiological correlates of human behavior* (Vol. 1, pp. 219–240). New York: Academic Press.

Posner, M. I. (1978). *Chronometric explorations of mind.* Hillsdale, NJ: Lawrence Erlbaum Associates.

Potter, R. F. (2000). The effects of voice changes on orienting and immediate cognitive overload in radio listeners. *Mediate Psychology, 2*(2), 147–177.

Potter, R. F. (2009). Double the units: How increasing the number of advertisements while keeping the overall duration of commercial breaks constant affects radio listeners. *Journal of Broadcasting & Electronic Media, 53*(4), 584–598.

Potter, R. F., & Choi, J. (2006). The effects of auditory structural complexity on attitudes, attention, arousal, and memory. *Media Psychology, 8*(4), 395–419.

Potter, R. F., Koruth, J., Bea, S., Weaver, A., Lee, S., Rubenking, B., & Kim, O. T. (2008). Correlating the motivation activation measure with media preference. Paper presented to the annual meeting of the International Communication Association.

Potter, R. F., Lang, A., & Bolls, P. D. (2008). Identifying structural features of audio: Orienting responses during radio messages and their impact on recognition. *Journal of Media Psychology: Theories, Methods, and Applications, 20*(4), 168–177.

Potter, R. F., LaTour, M. S., Braun-LaTour, K. A., & Reichert, T. (2006). The impact of program context on motivational system activation and subsequent effects on processing a fear appeal. *Journal of Advertising, 35*(3), 67–80.

Price, V., & Feldman, L. (2009). News and politics. In R. L. Nabi & M. B. Oliver (Eds.), *The Sage handbook of media processes and effects* (pp. 113–130). Newbury Park, CA: Sage.

Ravaja, N. (2004a). Contributions of psychophysiology to media research: Review and recommendations. *Media Psychology, 6*(2), 193–235.

Ravaja, N. (2004b). Effects of a small talking facial image on autonomic activity: The moderating influence of dispositional BIS and BAS sensitivities and emotions. *Biological Psychology, 65*(2), 163–183.

Ravaja, N. (2009). The psychophysiology of digital gaming: The effect of a non co-located opponent. *Media Psychology, 12*(3), 268–294.

Ravaja, N., Saari, T., Kallinen, K., & Laarni, J. (2006b). The role of mood in the processing of media messages from a small screen: Effects on subjective and physiological responses. *Media Psychology, 8,* 239–265.

Ravaja, N., Saari, T., Salminen, M., Laarni, J., & Kallinen, K. (2006a). Phasic emotional reactions to video game events: A psychophysiological investigation. *Media Psychology, 8,* 343–367.

Ravaja, N., Turpeinen, M., Saari, T., Puttonen, S., & Keitlkangas-Jarvinen, L. (2008). The psychophysiology of James Bond: Phasic emotional responses to violent video game events. *Emotion, 8*(1), 114–120.

Rawlings, D., & Dawe, S. (2008). Psychoticism and impulsivity. In G. J. Boyle, G. Matthews, & D. H. Saklofske (Eds.), *The Sage handbook of personality theory and assessment: Volume 1 personality theories and models* (pp. 357–378). Los Angeles: Sage.

Reeves, B., & Geiger, S. (1994). Designing experiments that assess psychological responses to media messages. In A. Lang (Ed.), *Measuring psychological responses to media* (pp. 165–180). Hillsdale, NJ: Lawrence Erlbaum Associates.

Reeves, B., Lang, A., Kim, E. Y., & Tatar, D. (1999). The effects of screen size and message content on attention and arousal. *Media Psychology, 1*(1), 49–67.

Reeves, B., & Nass, C. I. (1996). *The media equation: How people treat computers, television, and new media like real people and places.* New York: Cambridge University Press.

Reeves, B., Newhagen, J., Maibach, E., Basil, M., & Kurz, K. (1991). Negative and positive television messages: Effects of message type and message context on attention and memory. *American Behavioral Scientist, 34,* 679–694.

Reeves, B., & Thorson, E. (1986). Watching television: Experiments on viewing process. *Communication Research, 13,* 343–361.

Reeves, B., Thorson, E., Rothschild, M., McDonald, D., Hirsch, J., & Goldstein, R. (1985). Attention to television: Intrastimulus effects of movement and scene changes on alpha variation over time. *International Journal of Neuroscience, 27,* 241–255.

Roser, C. (1990). Involvement, attention, and perceptions of message relevance in the response to persuasive appeals. *Communication Research, 17*(5), 571–600.

Rothschild, M. L., Hyun, Y. J., Reeves, B., Thorson, E., & Goldstein, R. (1988). Hemispheric lateralized EEG as a response to television commercials. *Journal of Consumer Research, 15,* 185–198.

Roy, M., Mailhot, J. P., Gosselin, N., Paquette, S., & Peretz, I. (2009). Modulation of the startle reflex by pleasant and unpleasant music. *International Journal of Psychophysiology, 71*(1), 37–42.

Rubin, A. M. (2009). Uses and gratification: An evolving perspective of media effects. In R. L. Nabi & M. B. Oliver (Eds.), *The Sage handbook of media processes and effects* (pp. 147–160), Newbury Park, CA: Sage.

Rubin, R. B., Palmgreen, P., & Sypher, H. E. (1994). *Communication research measures: A sourcebook.* New York: The Guilford Press.

Russell, J. A. (2003). Core affect and the psychological construction of emotion. *Psychological Review, 110*(1), 145–172.

Russell, J. A., & Barrett, L. F. (1999). Core affect, prototypical emotional episodes, and other things called emotion: Dissecting the elephant. *Journal of Personality and Social Psychology, 76,* 805–819.

Ryan, K. J., Brady, J. V., Cooke, R. E., Height, D. I., Jonsen, A. F., King, P., et al. (1979). *The Belmont Report: Ethical principles and guidelines for the protection of human subjects of research.* Available from http://ohsr.od.nih.gov/guidelines/belmont.html.

Samoilov, V. O. (2007). Ivan Petrovich Pavlov (1849–1936). *Journal of the History of the Neurosciences, 16*(1/2), 74–89.

Saunders, J. B., & O'Malley, C.D. (1950). *The illustrations from the works of Andreas Vesalius of Brussels.* Cleveland: The World Publishing Company.

Sauseng, P., & Klimesch, W. (2008). What does phase information of oscillatory brain activity tell us about cognitive processes? *Neuroscience and Biobehavioral Reviews, 32,* 1001–1013.

Schachter, S., & Singer, J. E. (1962). Cognitive, social, and physiological determinants of emotional state. *Psychological Review, 69,* 379–399.

Scherer, K., & Ellgring, H. (2007). Are facial expressions of emotion produced by categorical affect programs or dynamically driven by appraisal? *Emotion, 7*(1), 113–130.

Schneider, W., Dumais, S. T., & Shiffrin, R. M. (1984). Automatic and control processing and attention. In R. Parasuraman & D. R. Davies (Eds.), *Varieties of attention* (pp. 1–25). Orlando, FL: Academic Press.

Schramm, W. (1971). The nature of communication between humans. In W. Schramm & D. F. Roberts (Eds.), *The process and effects of mass communications* (pp. 1–53). Urbana, IL: University of Illinois Press.

Schwartz, G. E., Fair, P. L., Salt, P., Mandel, M. R., & Klerman, G. L. (1976). Facial muscle patterning to affective imagery in depressed and nondepressed subjects. *Science, 192,* 489–491.

Shah, D. V., McLeod, D. M., Gotlieb, M. R., & Lee, N. (2009). Framing and agenda setting. In R. L. Nabi & M. B. Oliver (Eds.), *The Sage handbook of media processes and effects* (pp. 83–98). Newbury Park, CA: Sage.

Shannon, C. E., & Weaver, W. (1949). *The mathematical theory of communication.* Urbana, IL: University of Illinois Press.

Shapiro, M. A. (1994a). Signal detection measure of recognition memory. In A. Lang (Ed.), *Measuring psychological responses to media* (pp. 133–148). Hillsdale, NJ: Lawrence Erlbaum Associates.

Shapiro, M. A. (1994b). Think-aloud and thought-list procedures in investigating mental processes. In A. Lang (Ed.), *Measuring psychological responses to media* (pp. 1–14). Hillsdale, NJ: Lawrence Erlbaum Associates.

Sherry, J. L. (2004). Media effects theory and the nature/nurture debate: A historical overview and directions for future research. *Media Psychology, 6*(1), 83–109.

Shields, S. A., MacDowell, K. A., Fairchild, S. B., & Campbell, M. L. (1987). Is mediation of sweating cholinergic, adrenergic, or both? A comment on the literature. *Psychophysiology, 24,* 312–319.

Shiffrin, R. M., & Schneider, W. (1977). Controlled and automatic human information processing II: Perceptual learning, automatic attending, and a general theory. *Psychological Review, 84,* 127–190.

Shoemaker, P. J. (1996). Hardwired for news: Using biological and cultural evolution to explain the surveillance function. *Journal of Communication, 46*(3), 32–47.

Shoemaker, P. J., Tankard, J., James William, & Lasorsa, D. L. (2004). *How to build social science theories.* Thousand Oaks, CA: Sage.

Simons, R. F., Detenber, B. H., Cuthbert, B. N., Schwartz, D. D., & Reiss, J. E. (2003). Attention to television: Alpha power and its relationship to image motion and emotional content. *Media Psychology, 5*(3), 283–301.

Smith, L. D. (1996). *B.F. Skinner and behaviorism in American culture.* Bethlehem: Lehigh University Press.

Smith, M. E., & Gevins, A. (2004). Attention into brain activity while watching television: Components of viewer engagement. *Media Psychology, 6,* 285–305.

Sokolov, E. N. (1963). *Perception and the conditioned reflex.* Oxford, UK: Pergamon Press.

Sparks, G. G. (2002). *Media effects research: An overview.* Belmont, CA: Wadsworth.

Sparks, J. V., & Lang, A. (2010). An initial examination of the Post-Auricular Reflex as a physiological indicator of appetitive activation during television viewing. *Communication Methods and Measures, 4*(4), 311–330.

Stark, R., Walter, B., Schienle, A., & Vaitl, D. (2005). Psychophysiological correlates of disgust and disgust sensitivity. *Journal of Psychophysiology, 19*(1), 50–60.

Stayman, D. M., & Aaker, D. A. (1993). Continuous measurement of self-report of emotional response. *Psychology & Marketing, 10*(3), 199–214.

Stephens, D. L., & Russo, J. E. (1997). Extensions of the cognitive response approach to predicting postadvertisement attitudes. In W. D. Wells (Ed.), *Measuring Advertising Effectiveness* (pp. 157–178). Hillsdale, NJ: Lawrence Erlbaum Associates.

Stern, R. M., Ray, W. J., & Davis, C. M. (1980). *Psychophysiological recording.* New York: Oxford University Press.

Stern, R. M., Ray, W. J., & Quigley, K. S. (2001). *Psychophysiological recording* (2nd ed.). New York: Oxford University Press.

Stewart, D. W. (1984). Physiological measurement of advertising effects. *Psychology & Marketing, 1*(1), 43–48.

Strube, M. J., & Newman, L. C. (2007). Psychometrics. In J. T. Cacioppo, L. G. Tassinary, & G. G. Berntson (Eds.), *Handbook of psychophysiology* (pp. 789–811). New York: Cambridge University Press.

Sundar, S. S., & Kalyanaraman, S. (2004). Arousal, memory, and impression-formation effects of animation speed in Web advertising. *Journal of Advertising, 33*(1), 8–17.

Task Force of the European Society of Cardiology and the North American Society of Pacing and Electrophysiology (1996). Heart rate variability: Standards of measurement, physiological interpretation, and clinical use. *Circulation, 93,* 1043–1065.

Tassinary, L. G., Cacioppo, J. T., & Vanman, E. J. (2007). The skeletomotor system: Surface electromyography. In J. T. Cacioppo, L. G. Tassinary, & G. G. Berntson (Eds.), *Handbook of psychophysiology* (pp. 267–299). New York: Cambridge University Press.

Thelen, E. (1995). Time-scale dynamics and the development of an embodied cognition. In R. F. Port & T. van Gelder (Eds.), *Mind as motion: Explorations in the dynamics of cognition* (pp. 69–100). Boston: Massachusetts Institute of Technology.

Thelen, E., Schöner, G., Scheier, C., & Smith, L. B. (2001). The dynamics of embodiment: A field theory of infant perseverative reaching. *Behavioral and Brain Sciences, 24*(01), 1–34.

Thorson, E. (1989). Processing television commercials. In B. Dervin, L. Grossberg, B. J. O'Keefe, & E. Wartella (Eds.), *Rethinking communication, vol. 2: Paradigm exemplars* (pp. 397–410). Newbury Park, CA: Sage.

Thorson, E., & Lang, A. (1992). Effects of television videographics and lecture familiarity on adult cardiac orienting responses and memory. *Communication Research, 19*(3), 346–369.

Thorson, E., Reeves, B., & Schleuder, J. (1985). Message complexity and attention to television. *Communication Research, 12,* 427–454.

Thorson, E., Reeves, B., & Schleuder, J. (1987). Attention to local and global complexity of television messages. In M. L. McLaughlin (Ed.), *Communication yearbook 10* (pp. 366–383). Beverly Hills, CA: Sage.

Tranel, D. (2000). Electrodermal activity in cognitive neuroscience: Neuroanatomical and neuropsychological correlates. In R. D. Lane & L. Nadel (Eds.), *Cognitive neuroscience of emotion* (pp. 192–224). New York: Oxford University Press.

Tranel, D., & Damasio, A. (1994). Neuroanatomical correlates of electrodermal skin conductance responses. *Psychophysiology, 31*, 427–438.

Treleaven-Hassard, S., Gold, J., Bellman, S., Schweda, A., Ciorciari, J., Critchley, C., & Varan, D. (2010). Using the P3a to gauge automatic attention to interactive television advertising. *Journal of Economic Psychology, 31*(5), 777–784.

Tuch, A. N., Bargas-Avila, J. A., Opwis, K., & Wilhelm, F. H. (2009). Visual complexity of websites: Effects on users' experience, physiology, performance, and memory. *International Journal of Human Computer Studies, 67*(9), 703–715.

Tucker, D. M., Derryberry, D., & Luu, P. (2000). Anatomy and physiology of human emotion: Vertical integration of brainstem, limbic, and cortical systems. In J. C. Borod (Ed.), *The neuropsychology of emotion* (pp. 56–79). New York: Oxford University Press.

Valentini, R. P., & Daniels, S. R. (1997). The journal club. *Postgraduate Medical Journal, 73*, 81–85.

Vanman, E. J., Boehmelt, A. H., Dawson, M. E., & Schell, A. M. (1996). The varying time courses of attentional and affective modulation of the startle eyeblink reflex. *Psychophysiology, 33*(6), 691–697.

Varela, F., Lachaux, J., Rodriguez, E., & Martinerie, J. (2001). The brainweb: Phase synchronization and large-scale integration. *Nature Reviews Neuroscience, 2*, 229–239.

Vecchiato, G., Astolfi, L., Tabarrini, A., Salinari, S., Mattia, D., Cincotti, F., et al. (2010). EEG analysis of the brain activity during the observation of commercial, political, or public service announcements. *Computational Intelligence and Neuroscience*, 1–7.

Vrana, S. R. (1993). The psychophysiology of disgust: Differentiating negative emotional contexts with facial EMG. *Psychophysiology, 30*(3), 279–286.

Wager, T. D., Hernandez, L., Jonides, J., & Lindquist, M. (2007). Elements of functional neuroimaging. In J. T. Cacioppo, L. G. Tassinary, & G. G. Berntson (Eds.), *Handbook of psychophysiology* (pp. 19–55). New York: Cambridge University Press.

Wang, Z., Lang, A., & Busemeyer, J. R. (2011). Motivational processing and choice behavior during television viewing: An integrative dynamic approach. *Journal of Communication, 61*(1), 71–93.

Wartella, E., & Reeves, B. (1985). Historical trends in research on children and the media, 1900–1960. *Journal of Communication, 35*(2), 118–133.

Watt, J. H. (1994). Detecting and modeling time-sequenced processes. In A. Lang (Ed.), *Measuring psychological responses to media messages* (pp. 181–208). Hillsdale, NJ: Lawrence Erlbaum Associates.

Weber, E. J. M., Van Der Molen, M. W., & Molenaar, P. C. M. (1994). Heart rate and sustained attention during childhood: Age changes in anticipatory heart rate, primary bradycardia, and respiratory sinus arrhythmia. *Psychophysiology, 31*, 164–174.

Weinstein, S. (1982). A review of brain hemisphere research. *Journal of Advertising Research, 22*(3), 59.

Weinstein, S., Appel, V., & Weinstein, C. (1980). Brain-activity responses to magazine and television advertising. *Journal of Advertising Research, 20*(3), 57–63.

Weinstein, S., Drozdenko, R., & Weinstein, C. (1984). Brain wave analysis in advertising research. *Psychology & Marketing, 1*(3/4), 83–95.

Werner, K. (1979). Activation research: Psychobiological approaches in consumer research. *Journal of Consumer Research, 5*(4), 240–250.

Wetzel, J. M., Quigley, K. S., Morell, J., Eves, E., & Backs, R. W. (2006). Cardiovascular measures of attention to illusory and non-illusory visual stimuli. *Journal of Psychophysiology, 20*(4), 276–285.

Wickens, C. D. (1984). Processing resources and attention. In R. Parasuraman & D. R. Davies (Eds.), *Varieties of attention* (pp. 63–99). Orlando, FL: Academic Press.

Wight, R. (2010). Neuromarketing: useful or useless. *Admap,* 16.

Wilson, T. D., & Brekke, N. (1994). Mental contamination and mental correction: Unwanted influences on judgments and evaluations. *Psychological Bulletin, 116,* 117–142.

Wise, K., Bolls, P. D., Myers, J., & Sternadori, M. (2009). When words collide online: How writing style and video intensity affect cognitive processing online news. *Journal of Broadcasting & Electronic Media, 53*(4), 532–546.

Witte, K. (1994). Generating effective risk messages: How scary should your risk communication be? *Communication Yearbook, 18,* 229–254.

Woody, S. R., & Teachman, B. A. (2000). Intersection of fear and disgust: Normative and pathological views. *Clinical Psychology: Science and Practice, 7,* 291–311.

Yartz, A. R., & Hawk, L. W. (2002). Addressing the specificity of affective startle modulation: Fear versus disgust. *Biological Psychology, 59*(1), 55–68.

Young, D. G. (2008). The privileged role of the late-night joke: Exploring humor's role in disrupting argument scrutiny. *Media Psychology, 11*(1), 119–142.

Zaichkowsky, J. L. (1985). Measuring the involvement construct. *Journal of Consumer Research, 15,* 4–14.

Zechmeister, E. B., & Nyberg, S. E. (1982). *Human memory: An introduction to research and theory.* Monterey, CA: Brooks/Cole.

Zillmann, D. (1971). Excitation transfer in communication-mediated agressive behavior. *Journal of Experimental Social Psychology, 7,* 419–434.

Zillmann, D. (1983). Transfer of excitation in emotional behavior. In J. T. Cacioppo & R. E. Petty (Eds.), *Social psychophysiology: A sourcebook* (pp. 215–240). New York: Guilford.

Zillmann, D. (2003). Theory of affective dynamics: Emotions and moods. In J. Bryant, D. Roskos-Ewoldsen, & Cantor, J. (Eds.), *Communication and emotion: Essays in honor of Dolf Zillman* (pp. 533–567). Mahwah, NJ: Lawrence Erlbaum Associates.

Zillmann, D., & Bryant, J. (1974). Effect of residual excitation on the emotional response to provocation and delayed aggressive behavior. *Journal of Personality and Social Psychology, 30*(6), 782–791.

Zillmann, D., Hoyt, J. L., & Day, K. D. (1974). Strength and duration of the effect of aggressive, violent, and erotic communications on subsequent aggressive behavior. *Communication Research, 1*(3), 286–306.

Zillmann, D., & Johnson, R. C. (1973). Motivated aggressiveness perpetuated by exposure to aggressive films and reduced by exposure to nonaggressive films. *Journal of Research in Personality, 7*(3), 261–276.

Zillmann, D., Mody, B., & Cantor, J. R. (1974). Empathetic perception of emotional displays in films as a function of hedonic and excitatory state prior to exposure. *Journal of Research in Personality, 8*(4), 335–349.

Zuckerman, M. (1979). *Sensation seeking: Beyond the optimal level of arousal.* Hillsdale, NJ: Lawrence Erlbaum Associates.

Zuckerman, M. (1990). The psychophysiology of sensation seeking. *Journal of Personality, 58,* 315–345.

Zuckerman, M. (2008). The Zuckerman-Kuhlman personality questionnaire (ZKPQ): An operational definition of the alternative five factorial model of personality. In G. J. Boyle, G. Matthews, & D. H. Saklofske (Eds.), *The Sage handbook of personality theory and assessment: Volume 2 personality measurement and testing* (pp. 219–238). Los Angeles: Sage.